Rethinking the Medieval Senses

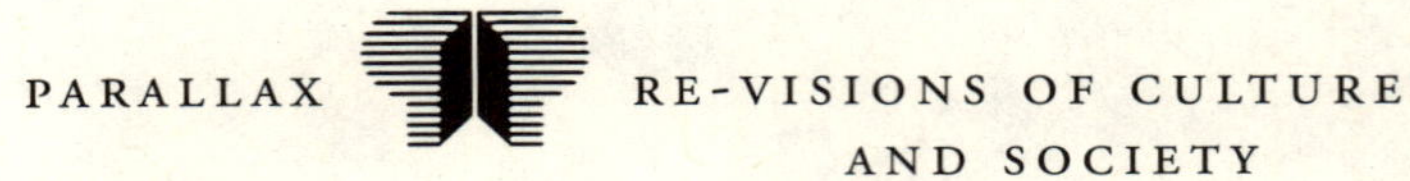

Stephen G. Nichols, Gerald Prince, and Wendy Steiner,
SERIES EDITORS

Rethinking the Medieval Senses

Heritage / Fascinations / Frames

EDITED BY

Stephen G. Nichols,
Andreas Kablitz, and Alison Calhoun

The Johns Hopkins University Press
Baltimore

Printed in the United States of America on acid-free paper
9 8 7 6 5 4 3 2 1

The Johns Hopkins University Press
2715 North Charles Street
Baltimore, Maryland 21218-4363
www.press.jhu.edu

Library of Congress Cataloging-in-Publication Data

Rethinking the medieval senses : heritage, fascinations, frames / edited by Stephen G. Nichols, Andreas Kablitz, and Alison Calhoun.
p. cm. — (Parallax)
Includes bibliographical references and index.
ISBN-13: 978-0-8018-8736-9 (hardcover : alk. paper)
ISBN-13: 978-0-8018-8737-6 (pbk. : alk. paper)
ISBN-10: 0-8018-8736-4 (hardcover : alk. paper)
ISBN-10: 0-8018-8737-2 (pbk. : alk. paper)
1. Middle Ages—Intellectual life. 2. Senses and sensation—History. 3. Senses and sensation—Religious aspects. 4. Senses and sensation in literature. 5. Literature, Medieval—History and criticism. I. Nichols, Stephen G. II. Kablitz, Andreas. III. Calhoun, Alison, 1979.
CB351.R455 2008
909.07—dc22 2007022614

A catalog record for this book is available from the British Library.

Special discounts are available for bulk purchases of this book. For more information, please contact Special Sales at 410-516-6936 or specialsales@press.jhu.edu.

The Johns Hopkins University Press uses environmentally friendly book materials, including recycled text paper that is composed of at least 30 percent post-consumer waste, whenever possible. All of our book papers are acid-free, and our jackets and covers are printed on paper with recycled content.

Contents

Prologue

Robert Grosseteste begins his commentary on the *Six Days of Creation* by asserting that when God utters the first command, *Fiat lux,* he means us to recognize that substance, word, and process are one and the same: Christ the creative principle. "Fiat lux," on this account, is the Ur-creation, the act from which all else comes into being. Grosseteste makes this claim by reading Genesis 1:3 through the combined lines of John 8:12: *ego sum lux mundi . . . ,* "I am the light of the world. Whoever follows me will never walk in darkness, but will have the light of life," and John 1:1–2: "In the beginning was the Word, and the Word was with God, and the Word was God. He was with God in the beginning." A Christ who is both light and Word, a Trinitarian force responsible for inventing the universe—and in the process sweeping away Hebrew primacy in this domain—offers compelling testimony to the importance of the physical senses in medieval culture.

If sight and hearing are the principal senses, it is not alone because of their association with Christ. They also constitute the chief vehicles for cognition, crucial conduits linking the external world to the soul and to reason. As the senses most intimately linked to soul and mind, they played a key role in forming the individual morally, intellectually, and above all in indoctrination to the faith. Purely bodily senses like taste, smell, and touch were suspect, but even sight, on the authority of St. Paul, followed by St. Augustine, was not above suspicion. "Faith cometh by hearing," says Paul, "and hearing by the word of God" (Romans 10:17). Guillaume de Deguileville, in his *Pèlerinage de la Vie Humaine* (1330 CE), succinctly, if intemperately, states the orthodox case for hearing when he condemns the four senses of sight, taste, smell, and touch: "these four senses are completely deceived and they are foolish. They are stupefied and they know nothing . . . but the sense of hearing alone informs the understanding. It knows more subtly and perceives more clearly than touching, tasting, smelling or seeing."

Hearing, of course, was the principal vehicle for learning by instruction. Since, as Grosseteste observes, "Scripture has a hidden and sealed up sense," it is difficult to reach without the aid of a teacher. He quotes St. Jerome's letter to Paulinus by way of making the case for hearing: "this 'living voice' teaches more vividly as it forces its way in through the ear, than does the 'dead voice' that slips in through the eyes." But if he pays lip service to the Patristic mistrust of all the senses but hearing, Grosseteste nonetheless did as much as anyone in the early years of the thirteenth century to foster scientific study of the bodily senses. He does so with a cunning worthy of Kierkegaard's "oblique approach" whereby he confronts conventional wisdom by taking it as a point of departure.

He prudently suggests that "certitudes about the various species in the sensible world fall under faith . . . and are more easily acceptable under faith," and that it is fitting that "the creation of the sensible world, on account of the way in which the world is imaginable and graspable by the external senses of the body, should be told [*ennari*] in the opening part of Scripture. This is in order that anyone, even among the uneducated, may be able to grasp a story [*narracionem*] . . . easily and through his imagination, through the images of corporeal things . . . and through the authority of the one who speaks."

Between the orthodox references to hearing (narration and authoritative speaking), Grosseteste deftly inserts a double reference to the data fed to the imagination by sensory perception and to the visual image they allow the mind to form. More importantly, it is this continual sensory feed from the external world that provides corroborating evidence allowing the hearer to concede authoritative status to the speaker. Credibility looms large in Grosseteste's exposition as a criterion; he stresses the necessity for an account to be "believable" in order to be authoritative, but rational processing of sensory data plays a major role for him in establishing believability. This reliance on verification by analysis of sense data sets him apart from earlier commentators on Genesis for whom faith sufficed.

We begin to understand why Grosseteste needed to reaffirm the preeminence of the scriptural narrative of creation before proceeding to focus on science—the technique of harnessing the bodily senses for the analysis of the physical world—as the most effective method for probing the mysteries of the physical world. His pupil, Roger Bacon—for whom vision, not hearing, was the queen of the bodily senses—praised Grosseteste repeatedly as a pioneer in the "scientific" study of phenomena in the physical world—including language—and the role of the senses in apprehending them.

Although far more radical than Grosseteste, and not uncritical of the cautiousness of his predecessor, Bacon credited him with embracing rather than rejecting the role of the corporeal senses in apprehending major physical phenomena—comets, light, sidereal manifestations of all sorts—which the mind could then contemplate in conjunction with scriptural accounts. Bacon applauds Grosseteste's boldness in stressing the primacy of vision for observational science, which then informed his theological commentary. This represents a sea change from theological speculation based on appeal to traditional (i.e., Patristic) wisdom to commentary based on direct observation: actually looking at and analyzing phenomena (with the result of correcting or even controverting received wisdom).

This focus on observational methodology resonated well beyond scholastic philosophy. Since language, as well as vision, formed an important part of the inquiry, an important subset of representational arts, particularly literature and painting, registered the effects of speculative philosophy. While the most exuberant and unruly early example might well be Jean de Meun's version of the *Roman de la Rose,* genres like the fabliaux, farce, and various forms of vernacular drama owe their existence in no small measure to the exploration of the corporeal senses' role in elucidating (or confusing!) external reality.

The effects were not only felt in the vernacular or secular world. Inevitably, the senses were harnessed to produce a rich—and richly satisfying—culture of devotional practice. Books of Hours, treatises like Grosseteste's own *Castle of Love,* or, in the fifteenth century, Nicholas Love's *Mirror of the Blessed Life of Jesus Christ,* hymns to the Annunciation like, *Angelus ad Virginem,* devotional images like the *Arma Christi,* all stress the mediation of "performative vision": intense contemplation of holy scenes in which the individual "actively" participates by a vivid exercise of the imagination.

The desire to explore different aspects of the corporeal senses as a cultural and intellectual force in medieval culture motivated the scholars represented in this volume to gather in Florence, Italy, in the spring of 2004. The settings of Johns Hopkins's Villa Spelman and the Stanford Center in Florence offered exceptionally supportive venues for lively discussions in each session and afterwards on the terrace looking out over Florence. I am not sure whether, like Beatrice speaking to Dante, we found that "the wings / Of reason to pursue the senses' flight / Are short" (*Paradiso* II), but we certainly found those magical hours all too short.

We would like to thank the Thyssen Foundation for its generous support of the conference (and publication of the papers), and the Deans of Arts and Sciences at the Johns Hopkins University and Stanford University for their contribution to the conference. Finally, the staff of the Villa Spelman, particularly Laura Di Poffi, provided the warmth and hospitality that made the occasion truly memorable.

Stephen G. Nichols

Rethinking the Medieval Senses

I

Introduction

Erudite Fascinations and Cultural Energies

How Much Can We Know about the Medieval Senses?

Hans Ulrich Gumbrecht

For what reasons we, a group of (full- and part-time) medievalists from Europe and the United States, decided to organize a series of colloquia on the medieval senses, I do not exactly remember. But it is obvious that our intellectual desire emerged from a certain epistemological climate and concern that was more hidden and less conceptually circumscribed back in the late 1990s than it is today. What I have in mind is of course the concern of identifying a dimension of cultural phenomena and of honing some scholarly skills and forms of analytic practice that would provoke an opening of the academic "Humanities and Arts" beyond and beside "interpretation," that is, beyond and beside meaning attribution, as it had been institutionally canonized as their central and only task. To concentrate on the "medieval senses," instead of, say, deepening our knowledge about the role of allegory in medieval literature, held an intellectual fascination similar to the fascination that had carried eighteenth-century materialism. This was—and is—the curiosity to see how humans in general and historical cultures in specific have been living and thinking their relation to the world of objects.

Now, professional medievalists and amateur lovers of the Middle Ages alike have long been under the impression that there had to be something about the role of the human senses in the Middle Ages that was profoundly different from the ways in which modern cultures relate to their material environments. Furthermore, it is astonishing to observe how this single fascination has produced two clearly distinct and even opposite images of medieval culture. On the one side, there is the both scholarly and popular conviction that the Middle Ages were a culture of high sensual intensity (das sinnenfrohe Mittelalter). But there is an equally strong scholarly and popular belief, on the other side, that the Middle Ages were a time of extreme sensual starvation (das asketische Mittelalter). While both these views of the Middle Ages obviously rely on problematic totalizations, it is clear—and quite interesting—that their respective backgrounds, hermeneutically speaking, are two opposite evaluations of contemporary culture, as either too puritanical (more precisely: as too much shaped by a drive toward abstraction, as Oswald Spengler, Martin Heidegger, Max Horkheimer, and Theodor W. Adorno would have had it), or as indulging in exuberant cascades of sensual gratification. The potential of interfering with those views of the Middle Ages, and through them with two of the more influential interpretations of our present, explains, I believe, the remarkable liveliness and the moments of true intellectual passion that characterized our discussions about the medieval senses.

These discussions took place at the Einstein Forum at Potsdam (1997), at Stanford University (2000), and at the Johns Hopkins and Stanford Centers in Florence (2004), and produced a much broader range of hypotheses, speculations, and historical quests than this volume—and any thematically coherent book—can possibly bring together. Indeed, however cautiously its fourteen authors present their observations and their (mostly tentative) conclusions, all of the essays from which I will try to cull a first mapping for the dominion of the medieval senses go back to our third and final meeting—which means that they presuppose a long preparatory process of philological and conceptual clarification.

Despite the richness and precision of the results achieved, it turned out to be unusually, not to say overwhelmingly, difficult to find points of convergence and shared contours between the different contributions, points of convergence that would confirm the hope that our initiative has produced a first mapping of the topic in question. For the medieval senses revealed themselves to be a stubbornly centrifugal topic—and one of the reasons for this experience must have been that our topic, while it was meant to undercut the Humanities' exclusive concentration on phenomena of text-based meaning production and reception, could only be accessed through a thick and intrinsically complex layer of medieval erudition. In other words, there was (and remains) an impressive plurality of discourses, dimensions of knowledge, and even ontological levels that all need to be taken into account although they do not show any immediately apparent order among themselves. Such a diverse plurality makes difficult any attempt to bring together philological materials and philosophical thoughts in a synthetic effort. From a historical standpoint, one might say that this is only fair because, rather than a homogeneous "discourse" or "system," the medieval senses seem to have been a field of often conflicting forces.

Here is, then, the structure within which I want to present the fourteen contributions to this book, and it implies the first rudimentary draft of a mapping for our topic as we can now begin to recognize it. I begin with a brief description of several philosophical conceptualizations, coming from Greek or Roman Antiquity and concerning the relation between the human mind and its material environment, conceptualizations of course whose influence can be traced in different times and different epistemological spaces of the Middle Ages. This is the classical *legacy* of the medieval senses.

In the process of its reception, medieval thinkers and authors developed two particularly *patent fascinations:* one of them is documented in the traces of countless attempts to fit the different human senses and the different models of their contact with the material world into all-embracing systems and representations of cosmological order. The other one, rather unexpectedly, lies in a focus on the specific motif of the "inner eyes" which, quite astonishingly, many, if not most, of our essays touch upon. This apparent metaphor referred to a capacity believed to be inherent to the soul or the spirit, which, in spite of belonging to the interior realm of the body, was supposed to enable humans to perceive (rather than to "imagine," as we moderns would immediately say) the material world in particularly intense ways.

I next deal with *hidden cultural energies* that can be reconstructed, at least in part, as the product of those classical models of conceptualization, after they have gone through the layers of medieval reception. I call them "hidden" energies because they lie behind or below that primary layer of explicit erudition and textual meaning, and while those hidden dynamics may well have set the tone of everyday life (and even holiday life) in medieval culture, our only retrospective way of accessing and of understanding them is by conjecture.

Finally, I address the distribution of certain phenomena and motifs belonging to the medieval senses within the *frames* of historical chronology and sociocultural hierarchy, especially between Latin culture and vernacular culture.

Legacy

Of course it was the proverbial tension between the "Aristotelian embrace" of the senses and their "Platonic scorn," supported and complexified by a large number of other authors from Greek and Roman Antiquity whose works belonged to the canon of medieval readers, that opened, determined, and inspired their reflection about the relations between human existence and the material world. The most compact way of describing the difference between the Platonic and the Aristotelian view of the senses might be to say that, for Plato, to experience the ideas as truth required an overcoming, a going beyond the physical surface as the world presents itself, whereas for Aristotle there could not be any truth experience unless it relied on the perception of the material world as its starting point and basis. During the Middle Ages, however, these two models were far from always (or mostly) finding themselves in contexts of neat separation, as had been the case, for example, with St. Paul, who never departed from his thoroughly Platonic premises. St. Augustine, in contrast, who, in some ways, may look like an even purer Platonist than St. Paul, did integrate the non-Platonic motif of the bodily resurrection of the dead into his theology and associated it with the hope for a corporeal vision of God after the end of our earthly life. In his circumspect assessment of Augustine's view, Eugene Vance (chapter 1) makes it clear how the insistence on the resurrected human body as a purified body must be read as a symptom for the saint's awareness of an epistemological tension that was inherent to this motif.

As a general rule, however, medieval reflections about the senses show a tendency to combine, quite freely and whenever it appeared convenient, concepts and arguments from different philosophico-theological traditions. What most medieval authors, independent of their authoritative reference texts, seem to have been concerned with, more concerned perhaps than comparable modern deliberations, is a stage of transition that would mediate between sensual perception and abstract thought. Mainly developed in St. Thomas's *De anima,* as Daniel Heller-Roazen impressively demonstrates in chapter 2, the medieval notion of *sensus communis* fits this very structural place. For Aquinas describes *sensus communis* as a sense that contributes to the transformation, a "vertical" transformation, so to speak, of (what we call) perceptions into (what we call) thoughts. But *sensus communis* is also supposed to serve, "horizontally," in determining the relations between the different types of perception that come from different senses.

On a higher level of typological abstraction, one might want to claim an affinity between *sensus communis* and the concept of the "soul," as St. Augustine uses it. For, like *sensus communis,* Augustine's notion of *anima* is located between the senses and the highest functions of the mind—but, more than *sensus communis, anima* implies, for St. Augustine, that the soul actively inspires and animates the senses. This could explain why, in clear contrast to most modern conceptions, medieval discourses often describe the senses as driven by an outward-going dynamic, a dynamic that flows toward the material world and addresses it, rather than merely and passively reacting to its impact. This trend becomes particularly apparent in certain medieval treatises about the sense of vision, some of which Stephen Nichols analyzes in chapter 14, with stunning results. Once, however, the senses are thought of as being active, such a conception seems to require that the function of the sense organs is doubled by other functions that are closer to the spirit. Roger Bacon, for example, in his book on *perspectiva,* distinguishes between the eye's perception (for whose description Bacon uses geometrical forms) and, on the other hand, acts of synthesis that Nichols characterizes as "visual judgment."

Visual judgment seems to have its historical and epistemological basis in a model that Gregor Vogt-Spira's chapter 3 traces in Greek and Roman source texts. This model hinges upon the concept of *phantasia,* whose Augustinian translation as *imaginatio* we can retrospectively identify as a decisive movement in intellectual history. Imagination will occupy the mediating position and function between the senses and human cognition. For like *sensus communis, phantasia* (*imaginatio*) had found its original discursive place between *aisthetis* and *noesis.* Emphasizing the active role played within perception by yet another mediating faculty, Vogt-Spira goes so far as to attribute, convincingly, I think, the task of meaning attribution to *phantasia.*

Patent Fascinations

There is ample reason to believe that the ancient concern with mediating levels in the process of cognition turned into a medieval fascination with the motif of "the eyes of the mind," as we can find it, with a high degree of variation, in multiple discourses and individual texts. Let me underline, once again that the "eyes of the mind" (or the "eyes of the heart"), from a medieval point of view, were not just a metaphor. Adulterous thoughts and imaginations, therefore, as Marina Brownlee shows in chapter 4, were not as categorically different from adulterous acts—as we tend to see it today. Now, the most interesting question may be why it is so difficult for us moderns to concede to the inner sphere of human existence and human cognition certain functions and effects that are—to say it again—not categorically different from sensual perception. My tentative answer is that the modern astonishment about the "eyes of the mind" comes from our self-reference as "subjects," that is, from our self-reference as immaterial outside observers of a material word. We see ourselves as standing outside Nature and not in a situation of immersion into or fusion with Nature, as Michel Zink claims for medieval culture in chapter 5. As long as we think that, as humans, we are "outside Nature," it would be incoherent to claim that our psyche can have an immediate contact with Nature. Immersed into and fused with Nature, in contrast, it is no longer out of the question that our psyche may be thought of as having "eyes" that function like sense organs. Chapters 1, 3, 6, and 14 document how fruitful indeed and how central the motif of the "oculi mentis" became since the transition from classical Antiquity to medieval times.

Another fascination that becomes explicit in medieval texts, a fascination indeed bordering on obsession, stems from the presupposition that any object of experience is not only necessarily a part of the order of divine Creation but must show signs of its inscription into this order. It was above all during the first and second of our three colloquia about the medieval senses that we became familiar with the tenacious medieval debates about the number of the human senses and, also, with the efforts of finding a symmetry and a mutual correspondence between the five senses and the (unfortunately only) four elements. But none of these attempts at fitting the senses into a cosmological order ever achieved any discursive or institutional stability. Nor did those more ambitious arguments that tried to prove that a hierarchical order existed among the different human senses. Rainer Warning, in chapter 6, one of the conceptually richest contributions to this volume, suggests that epiphanic events, in their classical ontology, were predominantly visual, then became primarily acoustic in Christian Late Antiquity and in the Middle Ages (within a topology that staged the word of God as a word to be heard by the "ears of the mind"), to end up turning back to visuality in the early modern period. As far as the change in the predominant patterns and motifs of epiphany is concerned, I certainly agree with Warning. But there is particular reason to be reluctant with general and rather abstract descriptions of the historical transformations in question. For while Warning is most likely right in the historical thesis suggested by his narrative, there was a truly striking openness and variety to the medieval senses as an intellectual field that we should elaborate and highlight rather than level through any totalizing claims.

Hidden Energies

"Under the surface" of all those discourses whose authors were struggling (but never ultimately successful) to draw a coherent picture of how humans were supposed to establish their relations with the world of objects, a proliferation of thoughts and concepts were producing tensions that had a powerful—indirect—impact on the ways people were living in medieval societies. This impact was not a direct consequence of any specific arguments or conceptions. Rather, I imagine, it was an involuntary effect coming from the interference of certain claims and promises, pressures, and hopes, an effect that escaped the control of the historical agents. Without any doubt, one of the breakthrough discoveries of our debates is marked in chapter 7 by Joachim Küpper's characterization of medieval culture's relationship to the dimension of the senses as "hysterical"—however strong this word may sound at first. In his symptomatological reading of a Castilian text from the fifteenth century, Küpper develops the insight that medieval behavior was trapped between the conflicting premises of, on the one hand, an (Aristotelian) worldview within which a sense-based approach to the material world was a necessary condition for survival; and, on the other hand, the Christian-Paulinian condemnation of the senses as making permanently present the original sin as an unavoidable road to perdition. It is my impression that Küpper's description of this medieval "hysteria" corresponds to the modern definition of the "double-bind" situation, that is, the situation of an obligatory choice that always already implies an illegitimate transgression—which is one reason why his thesis offers a truly innovative master key for the understanding of certain behavioral patterns in medieval societies.

I can also see a possibility of connecting his thesis, on a (more or less) psychoanalytical basis, with David Nirenberg's historical demonstration in chapter 8 of how the Paulinian motif of the "dead letter" became a central resource of energy for Christian anti-Semitism. For, is it not plausible to imagine that making the Jews responsible for humankind's material-based, sensual relationship to the world, was a preconscious attempt, on the Christian side, of cutting through the hysterical ambiguity of its own relation to the material world? Was anti-Semitism not a way of dissolving this ambiguity by just isolating one half of the double bind that was associated with original sin?

Andreas Kablitz's both provocative and persuasive argument in chapter 10 about the (again: largely implicit) attitude in which medieval culture may have lived (rather than "experienced") the temporality of Christ's redemption, fits, in an almost uncanny fashion, the double-bind panorama suggested by Küpper and Nirenberg. For if the original sin was perceived as a presence, as a sensual presence indeed that neutralized temporal distance, then the drastic cruelty of the crucifixion needed to be equally present, sensually present, in order to keep available and open the hope and the possibility for salvation. This "keeping present" of Christ's passion was of course institutionally shaped and condensed in the sacrament of the Eucharist—which ritual, I believe, offers the strongest support for Kablitz's bold thesis. Within the range of medieval culture, the theological need to keep the act of Christ's passion present echoes what Michel Zink describes as the temporal logic of the *locus amoenus*—however far apart these two motifs and the emotions that they triggered must have been.

For the eternal spring that permeates the *locus amoenus* and its never-ending sensual gratifications is also based on a "suspension of temporal progress," together with a "dilation of the moment of perception." The seasons do not change, in the *locus amoenus,* as the presence of the original sin and the presence of the act of redemption do not fade; and gratification is eternal, just as the pain of Christ's passion and the seduction of the both sensual and sinful desire from the original sin in Paradise will never cease.

There is a danger, however, to push too far such attempts at bringing together, in a reconstruction resembling a "system," the different vectors and energies that sprang from living and from thinking the senses in medieval culture. This is why we should not forget our characterization of their interplay as a "field of forces"—which certainly implies that there were fascinations and obsessions that appeared in seeming isolation. Jan-Dirk Müller and Hildegard E. Keller deal with such decontextualized motifs, in chapters 11 and 12, respectively. Analyzing the exuberant thirteenth-century narratives attributed to Konrad von Würzburg, Müller discovers an unbridled display of rhetorical effects in the descriptions of bodies and objects that produce, as the text itself describes, a splendor that "blinds" both protagonists and readers. It is as if an exclusive concentration on the material world had left behind all the warnings against its seductive powers. Keller, in contrast, returns to the familiar scenes of "invisibilization" in medieval romance—where knowing about a presence that has no perceptive equivalent produces moments of confusion and panic. In this case, it is as if the other side of the sensual double bind, the empirical relation to the material world, had been lost, and the loss had triggered all kinds of textual reflections about the world order and why it can or cannot be grasped by human intuition.

Once we compare these first impressions about how the senses and their functions were experienced in medieval culture to a modern worldview, the one unifying characterization that comes to mind for the Middle Ages is "insecurity." Invariably, the medieval senses appeared to be much less reliable than today, they caused endless deceptions and uncertainties, and this must have had to do with the fact, at least in part, that the Sciences' view of phenomena of nature had not yet differentiated itself into an exclusive view. Sensual perception, myth, and freewheeling speculations, therefore, were still tied together, without any generally accepted hierarchy between them.

Frames

This insecurity about the senses within medieval culture is still—and perhaps forever—doubled by our scholarly uncertainty about the conditions and the extent to which the border between the Latin world of learning and the sphere of vernacular writing and thinking was permeable (or not) for concepts, arguments, and existential energies. Can we assume, for example, that troubadour poetry was informed by the Aristotelian view of the senses and of their relation to the material world? Of course there are individual cases, like that of Jean de Meun, author of the second part of the *Roman de la Rose,* where biographical knowledge encourages us to count on a learned background for a vernacular text. As a general rule, however, I would go with the more skeptical view that Michel Zink advocates. We may well juxtapose vernacular texts and the "learned apparatus" that modern scholarship has established about the worldviews of medieval scholars; we may then engage in endless debates about possible parallels and influences—but we will never reach a level of certainty regarding the relationship between these two discursive dominions within medieval culture.

We encounter similar problems when we try to delineate and to limit the medieval senses as a complex historical phenomenon, along somewhat vague chronological lines. Does their dominance begin with the writings of the Church Fathers, or do their concepts, arguments, and models still belong to the intellectual realm of classical Antiquity? It is certainly much easier to pinpoint at least some symptoms for the historical vanishing of typically medieval speculations and fascinations about the senses during the waning of the Middle Ages. Heather Webb's beautiful reconstruction in chapter 13 allows us to discover the fully developed "cardiosensory" model, as it had emerged in the thirteenth and fourteenth centuries, based on a combination of elements from

Galen's and from Aristotle's topologies of the human body. At a considerable level of complexity, this system claimed to explain the origin and the effects of allsensory phenomena, both spiritual and physical, through the action of the heart. Taking up a suggestion from Niklas Luhmann, we might consider this cardiosensory view as an "involutionary" symptom, that is, as a full, almost obsessive development of the possibilities offered by a conceptual repertoire, a development whose push toward perfection, paradoxically somehow, announced its imminent vanishing. Rather than as a syndrome of involution, Stephen Nichols makes us understand in chapter 14 that the multiple mirror scenes and mirror images that characterize the *Roman de la Rose,* and also the text's indulging in many forms of observer reflexivity, were the beginning of a transitional stage between medieval and early modern paradigms of world observation.

With Petrarch's "differential" staging, as Rainer Warning describes it, of epiphanies that now become secular epiphanies experienced by lovingly admiring eyes and, even more obviously and solidly, with the new shaping of the world observer position in Galilei's science and in Descartes's philosophy, we find ourselves on the side of a modern epistemology of the senses. This also was the beginning of an era whose anti-Semitism had to discover new sources of energy in biologically, rather than theologically, based forms of prejudice. But can we finally say that the modern age is a time of liberation from the "hysterical" lock into the dimension of the senses, into the double bind that held the senses trapped between original sin and redemption, into the double bind, too, that had paralyzed and, at the same time, energized medieval culture? Michel Foucault, among others, has shown that the "liberation of the senses" was indeed one of the self-entitling claims formulated by the discourses of the Enlightenment and advocated by science and politics since the nineteenth century.

At the beginning of the twenty-first century, we have become weary of similar premises—and such skepticism may well have been the mood, an ambiguous mood, that first triggered, somehow preconsciously, our interest in the medieval senses. Are we not once again torn between an aesthetic desire and an ascetic repulsion of the material world? Today the number of those is growing who make this double bind plausible to themselves by seeing it as the play between the religious concepts of "redemption" and "original sin." For some others among us who continue to experience secularization as a point of no return, the same function is now covered by the tension between sports as an array of health care and sports as erotico-hedonistic excess. And there are more variations for the same structural pattern at hand.

PART ONE
Heritage

1 Seeing God

Augustine, Sensation, and the Mind's Eye

Eugene Vance

To speak of "the medieval senses" compels us to turn upside down and to complicate a mechanistic model of cause and effect that prevails broadly in the unscientific discourses of modern culture: namely, the supposition that sensation originates with stimulations or movements of the bodily organs of sight, sound, odor, taste, or touch. In this brief essay, I'll first summarize Augustine's very different understanding of the dynamics of sensation, and then explore some of its ramifications. One should bear in mind, though, that even though Augustine carefully studied the painful lessons of his own youthful indulgences and yearnings, and later brought to bear on them the best scientific and medical theories of sensation available to him, his purpose was never to valorize the phenomenon of sense experience as an end in its own right.[1] To the contrary, his goal as a Christian Neoplatonist was theological: to discover how his mind (*mens, intellectus*) might be liberated from its servitude to material bodies (*sensibilia*) so that it may pursue its preordained trajectory toward wisdom (*sapientia*) that might culminate in the knowledge, love, and sight of God.

The Structure and Physics of Sensation

Augustine held that feeling (*sentire*) could not originate or occur in the body but only in the soul.[2] Nothing, including a plant or animal, can be alive unless it is first vivified by soul (*anima*), which "animates" the body and provides for its survival, nutrition, and processes of growth and reproduction.[3]

Otherwise, Augustine asks, how could sensation possibly begin in the body if a dead body can sense nothing?[4] Etymologically, *anima* derives from a Greek root (*anemo*) signifying a wind, or breeze, and in that sense it is nearly synonymous with *spiritus,* and is a figure of the psychological processes of movement and emotion.

> [T]he nature of the human soul is not of earth nor of water nor of air nor of any kind of fire; but all the same it administers [*administrare*] the coarser material of its body, namely a kind of moist earth which has been given the quality of flesh, by means of the finer kinds of body, that is by means of light and air; without these two, you see, there is neither any sensation in the body, nor any deliberate movement of the body by the soul. . . . The soul, therefore, being something non-bodily, first activates the kind of body which is nearest to being non-bodily, like fire (or rather light) and air; and then through the other coarser elements of the body, like moisture and earth, which constitute the solid mass of the flesh, and which are more subject to being acted on than equipped to act.[5]

The hierarchal levels of Augustine's subjective being as "soul" were homologous with his understanding of the objective hierarchy of cosmic being, extending upward from the lowest order of material things to God. Thus, the human soul infuses not only biological life into the highest of all corporeal forms, but spiritual life into an intellect that has the capacity to free itself from sensible knowledge in order to ascend in a hierarchy of incorporeal beings by learning truly to know (*scire*) it.[6] We should perhaps bear in mind from the start that Augustine constantly revised and refined his theories of the human soul, concluding after three decades of speculation that the human soul exists as an image of the Holy Trinity, in *On the Trinity* (*De trinitate*).[7]

In Augustine's psychology, the notion of sensation involves what transpires across the threshold between the material body and the vital principle—or the immaterial being of the soul. The sense organs are corporeal, but sensation occurs in what some of Augustine's sources Aristotle and the Neoplatonists Porphyry and Victorinus (but not, apparently, Augustine himself) called the "sensitive" soul. Augustine called it the "passive" soul because at the level of basic reflexes the human soul does not respond to sensations "actively," that is to say, intellectually or rationally.[8] Rather, the passive soul merely experiences or "undergoes" (*pati*) as passions (*passiones*) the data of whatever in the realm of corporeal things strikes the five body's sense organs. Augustine commonly used the term *anima* to signify the lower levels of the soul's range of being—that is to say, its life as an embodied yet sentient and knowing soul. The souls of animals (but not, of course, those of plants) share that human potential of being and knowing, though only in a limited way: for instance, like humans, animals certainly know material things; so too, their souls are "moved" (*movere*) according to that material knowledge; but what is crucial is that, unlike humans, animals cannot *know* that they are knowing.

When Augustine wishes to refer more specifically to the higher operations of the animal (and human) soul, he uses the word *animus,* and the shared Greek etymological roots of both *anima* and *animus* express the movements of "wind" (*anemos*) or breathing.[9] This movement begins with the soul's experience of material things (*sensibilia*), including that of its own body, and then with an understanding of how it "moves" or is "moved" (*movere*) according to that knowledge. Such movements are also called "passions" (*passiones*) or "affections" (*affectiones*). Following the Stoics, Augustine held that the four basic human passions or emotions (or "movements") of the passive soul are fear (*metu*), desire (*cupiditas*), grief (*dolor*), and joy (*gaudium*).[10]

If the male gender of *animus* names the higher, rational faculty of the soul, and the female gender of *anima* names the passive and irrational faculties of the soul, the very foundations of Augustine's psychology imply what might seem like a hierarchal gender model, though in fact it can be expressed equally by men and women. Thus, Augustine praises his mother Monica as someone who was "by form a woman, by faith a man" (*muliebri habitu, virili fide,* IX. vii. 8). Males, in other words, have no monopoly over virility.

Augustine uses the word *mens* (which we commonly translate as "mind") to imply all levels of the soul's inner life, but more specifically its capacity to know immaterial things, whose status is commensurable with that of the soul itself as an immaterial, or spiritual, entity. However, he reserves the word "intellect" (*intellectus*) to refer only to the soul's highest power: specifically, that of attaining rational understanding (*intellectio*) of what is true, including knowledge of its own truth *as* soul. The soul's power to attain true knowledge (*scientia*) extends upward to the final threshold of understanding, which lies between the order of eternal beings (or forms), and God as infinite Being. Beyond this threshold, all higher knowledge comes only with *ecstasis* or illumination.

In a word, the bodily sense organs are necessarily the instruments that inform the soul about the world so long as it remains incarnate in its human body: "The sense of the eyes . . . is called a sense of the body precisely because the eyes too are parts of the body; and although an unconscious or lifeless body does not sense anything, yet it is through a bodily instrument [*instru-*

mentum] that the conscious soul [*anima]* is mixed with the body senses, and it is this instrument that is called a sense."[11] It follows that the body's organs can sense nothing by themselves. For instance, sight is made possible by the bodily eye; but the act of *seeing* occurs only in the soul. Thus, the faculty of sight, the phenomenon of seeing and the object seen are three separate and ontologically distinct components of a triad constituted by visual perception as a *process.*[12] As he explains in *On the Trinity,*

> When we see some particular body, there are three things that we can very easily remark and distinguish from each other. First of all there is the thing we see, a stone or a flame or anything else the eyes can see, which of course could exist even before it was seen. Next there is the actual sight or vision [*visio*], which did not exist before we sensed that object presented to the sense. Thirdly there is what holds the sense of the eyes on the thing being seen as long as it is being seen, namely the conscious intention [*animi intentio*].[13]

Since sensation occurs in the soul, one might think or speak of the passive soul as having five discrete inner senses, each pertaining to a single sense organ located in the various parts of the body. However these multiple discrete sensations are all enabled by a single higher or collective power of the soul, which Augustine also called the inner sense (*sensus interioris*).[14] The soul (*anima*) can feel a discrete bodily pain in only one location of the body—in the foot, for example, and not everywhere else—but the sensitive soul, by contrast, must be simultaneously present to the whole body and all of its parts. Augustine once empirically demonstrated this point to his young friends by cutting a centipede in two and watching how the separate pieces squirmed at once.[15] Even though the passive soul pervades the whole body, we must think not in terms of five autonomous inner senses, but of five potentialities of a single inner sense.

Augustine held that together, the five bodily organs of sight, sound, smell, taste, and touch express a hierarchy based on how the four physical elements (fire, air, earth, and water) engage the human soul. Earth is the lowest and grossest of the four elements, and it affects the sense of touch. Because touch can affect the whole body all at once, both outside and inside, this sense most threatens to degrade the soul and estrange it from the spiritual realm that is proper to it.[16] Augustine singled out not earth, but the bodily touch of women as the most pervasive and overwhelming form of (male) sensuality, and on that score Augustine knew all too well what he was talking about: "The word lust [*libido*] usually suggests to mind the lustful excitement of the organs of generation. And this lust not only takes possession of the whole body and outward members, but also makes itself felt within, and moves [*commovere*] the whole human [*homo*] soul [*animus*] with a passion [*voluptas*] in which mental emotion [*affectus*] is mingled with bodily appetite [*carnis appetitus*], so that the pleasure which results is the greatest of all bodily pleasures."[17] Taste requires water, while smell requires only moisture; and hearing requires air. Because sight functions only by means of light, it entails no physical contact between the seer and the seen, and on that ground, sight is the highest of the five senses. Vision, Augustine says, is the bodily sense most compatible with the rational life of the active soul: "So let us use for preference the evidence of the eyes; this is the most excellent of the body's senses, and for all its difference in kind has the greatest affinity to mental vision [*visio mentis*]."[18]

The discrete five senses can perform their mandated purposes, but cognitively nothing more:

> Now when we perceive [*sentire*] color, we do not by that same sense [*sensus*] perceive [*sentire*] that we are perceiving [*sentire*]. When we hear a sound, we do not hear our sense of hearing. When we smell a rose, we do not smell our sense of smell. When we taste something, we do not also taste the sense of taste. When we touch something, we cannot also touch the sense touch. It is therefore obvious that none of the five senses can perceive itself, although all of them can perceive material objects.[19]
>
> We see bodies through our bodily eyes because the rays of our mind [*radii mentis*] which shoot out of them touch whatever they observe; but we cannot snap off these rays and bend them back into our own [seeing] eyes except when we look in a mirror.[20]

If sensation does not occur in the sense organs but in the soul, where in the body does the soul feel the effects of the separate and local bodily senses? Plotinus, who was Augustine's major primary source of Neoplatonic doctrine, had located the "source or principle [*arche*]" of sensation in the head, according to H. J. Blumenthal, because the nerves that are the locus of sensation lie there. Therefore, the combined data of several sense organs can activate the intellectual powers of imagination and of movement lying adjacent to them in the "active" rational soul, which resides in the brain.[21] For his part Augustine believed, more precisely, that while the vital soul permeates the entire body, the data of the five bodily senses that affect the passive intellect senses converge and are united in the forward chamber (*ventriculus*) of the brain. As his disciple Evodius puts it in *On the Free Choice of the Soul* (*De libero arbitrio*):

> I think that by reason we understand that we have a kind of inner sense [*quisdam sensus interioris*] to which everything is conveyed from those five familiar senses. An animal's sense of sight is one thing; the sense by which it either avoids or pursues what it sees is quite another. Sight is in the eyes, the other [inner] sense is in the soul. By it animals either pursue and accept what gives them pleasure [*delectare*] or avoid and reject what gives them pain [*offendere*], whether these things are the objects of sight or of hearing or of the other bodily senses. This inner sense is itself neither sight nor hearing nor smell nor taste nor touch. It is the same other thing that presides over all of them.[22]

However, the capacity of the inner sense to recognize the data of more than one sense and respond to several senses with the appropriate bodily reflexes implies the participation of our memory as well. These three nearly simultaneous operations—sense perception, recognition, and bodily movements—imply three different lobes of the brain:

> since bodily movement [*corporalis motus*], which follows upon sensation [*sensus*], always involves intervals of time, and since we cannot perform deliberate movements [*spontanei motus*] over intervals of time without the aid of memory [*remiscentia*], that is why the brain is shown to have three ventricles [*ventriculi*], one in front, at the face, from which all sensation is controlled; a second behind at the neck, from which all movement comes; the third between the two, in which they demonstrate that memory is active; otherwise, since movement follows upon sensation, you may fail to link your perceptions to what has to be done, if you have forgotten what you have done on previous occasions.[23]

The soul (*anima*) itself is distinct from the brain's operations, but makes the latter possible by vivifying (*vivificare*) the body, and so it mobilizes the functions of the brain in the same way as it does the other bodily organs, and by doing so it rules over them (*regere*).[24]

In short, the faculty of inner sense is what empowers the passive soul to undergo sensations, though the inner sense itself cannot be considered as properly active or rational in its fullest sense, if only because animals (who are not rational) share it with us too: "An animal would not move to pursue or flee from something unless it perceived the fact that it was perceiving, and cannot perceive that fact by any of the five senses. This perception does not amount to knowledge [*scientia*], since only reason [*ratio*] can produce knowledge; but it does suffice to move the animal."[25]

Although it is prerational and not properly intellectual in its own right, the inner sense still presides over the body's senses and its reflexes, and it should therefore keep their operations orderly. The inner sense functions as a sort of soul's street-cop whose beat includes the bodily senses:

> the inner sense is a kind of controller [*moderator*] and judge [*iudex*] of the bodily sense. If the sense falls short in performing its duty [*officium*], the inner sense demands that its agent [*minister*] make good on this debt. . . . The sense of the eye does not see whether it is seeing or not, and so it cannot judge what it lacks or what is enough. That is the job of the inner sense, which warns even the soul of an animal to open its eyes and make up for what it perceives is missing.[26]

When the human will impels it, the inner sense can either block unwanted or improper sensations, or (just as importantly) *incite* desired bodily sensations and reflexes. Augustine gives several examples. The inner sense can block pain associated with the touch of fire and prevent the bodily reflexes that burning would normally summon—just as if the person who is being burnt were already dead.[27] There are other people who can vomit not only when they wish, but expel whatever element they wish, as if they were taking it out of a sack; others can fart and even sing by doing so; one man, whom Augustine claims to have known, could sweat on demand; and elsewhere Augustine recalls hearing of another man who could think so hard about embracing a woman that he could spontaneously ejaculate.[28]

Though not rational in its own right, the inner sense nevertheless organizes and conveys information about the world of sensible things in such a manner as empirically to support the higher rational operations of Platonic dialectics. These are division (or definition) and synthesis.[29] The first corresponds to the mind's need to perceive discrete objects as they are apprehended in a distinct or "specific" aspect; the second corresponds to the ability of the several inner senses to combine the data of things perceived by several senses so as to find in them a generic or "common" sense: "The inner sense . . . perceives [*sentire*] material objects through the bodily senses and perceives the bodily senses themselves. And by reason all of these things, as well as reason itself, become known [*nota*] and are part of knowledge [*scientia*]."[30] This higher power of synthesis came to be known as the "sixth" sense, or what Augustine commonly called the "eye of the mind" (*oculus mentis*).[31] In other words, "eye of the mind" provides to the mind a perceptual ground that can initiate a journey that extends beyond the data of corporeal species and genres, beyond a hierarchy of eternal or spiritual forms akin to the human soul's own being, and concluding (during rare moments during this lifetime) in an intellection of the one (or "simple") and all-transcending God.[32]

When the inner sense appears to fail in its duty, where, one may ask, does the fault lie? In the bodily senses? In the inner sense itself? In the intellect? Augustine's answers to all of these questions are based on the single principle: that whatever is lower in the hierarchy of being has no power to affect what is higher. Therefore, the bodily sense organs are not inherently bad: they become harmful only when the inner sense fails to control them. As the next power of the soul, the inner sense, in turn, is not bad either, so long as it remains subordinate to the higher faculty of reason. But can reason itself ever be bad? No—though the last answer is not simple, since reason itself is subject to the human will, and the will is corrupted by original sin, from which it cannot be freed unless by the wisdom of Christ, the soul's interior "teacher,"[33] or by God's grace, which directly illuminates the human mind with true wisdom.[34]

Soul, the Inner Sense, and Sensation

So far, we have considered the phenomenon of sensation mainly in an upward trajectory that begins when the inner sense first apprehends and organizes the data of the bodily sense organs in order to enable the soul's quest for rational knowledge and spiritual illumination. However, Augustine also deplored the fact that sensual impulses could subvert the goals of his mind as well as propel them. Moreover, the early Augustine was also intrigued by an inverse principle: that every act of the human mind exerts some kind of downward effect upon the bodily senses. Do higher mental acts always inevitably provoke in some way the inner sense to somatize the life of the mind?

Such was Augustine's claim in one of his earliest letters, written soon after his conversion to Christianity to his close friend Nebridius in 386. In this letter, he responds to Nebridius's question as to how supernatural beings (*superiores potestates*) or demons (*daimones*) can provoke thoughts and dreams in us: "I am of the opinion that every act of our mind [*motus animi*] produces some effect in the body, and that, however heavy and slow our senses may be, they feel this effect, in proportion to the intensity of the mental act, as when we are angry or sad or joyful."[35] So too, he believed that bodily sensations can be stirred up from *outside* the soul by the intrusions of divine and demonic beings upon the perceptive life of the inner sense:

From this it may be concluded that, when we think something which has no apparent effect on the body, it can nevertheless be apparent to the supernatural [*aerius*] and heavenly [*aetherius*] spirits, whose perception [*sensus*] is so very keen that ours does not deserve the name of perception in comparison with it. Therefore, those traces [*vestigia*] of its activity which the mind imprints [*figere*], so to speak, on the body can both remain and take on a certain appearance; and when they are subconsciously [*latere*] aroused [*agitare*] and activated [*contrectare*], they easily produce in us thoughts and dreams according to the intention [*voluntas*] of the arouser [*agitans*] and activator [*contrectans*].[36]

Augustine gives many examples of this phenomenon in his writings, especially in the final book of the *City of God*, with stories of demonic possessions of the bodies and minds of pathological people, as well as examples of miraculous cures wrought by divine intervention through the advocacy of the saints. Thus, whether the inner sense and the bodily senses are moved by intramental acts or by external beings (demonic or divine) that possess the soul, the body undergoes what we would now call "psychosomatic" sensations, and these are "true" in the same way that modern psychiatrists hold that psychosomatic sensations are experienced no less "truly" than those arising from the body itself.

Thus, just as Plotinus taught that the beauty of intelligible forms can stir up sensual pleasure that is more sublime and intense than that caused by sensible objects,[37] so too, Augustine affirmed that God's presence in the higher soul could excite both the inner sense and the bodily senses according to his scheme of divine justice. Thus, he tells in the *Confessions* how the tempest of his own divided will tormented his entire body during his struggle in a "monstrous state" while poised on the threshold of conversion in Milan: "Finally, in the shifting tides of my indecision, I made many bodily movements, whether because they lack certain members or because those members are bound with chains, weakened by illness or hindered in one way or another. If I tore my hair and beat my forehead, if I locked my fingers together and clasped my knees, I did so because I willed it."[38]

Augustine also tells in the *Confessions* how, after his conversion, his soul *and* his body could rejoice simultaneously in their spiritual pleasure at God's presence as it flooded the five senses, both outer and inner, of his being:

What is it then that I love when I love you? Not bodily beauty, and not temporal glory, not the clear shining light, lovely as it is to our eyes, not the sweet melodies of many-moded songs, not the soft smell of flowers and oint-

> ments and perfumes, not manna and honey, not limbs made for the body's embrace, not these when I love my God.
>
> Yet I do love a certain light, a certain voice, a certain odor, a certain food, a certain embrace when I love my God: a light, a voice, an odor, a food, an embrace for the man within me, where his light, which no place can contain, floods into my soul; where he utters words that time does not speed away; where he sends forth an aroma that no wind can scatter; where he provides food that no eating can lessen; where he so clings that satiety does not sunder us. This is what I love when I love my God.[39]

By themselves, bodily sensations obviously cannot reveal anything about a God who transcends the intelligible as well as material world, but when our senses apprehend the beauty of the creation, these can certainly incite the soul's inner sense to participate and rejoice, to the limit of its capacity, in the truth of God as its Creator:

> Better indeed is that inner being. For to it, as that which rules over other things and passes judgment upon them, all those bodily messengers reported back answers of heaven and earth and all things that are in them, as they said: "We are not God!" and again, "He made us." The inner man knows those things through the ministry of the outer man.[40]

By virtue of its status as a spiritual or "intelligible" substance, the human soul is eternal; however, during this present life the soul must rely on the data of the sense organs, as a basis for immediately apprehending its own body, as well as for intellectual knowledge of the bodily world around it during this earthly life. However much its involvement with the perishable world makes the soul subject to accidental degradation, the soul remains an imperishable substance in its own right. And because it is imperishable, it is also "capable of sharing in that wisdom which is changeless."[41]

Because what exists *truly* exists, it follows that "falsity is not in things, but in the senses."[42] More precisely, he writes, a misperception does not arise in the sense organs themselves, rather, "it is the soul that either causes or cooperates in causing it."[43] Thus, the bodily senses do not lie. For instance, "the image of a crow may be, as it were, set before the eyes, recognizable in all its features; but by subtracting or adding certain details it may be changed into something never seen anywhere."[44]

If, by its innate rational powers, the soul may truly distinguish between perishable and imperishable things, more importantly, it can then also recognize its own power to *know* that truth. With the knowledge of that knowledge, the soul may then grasp *the* truth of itself as a spiritual and eternal being. Thereafter, the soul must will to cherish and *cling* to that truth so that it will govern the life of the senses. The soul that senses most fully the truth of its own being finally becomes capable of recognizing—and perhaps of momentarily seeing—God himself (in whose image humans were created) as the indivisible and eternal truth and being of all that exists.[45] Such, then, is Augustine's Neoplatonic trajectory from sensual knowledge to spiritual knowledge that is capable of knowing even God.

Though God is ultimately intelligible to the pure soul,[46] the early Augustine believed that for the human soul to know either the material and sensible world intellectually, it must first become trained in the disciplines of the liberal arts. By contrast, the later Augustine believed that ultimately, all spiritual truth is immediately revealed.

The Senses and the End of Vision

Augustine's final goal (and that of all Neoplatonizing Christians) was not merely to know and love God, but ultimately to contemplate, indeed, to *see,* him eternally.[47] Scripture, of course, had variously both denied and affirmed that very possibility, whether as a recorded event, a human wish, or divine promise. On the one hand, God had told Moses, "You cannot see my face; for no man can see my face and live."[48] On the other hand, Isaiah claimed that he "saw the lord of hosts sitting on a throne."[49] Christ assured his disciples that "[b]lessed are the clean of heart, for they shall see God."[50] So too, Christ had preached that "[h]e that sees me sees the Father also."[51]

Moreover, the apostles John and Paul prophesied that humans might not only see, but even *resemble* God. "We know that when He shall appear, we shall be like to Him, because we will see him as he is."[52] "But we, beholding the glory of the Lord with open face, are transformed into the same image from glory to glory as by the spirit of the Lord."[53]

The promise that humans might contemplate and, by so doing, resemble God[54] rested on a direct analogy with the so-called extramissive model of bodily vision that prevailed in Classical and Early Christian culture. According to this model, vision occurs when "rays" of the mind (*mentis radii*) are emitted from the bodily eyes. When these rays strike and conform to some material object, they simultaneously convey its image back to the perceiving mind.[55] The sensory image of the thing perceived through the inner senses is imprinted as a phantasm or image (*phantasia, visum, imago*) in the seer's memory, or imagination, and it dwells there as a basis of future recollection and cognition. Humans are free to choose whether or not their soul will conform to this or that higher or lower image. Images, the early Augustine believed, are the basis of all cognition, and even incorporeal or "intelligible" things (including numbers, dimensions, and forms) that do not exist materially at all may be perceived by the inner senses as images through the mind's "eye" (*oculus mentis*) when it actively seeks or "looks for" (*aspicere*) them, and later in this chapter we will study Augustine's earliest exploration of that potential. The later Augustine, by contrast, would substitute the model of the Word/word for that of the image as a foundation of cognition and intellection.[56]

In short, three different classes of image (that sensed by the body, that supposed by the imagination, and that which is intelligible) may reside in the imaginative area of the human memory.[57] Their common presence and availability imply that the seer's soul will be potentially degraded or reformed according to the *kind* of image that the soul wills and summons to mind during its cognitive activity. Like his mentor Victorinus,[58] Augustine understood that, despite the fact that the sensitive intellect is a property of a soul that dwells in a material body, that same still remains free *intellectually* to judge and use images of sensible objects when it so chooses. So too the mind can freely lust after—and worse, proliferate in itself—images of sensuous things. The soul that does so punishes itself, however, because by doing so it has willfully forsaken the true happiness that lies only in the contemplation and enjoyment of intellectual (and eternal) substances because these are the soul's proper habitat. As Augustine put it in his treatise, *On the Free Choice* of the will:

> Only something that is seen can incite the will to act [*facere*]. It is in our power [*potestas*] to control what we summon [*sumere*] or reject [*respuere*] what we see, but we have no power to control what is seen [*tangere*]. Therefore, we must acknowledge that the soul as a rational substance [*substantia*] sees both superior and inferior things; and according to the merit of what is summoned, the soul suffers either misery [*miseria*] or happiness [*beatitudo*].[59]

Thus, for Augustine as for Plotinus, the primordial fall of the soul begins not in the bodily senses, but within the soul itself when it first directs its attention away from its search to know spiritual or intelligible things, and chooses instead to entertain and indulge in the images of material things.[60] Evil, in this sense, consists in a subversion of the soul's high place and purpose in the hierarchal order of being. In other words, when an impious or unhealthy (*insana*) active soul is enslaved by bad physical habits which cause it to recall and then proliferate, as a kind of mental cinema, phantasms of sensuous things (including its own body), these incite involuntary frenzies in the body.[61] Inversely, the inner sense that willfully blocks or purges corporeal images keeps the soul free to embrace spiritual truths with all its being, and sometimes to glimpse even God himself during a moment of *ecstasis*.[62] Moreover, for the soul to attain this vision is momentarily to recover its supreme and inaugural status as God's image, according to which humanity was first created, "in the beginning."[63] This exalting instant of restored *mimesis*—that of the seer to the Seen—"deifies" the human soul, a term that the Neoplatonists and Greek Fathers readily used, though a term that Augustine himself used only occasionally, and with extreme caution: for example, in his Commentary on Psalm 49, Augustine writes that deification is accorded only by God's grace, and cannot be achieved by any human power.[64]

As for the hope of seeing God eternally in the future life, Augustine always bore in mind Paul's prophecy that the saved would see God face to face in eternity: "We see now through a glass darkly, then, however, face to face."[65]

However, this irreducible question never ceased to preoccupy Augustine: how can finite human vision, whether physical or spiritual, possibly be commensurable with an all-transcending, infinite, and invisible God? More radically, how, as both testaments of Scripture record, proclaim, or at least imply, might humans be able to see God face to face in this present life with their bodily eyes?

Augustine revisited the latter question many times during his four decades as a theologian and writer. Each time, however, he did so with a different rhetorical goal and method, without ever affirming that it was indeed possible. His most careful statement on the question is stated in a treatise written as a long letter in 413 to a high lady named Paulina, where Augustine concluded that humans cannot see God either corporeally or mentally in this present life, and that only a very few among the saved in heaven will see God.[66] Only near the end of his life did he answer the question definitively, and affirmatively, and he did so to his entire satisfaction: if seeing God with bodily eyes is not presently possible, it certainly will be so in the life of the future. As he concluded in the final book of his most laborious and exalted lifework, the *City of God*, the old bishop triumphantly prophesied that after death, the human souls of the saved would indeed contemplate God. What is more, he believed that when the resurrected bodily eyes are restored to the souls of the saved after the Last Judgment, all of these souls will even more perfectly see God, love him, and praise him eternally.[67]

Such are the broad parameters of the relationship between the bodily senses, the human mind, and the sight of God. However, to summarize Augustine's premises thus is drastically reductive, and even misleading to the extent that it implies the steady and coherent growth of doctrine in an orthodox mind—as if (in retrospect) this progress had been inevitable, and as if his "errors" were not also precious for what they reveal both to him and his readers. Any doctrinal synopsis of Augustine's theology can only occult the radical ups and downs, the rhetorical vitality, and the aleatory insights and lapses of Augustine's boldness as a student of the human soul, starting with his own. Augustine was always as interested in exploring the search for understanding as he was in adhering to its truth. But what kinds of sufferings, sacrifices, and personal choices does that search necessarily imply? To fortify both himself and his readers, Augustine recited (often only indirectly) over and over again this verse of Matthew: "Ask, and it will be given you; seek, and you will find; knock, and it will be opened to you."[68]

Notes

1. A partial exception to this generality is a treatise he appended as Book XII to his commentary, *The Literal Meaning of Genesis* (*De Genesi ad litteram*), included in *On Genesis,* trans. Edmund Hill, The Works of St. Augustine: A Translation for the 21st Century (Hyde Park, NY: New City Press, 2002), 464–506.

2. *De Gen. ad lit.* III. v. l; Augustine, *Soliloquies* (*Soliloquia*), trans. Gerard Watson, *Soliloquies and Immortality of the Soul* (Westminster: Aris and Phillips, 1986), II. i. 1.

3. *On the Greatness of the Soul* (*De quantitate animae*), xxxiii. 70.

4. *Sol.* II. iii. 3.

5. *De Gen. ad lit.* VII. xv. 20.

6. Ibid., xxxiii. 70–76.

7. For a concise and helpful schema of the human soul's homologous functions with respect to the hierarchy of being, see the diagrams and explanations offered by Edmund Hill in his preface to the last four books (IX–XIV) of *De Gen. ad lit.*

8. For a discussion of the "active" and "passive" dimensions of the human intellect in Porphyry and Victorinus, who were Augustine's most immediate sources of Neoplatonic theories, see Pierre Hadot, *Porphyre et Victorinus* (Paris: Etudes augustiniennes, 1968), I. 190–200. To my knowledge, Augustine himself used the term "passive" in that sense only twice in *The City of God* (*De civitate Dei*), VIII. xv and IX. viii, though the concept was implicit in his mind from his first days as a devout initiate to Christian Neoplatonism.

9. See *anima* and *animus* in www.perseus.tufts.edu.

10. *De civ. Dei* XIV. ix. 1. He often named these same things in other ways, depending on the context.

11. Augustine, *The Trinity* (*De trinitate*), trans. Edmund Hill, The Works of St. Augustine: A Translation for the 21st Century (Hyde Park, NY: New City Press, 1993), vol. 5, XI. i. 2.

12. *Sol.* I. vi. 12.

13. *De trin.* XI. i. 2.

14. Augustine, *On Free Choice of the Will* (*De libero arbitrio voluntatis),* trans. Thomas Williams (Indianapolis: Hackett, 1993), II. iii. viii.

15. *On the Greatness of the Soul* (*De quantitate animae*), xxxi. 63.

16. *De Gen. ad lit.* III. iv. 6.

17. *De civ. Dei* XIV. xvi. 1. I have changed the word "man" used by the translator for *homo* to "human."

18. *De trin.* XI. i. 1.

19. *De lib. arb.* II . iii. 9–iv.10, *On Free Choice of the Will,* trans. Thomas Williams (Indianapolis: Hackett, 1993).

20. *De trin.* IX. ii. 3. Brackets mine.

21. H. J. Blumenthal, *Plotinus' Psychology: His Doctrines of the Embodied Soul* (The Hague: Martinus Nijhoff, 1971), 33.

22. *De lib. arb.* II. iii. 8.

23. *De Gen. ad lit.* VII. xviii. 24.

24. Ibid.

25. *De lib. arb.* II. iv. 10.

26. *De lib. arb.* II. v. 11.

27. *De civ. Dei* XIV. xxiv.

28. Ibid. Regrettably, I am unable to recall the textual reference for that last detail.

29. Plato, *Phaedrus,* 265c–266b.

30. *De lib. arb.* II. iii. 8

31. For an overview of the history of the notion of the "common," or "sixth" sense, see Peter von Moos, "Le sens commun au moyen âge: sixième sens et sens social. Aspects épistémologiques, ecclésiologiques et eschatologiques," *Studi medievali,* 3rd series, vol. 43, fasc. I (2002): 1–55.

32. This is precisely Augustine's lofty (but failed) philosophical project in *Sol.* I. 15.

33. Augustine, *On the Teacher* (*De magistro*), xiv. 46.

34. *Sol.* I. vi. 12; *Retractations* (*Retractationes*), I. xii. 11.

35. Augustine, *Letters* (*Epistolae*), trans. Wilfrid Parsons, The Fathers of the Church, A New Translation (New York: Fathers of the Church, 1951), vol. 1, Letter 9, to Nebridius (389).

36. Ibid. See also, *De trin.* IV. xi. 14.

37. Pierre Hadot, *Plotin, ou la simplicité du regard* (Paris: Plon, 1963; rpt. Folio, 1987), 51.

38. Augustine, *Confessions* (*Confessiones*), trans. John K. Ryan (Garden City: Doubleday, 1961), VIII. viii.

39. *Conf.* X. vi. 8.

40. *Conf.* X. xxvii. 38.

41. De *trin.* III. i. 8.

42. *Sol.* II. iii. 3.

43. Ibid.

44. Augustine, Letter 7, to Nebridius (389), 18.

45. Such was Augustine's claim in *Conf.*

46. *Conf.* VII. xvii. 23.

47. For two basic studies on the question of seeing and contemplating God, see Fulbert Cayré, *La contemplation augustinienne* (Paris: A. Blot, 1927), and J. Maréchal, "La vision de Dieu au sommet de la contemplation d'après saint Augustin," *Nouvelle revue théologique* 2 (1930): 89–109; 191–214. The very notion of *sapientia* is indissociable from the knowledge and sight of God in contemplation. See Henri-Irénée Marrou, *Saint Augustin et la fin de la culture antique* (Paris: Boccard, 1983), 363. The later Augustine, by contrast, held that the sight of God may only be achieved through the Holy Spirit (*De trin.* XV. v. 27).

48. Exod. 33:20.

49. Isa. 6:1.

50. Matt. 5:8.

51. John 14:9.

52. 1 John 3:2.

53. 2 Cor. 3:18.

54. Jean-François Pradeau, *L'image du principe: Plotin et la participation* (Paris: Vrin, 2003), 97–103.

55. See David C. Lindberg, *Theories of Vision from Al-Kindi to Kepler* (Chicago: University of Chicago Press, 1976), 1–16.

56. See, e.g., *De trin.* IX. x. 15.

57. Augustine revised that triad in 413 in Book XII of *De Gen. ad lit.* (XII. vi. 15–xxxvi. 69), which is his most sustained "scientific" treatise on the faculty of vision in the human soul: here they are called corporeal, spiritual, and intellectual.

58. Hadot, *Porphyre et Victorinus,* I. 198.

59. *De lib. arb.* III. xxv. 74.

60. Paul, 1 Cor. 13:12. The importance of this doctrine to Augustine was its congruence with the Plotinian notion that contemplation implies a mimetic relationship between the human soul that sees and the One that it contemplates. See Pradeau, *L'image du principe,* 106–147.

61. Pradeau, *L'image du principe,* 127.

62. *Conf.* VII. vii. 23.

63. Gen. 1:26.

64. For a list of occurrences of the word in Augustine's writing, consult the search engine CETEDOC, or the Web site www.sant-agostino.it/latino.

65. 1 Cor. 13:12.

66. Augustine, "On seeing God," trans. Mary T. Clark, *Augustine of Hippo, Selected Writings* (New York: Paulist Press, 1984), 365–402.

67. *De civ. Dei.* XXII. xxx. 5.

68. Matt. 7:7. He quotes it some nineteen times in *Conf.* alone, according to James J. O'Donnell's count in his edition and commentary, in Augustine, *Confessions* (Oxford: Clarendon, 1992), vol. 3, 470.

2 Common Sense

Greek, Arabic, Latin

Daniel Heller-Roazen

Another Common Sense

Little seems more obvious than common sense. Before the undeniable differences between the idioms, beliefs, cultures, and traditions of individuals and communities, little seems more likely to be assumed, affirmed, and reaffirmed than this simplest of senses, which everyone, in principle, can share. On the surface, of course, the terms for the phenomenon are many. To the contemporary sensibility one may attribute a number of names, which imposed themselves with increasing force in the course of the development of the technical and conceptual vocabulary of the aesthetic, moral, and political philosophy of the modern age. At the inception of that development, Descartes identified common sense as simply "good sense" (*bon sens*), that with which no rational being would disagree, and which every demonstration must presuppose. In the *Discours de la méthode,* we thus encounter the sense as the most fundamental of the faculties of reasoned reflection, which precedes and conditions the many forms of argument and proof learned in the schools: it is merely the capacity "to judge well, and to distinguish the true and the false" (*de bien juger, & distinguer le vray d'auec le faux*).[1] From Chanet, who explained that in its regular use, "common sense" signified "nothing other than the Reason common to all men,"[2] to Fénelon, for whom it was a matter of the "first notions that all men have equally of the same things,"[3] to Buffier, Condillac, Helvétius, and Voltaire, the shared sensibility remained in modern French thought an often named and much discussed phenomenon, a datum repeatedly presupposed, to be lauded as a *lumen naturale* or, instead, to be condemned as a crude form of reason (*raison grossière, état mitoyen entre la stupidité & l'esprit,* in the terms of Voltaire).[4]

The philosophical literatures of the modern European languages contain abundant references to the common sense in this modern acceptation. In the tradition of the English language, the first attestations of the expression in this meaning date from the time of the Cartesian formulation of the phenomenon. It seems that it was not long before the usage grew frequent, giving rise to an intellectual tradition to which the notion of common sense proved in every sense decisive. Thomas Browne already invoked sound "common sense" in opposition to unfounded metaphysical "speculations and subtilities"; E. Herbert of Cherburg considered its perceptions to be the fruits of the *instinctus naturalis* of all men; J. Toland assimilated it to "reason in general"; and, beginning with the inception of the eighteenth century, "common sense" functioned in English philosophical parlance, from Berkeley to Shaftesbury, Hutcheson, Hume, and Reid, as a synonym of "judgment," "reason," and "right understanding."[5] In modern German thought, the notion later came to provoke greater controversy, but it retained a central role in the elaboration of the doctrine of the good and the beautiful, as well as the theory of the human cognitive faculties as a whole. It suffices, in this setting, to note that Kant's opposition to the Scottish common-sense philosophers did not keep him from assigning to *sensus communis* a capital role in the fortieth section of the *Critique of Judgment.*[6] One may also recall Herder's pronouncement, whose philosophical consequences are great: "We are a thinking *sensorium commune,* which is merely touched at various sides."[7]

It is well known that the early modern debates about the shared faculty of judgment had a rich and widely contested afterlife in nineteenth- and twentieth-century thought. More modern thinkers repeatedly returned to the question of the conditions, limitations, and promise of a common sense, in discussions which involved moral, social, political, and aesthetic theory, as well as the philosophy of science. After Hegel, Marx, and Nietzsche, who aimed in different ways to call into question the immediate evidence of any "sound common sense" (*gesunden Menschenverstand*), such diverse philosophical figures of the last century as Bergson, Arendt, G. E. Moore, Gadamer, and Lyotard all sought to rehabilitate the notion alternately with and against the modern tradition in which it had played such a prominent role.

It has less often been observed that the modern notion of common sense as a cognitive faculty shared by all men is of ancient origin, a conceptual invention to be attributed, more precisely, to the classical Roman tradition. Before Vico and Shaftesbury, the phrase *sensus communis* already appears in the prose of Latin authors, where, as in the early moderns, it designates a sensibility shared by all, from which one may deduce a number of fundamental judgments that need not, or cannot, be questioned by rational reflection. It has been remarked that Cicero, for instance, writes in these terms of the necessity of a common sense (*pincipio necesse erat sensu exsistere unum communemque omnium*),[8] that in the *De rerum naturae* Lucretius founds certain truths on the self-evidence of the *communis sensus,*[9] and that Quintilian and Seneca both invoke a *sensus communis hominum* as a faculty by which all men can determine which of their principles they may take for granted.[10]

There is, however, another common sense. It is far less familiar to the modern epoch, but it was for a long time the principal philosophical concept signified by the expression "common sense," whose meaning we now so unhesitatingly take to be, if one may say so, a matter of common sense. In the philosophical vocabulary of the Arabic, Hebrew, and Latin Middle Ages, the term *sensus communis* (like the corresponding *koinē aisthēsis, al-hiss al-mushtarak,* and *hush* or *da'at meshutaf*) designates not a sensibility common to men, by which all can agree on certain judgments more fundamental than those of rational argument, but a mode of sensation in the most literal sense: a power of perception to be classed among the primary faculties of the soul, whose role in the doctrine of sensation is at least as decisive as that of the five senses of sight, hearing, touch, taste, and smell. The common sense, in this "second sense," was not the invention of the medieval thinkers. Like the notion of the shared sensibility that remains current today, the concept of common sense known to the philosophers of the Middle Ages had its roots in classical antiquity. It hearkened back, however, to a period prior to the emergence of the Roman doctrine of the *sensus communis hominum* that has held sway, in a revised and amplified form, in modernity. The medieval theory of common sense found its roots, like so much else of the psychology of the Middle Ages, in Aristotle's doctrine of the soul, as it was transmitted to literary posterity by the *De anima* and the lesser philosophical and medical treatises known to modern Europe as the *Parva Naturalia.*

These works on the nature of life approach their object, in accordance with the classic Aristotelian procedure, by means of a series of definitions of increasing specificity: the Philosopher characterizes the soul by its parts, its parts by its functions, and its functions, in turn, by the various phenomena with which they are concerned.[11] At the start of the second book of the *De anima,* Aristotle thus pauses to distinguish the faculties of the soul (*dynameis*), which constitute the structurally distinct dimensions of its operation. In human beings, they appear to be five: nutrition (*threptikon*); appetite (*oretikon*); sensation (*aisthētikon*); movement (*kinētikon kata topon*); and thought (*dianoētikon*).[12] The enumeration proposed by Aristotle moves from the most fundamental of the faculties of the soul, the nutritive faculty, which is shared by all living beings, vegetative and animal, to the most rarefied of them, the intellectual faculty, which man alone among animals seems to possess. At its center lies sensation: "the first characteristic of the animal,"[13] according to the Stagirite, which may be defined in general terms as a form of "being moved upon and acted upon" (*hē d' aisthēsis en tōi kineisthai te kai paskhein symbainei*).[14]

According to the second book of the *De anima,* the sensitive faculty in turn operates by means of five proper senses: sight, hearing, smell, taste, and touch. To each sense, Aristotle maintains, there corresponds a proper object, which affects the soul through each of the five forms of sensation. They are, respectively, the visible, the audible, the odorous, the gustative, and the tangible.[15] In each case, Aristotle writes, sensation takes the form of "a kind of mean [*mesotētos*] between two objects,"[16] for the actual object of sensation always presents itself as situated at a certain point on a continuum between two opposed sensible qualities. Take, for instance, the sense of sight: the visible object that is seen falls invariably between the extremes of the bright and the dark. So, too, Aristotle reasons, the tangible that is the object of the sense of touch must fall between the rough and the smooth, or the hard and the soft; and, in the same way, the gustative that is the object of taste can always be situated between the extremes of the sour and the sweet, and so forth.[17] To each of the five senses, there correspond, therefore, a proper object as well as a proper spectrum of perception, and in the event of actual sensation, the two phenomena remain inseparable: one always perceives the visible at a point between the extremes of dark and light, and one always encounters the tangible at some point between the extremes of rough and smooth.

Aristotle shows no signs of doubting that the proper senses are five, and only five.[18] But his account of sensation does not end with their enumeration, classification, and analysis. For the Philosopher is acutely aware of the existence and importance of experiences of sensation that far exceed the competencies of the individual senses. The first among them involves those perceptual phenomena considered by Aristotle to form the set of "common sensibles": motion, rest, figure, magnitude, number, and unity.[19] When, for example, we perceive that something is moving, or at rest, or square, or large, or three, or one, by means of what sense do we do so? Aristotle makes it clear that such sensibles cannot impress themselves upon the soul through any one of the five senses; on the contrary, they are "common" in that they remain perceptible by any, and by all, of the senses as a whole. We may, for example, sense by the faculty of vision that there are many leaves on a tree, perceive by the sense of hearing or by that of smell that something is approaching or moving away, sense by taste that something is composed of two ingredients, or sense by touch that an object is round. In each case, the perception of the common sensible cannot be conceived as the activity of any one of the proper senses. To explain it, one must go further.

A second phenomenon that clearly exceeds the bounds of the proper senses is that of complex sensation, in which we perceive, in a single moment, a number of sensible qualities of different types. As we have seen, the second book of the *De anima* establishes that each sense "discerns differences in its sensible object" (*krinei tas tou hypokeimenou aisthētou diaphoras*).[20] The principle is fundamental to the Aristotelian theory of sensation, but on its own it can hardly do justice to sensory experience, as the Stagirite himself indicates toward the inception of the third book of the treatise on the soul. "Vision discriminates between white and black," he writes,

> and taste distinguishes between sweet and bitter, and similarly in all other cases. But, since we also distinguish white and sweet, and compare all objects perceived by each other, by what sense do we perceive that they differ? It must evidently be by some sense that we perceive the difference; for they are objects of sense.[21]

Here the limitations of the proper sense, as Aristotle defines it, come fully to light. The sense of sight can clearly distinguish between the bright and the dark, even as the sense of taste can tell the sweet from the sour. But how can one explain the sense that something is bright and also sweet, or, alternately, the sense that something is bright but not sweet? The particular sense can perceive the difference that defines its own proper object, but it can do no more; the sense of the conjunction and disjunction of the qualities of the senses cannot be attributed to the activity of any one of them. There must be yet another sense, which coordinates, unifies, and distinguishes the five senses, while coinciding, at the same time, with none.

Aristotle devotes particular attention to a third sensory phenomenon that he considers to lie within the province of sensation and yet to exceed the terrain of the five senses. It is the "perception of perception," the bare sense that something at all is sensed. The Stagirite clearly indicates that the existence of such a perception, which he presupposes as evident, implies a substantial theoretical difficulty (*aporia*). "Since we perceive that we see and hear," Aristotle reasons, "it must be either by sight itself, or by some other sense."[22] Both possibilities lead to perplexity. If it is by the sense of sight, for instance, that we perceive that we see, then the sense of sight has not one but two objects: the proper object of vision will be not only the visible but also the mere fact of vision, and it will be necessary to reject the doctrine developed in the preceding sections of the treatise, according to which to every particular sense there corresponds a particular object, situated at a point in a continuum between two extremes. But if, instead, it is by a sense other than sight that we perceive that we see, the problem cannot be said to be solved. For what will one say of this second sense: does it, too, perceive that it perceives the fact of vision? "Either the process will go *ad infinitum,*" Aristotle writes, "or a sense must perceive itself."[23] To avoid an infinite regress, the Philosopher must therefore accept that a sense may refer to itself, that it may, in other words, perceive its own perception. He thus finds himself obliged not so much to revise his doctrine of the five proper senses as to complete it, through the introduction of a further faculty of sensation, by which not only the sense of sense but also common sensibles and complex sensations may all be perceived.

Aristotle calls this faculty of sensation "common sense" (*hē koinē aisthēsis*).[24] In the terms of the *De anima,* this "sense" constitutes a power of perception that is common to all the five senses yet reducible to none of them. Strictly speaking, the common sense is for this reason not a sixth sense, for it is nothing other than the sense of the difference and unity of the five senses as a whole: the perception of the simultaneous conjunction and disjunction of sensations in the common sensible, the complex sensation, and, finally, the self-reflexive perception. To be sure, the discussion of the matter in the *De anima* is elliptical, and it is not easy to interpret; the terms of the Aristotelian corpus as a whole, moreover, are varied and can be read in several ways. The *De anima* contains the expression "common" or "shared sense" (*hē koinē aisthēsis*);[25] the *De memoria* refers instead, in a treatment of a similar phenomenon, to "the primary sense" (*to prōton aisthētikon*);[26] the *De sensu* contains a discussion of "the total sense" (*to aisthētikon pantōn*);[27] and in the *De somno* we read of "a common power" (*tis koinē dynamis*) among the faculties of the soul.[28] Modern scholars of Aristotle have therefore differed in their interpretations of these expressions. Some have sought to refer the many terms of the

De anima and the *Parva Naturalia* to a single perceptual faculty, of which Aristotle gave fragmentary, if precious, indications; others, by contrast, have wished to separate them, and to distinguish all the terms of the lesser treatises from the "common sense" (*koinē aisthēsis*) of the *De anima.*[29]

The medieval tradition developed its own responses to the question. For in the period that followed the dissemination and reception of the peripatetic doctrine of the soul, the diverse terms of the Aristotelian treatises came to be read together as the elements of a complex theory of common sense that remained only implicit in the works of the Stagirite himself. In different ways, the philosophers of the medieval Arabic and Latin tradition, from Al-Fārābī to Avicenna, Averroës, Albert, and Thomas, found in the *De anima* and the *Parva Naturalia* the scattered elements of a coherent doctrine of the "central" faculty of the sensuous soul; and, over the course of the centuries that witnessed the transmission, translation, and transformation of philosophy from Greek to Arabic and from Arabic to Latin, they made of the Philosopher's enigmatic remarks on the "shared sense" the basis for far-reaching and original accounts of the relations between perception and intellection and between sensation and thought.

Régimes of Sensation after Aristotle

According to the doctrine proposed by the Stagirite, the common sense is but one of several faculties of the soul whose operation transcends the activity of the five proper senses. Aristotle discusses them, in programmatic fashion, after having treated sight, hearing, smell, taste, and touch, in the pages which are considered today to compose the opening of Book Three of the *De anima* but which, in the medieval edition of the treatise, were appended to the discussion of the senses in Book Two. After the brief discussion of the "shared" power of the soul, the Philosopher offers an extended discussion of the faculty of the "imagination" (*phantasikon*), by which the mind retains and represents to itself actual sensation in the form of the "phantasm," as it assumes the position of a "spectator looking at something dreadful or encouraging in a picture" (*hōsper an hoi theōmenoi en graphē ta deina ē tharraleia*).[30] The discussion of imagination, in turn, leads logically in the *De anima* to a consideration of the power of "cognition" (*dianoētikon*); for it is by means of the apprehension of sensibility in "images" that the soul moves to the abstraction that defines the intellectual act.[31] Finally, to the imagination and cognition, the commentators of the peripatetic doctrine could add a further postsensory power, which the

Philosopher considered at some length in the *De memoria,* namely, "memory" (*mnēmoneutikon*).[32] Together, the three faculties formed a class to which the classical and late ancient thinkers could add, or not add, the common sense. Galen, whose influence in the late ancient and medieval account of the powers of the soul can hardly be overestimated, thus considered imagination, cognition, and memory as the elements of a single set of postsensitive faculties.[33]

All these capacities of the soul are known in the historical lexicon of philosophy as "internal senses," presumably because the medical tradition, beginning with Galen, locates the seat of their power within the brain and believes them to function without the use of bodily organs.[34] The term "inner sense," however, is not to be found in the Aristotelian corpus; and there is no evidence that it was used by the commentators of the Stagirite in their accounts of the peripatetic doctrine of the soul. The earliest attested application of the predicate "internal" to designate one of the Aristotelian postsensory faculties appears to have been the work of the Stoics, who according to an ancient source held that "the common sense is kind of inner touching, by which we are able to grasp ourselves" (*Hoi Stōikoi tēnde tēn koinēn aisthēsin entos haphēn podagopeuosi, kath' hēn kai hēmōn autōn antilambanometha*).[35] It was perhaps this Stoic usage that constituted the point of departure for Augustine, who was the first Latin writer to make use of the expressions "inner sense" and "internal power," and to do so repeatedly. In Book One of the *Confessions,* Augustine wrote of an *interior sensus* "that preserves the fullness of the five senses" (*custodiebam interiore sunsu integritatem sensuum meorum*);[36] in Book Seven of the same work he referred to an *interior vis* that reproduces external objects within the soul (*interior vis, cui sensus corporis exteriora nuntiaret*),[37] and in the second book of *De libero arbitrio,* he assigned to a power he called *sensus interior* all the functions of Aristotle's common sense: the perception of common sensibles, the unification of sensory data, self-reflexive perception, and the "judgment and measurement of the external senses."[38] After Augustine, "inner sense" gradually became an accepted term in the conceptual vocabulary of the Latin Church Fathers. As H. A. Wolfson has shown, in Gregory the Great one finds references to a "sense of the brain" (*sensus cerebri*) that "presides within" (*qui intrinsecus praesidet*) and that performs several of the activities of the Aristotelian common sense, and in Eriugena we learn that the Greek term *dianoia* ("cognition") signifies an "internal" (*interior*) power of the soul.[39]

Classical Arabic and Hebrew philosophy includes the term "internal senses" (حواس باطنة, חושים פנימים) in its technical lexicon from its inception.[40] The thinkers of the tradition, who were both physicians and philosophers, classified these powers of the soul in a variety of ways, which, as Wolfson demonstrated, can be reduced for the purposes of economy to two taxonomies. According to one school, which includes Hunayn ibn Ishāk, Razi, Isaac Israeli, and Pseudo-Bahya, the internal senses include imagination (*khayāl*), cognition (*fakr*), and memory (*dhikr*); according to the other, which includes Ibn Gabirol, Abraham ibn ᶜEzra, and Maimonides, they are instead imagination, thinking and "comprehension" (as in Ibn Gabirol and Maimonides, who employ the term *fahm*) or "wisdom" (as in Ibn ᶜEzra, who has *hikma*).[41] Both sets seem traceable to a Galenic source.[42] It is remarkable that in both the classifications of the early Arabic and Hebrew thinkers, common sense finds no place among the "internal powers" of the soul. Although the Aristotelian shared sense appears to lie at the origin of the formulation of the concept of the internal sense in both Greek and Latin, it is excluded from the first systematic accounts of the inner powers in Arabo-Islamic thought. It is as if common sense could be no more easily assimilated to the higher perceptual powers of the soul than to the lower ones; it is as if the "shared" faculty of sense were not, in short, a sense among others, be it "external" or "internal."

This impression is confirmed by one of the earliest surviving considerations of common sense, a discussion of the faculty by the early tenth-century Egyptian philosopher and physician Isaac ben Solomon Israeli. Often considered the first medieval Jewish philosopher, Isaac Israeli wrote in Arabic; but his works were translated into Hebrew and into Latin, circulating in the centuries after his death in Christian Europe as well as the Islamic world. In *The Book of Elements* (*Kitāb al-Ustuqsāt*), which survives only in fragmentary form in Hebrew and Latin translations, the original Arabic being lost, Isaac devoted several pages to the psychological conditions of prophecy. Reconstructing the teaching of the "Ancients" on the nature of sleep and dreams, he offered the following characterization of the place of common sense within the order of the human faculties:

> The common sense is intermediate between the corporeal sense of sight and the imaginative faculty, which resides in the anterior ventricle of the brain and is called *fantasia.* It is for this reason that it is called "common sense," for it receives from corporeal sense, i.e., that of sight, the corporeal aspects of things and transmits them to the spiritual sense mentioned before, i.e., the imaginative faculty [*cum sit medius inter sensum visibilem scilicet corporeum et informatum qui est in anteriori parte cerebri nominatuum phantasia*].[43]

Isaac Israeli's claims for the singularity of the faculty are striking. The sense of the peripatetic tradition appears here as the intermediary faculty between the many powers of the soul: neither corporeal nor incorporeal, neither external nor internal, neither sensible nor intellectual. It is said to be "common," therefore, in a new sense: not because, as in Aristotle, its power can be attributed to each of the senses, but precisely because it differs from them all, as the medium can be distinguished from that which it mediates. The common sense of the Judaeo-Arabic thinker constitutes a sense of the threshold between all the senses, a sense of the lines at which each fades into the next and the lower powers of the soul border upon the higher.

If one turns to the surviving works of the first of the great Arabic philosophers, the contemporary Abū Nasr al-Fārābī, one finds that the position of common sense among the sensible and cognitive powers of the soul is no less singular. The "second master" left us two classifications of the internal senses. The first, to be found in the *Epistle on the Classification of the Sciences,* consists of a description as well as an enumeration, while the second, to be found in one of the lesser works, contains only an enumeration.[44] Both omit all reference to common sense. But in the twentieth chapter of *The Book of the Views of the Inhabitants of the Virtuous City,* which is dedicated to parts and powers of the human soul, the "shared power" of the Aristotelian tradition is clearly present. After having described the nutritive faculty as composed of a "main power and others that are servants and nursemaids," Fārābī turns to the sensitive faculty. He writes:

> The sensitive faculty is also composed of a main power [*ra'īs*] and nursemaids [*riwāda*ʿ]. The latter are the five senses known to everyone, and they are located in the eyes, the ears and the rest. Each of the five senses perceives the sensible that is proper to it. The main power is the one in which all the perceptions of the five senses are gathered together, the five senses being like its reporters. It is as if the five senses were all its advisors, each responsible for a different kind of information from one of the regions of the kingdom. The main power is like the king at whose court the advisors gather the news from all the regions of the kingdom.[45]

Fārābī invokes a trope that finds its classic formulation in Plato's *Republic:* the order of the soul appears as that of a political unity. But the Platonic metaphor functions in the *Virtuous City* to reformulate the Aristotelian doctrine of the powers of the soul. The *politeia* of the Arabic philosopher, to be sure, is not a city, but a kingdom (*mamlaka*); yet behind the masks of its characteristic personages it is not difficult to see the faculties of the Aristotelian treatise on the soul. Just as to every sense, according to the second book of the *De anima,* there corresponds a particular object, to each of the five "advisors," there belongs a single region; and just as the individual senses, in the account of the Stagirite, are said to receive their sensible objects at a given position in the spectrum that defines its appearance, so each of Fārābī's "advisors" is entrusted with the task of relaying to the capital news drawn from his own terrain.

The striking invention of the Arabic philosopher consists in the elevation of the one Aristotelian faculty now said to be "king" (*malik*), which is no less unmistakable in this chapter for remaining unnamed and unqualified as either outer or inner: it can be none other than common sense. Here the classical capacity is no longer said to be merely "shared" among the faculties of perception, nor is it characterized as "intermediary" in the order of the soul; it is neither external nor internal but, instead, capital, the "main power" with respect to which the proper senses are but "nursemaids." Even as it is the ruler who establishes the law that divides and unifies the territories of a single kingdom, so it is common sense, in the allegorical fable of the *Virtuous City,* that secures the order of the powers of the sensible soul, allotting to each its terrain as well as the responsibility of drawing from it the "kind of information" proper to it. It follows that the disappearance of common sense would inevitably bring about the demise of the entire régime of sensation: in the absence of the king, after all, there can be no kingdom, and without this "ruler" and his court, the second master suggests, the sensible soul would not be one.

Avicenna's Central Faculty

Only with Avicenna, the great Persian philosopher of the early eleventh century, did common sense find a fixed place within the classification of the internal senses.[46] The early Arabic thinkers, as we have seen, proposed a threefold account of the higher powers of the sensible soul, which, although variable in its details, can be understood as the reproduction of a Hellenistic adaptation of the Aristotelian distinction between "imagination" (*phantastikon*), "cogitation" (*dianoētikon*), and "memory" (*mnēmoneutikon*). To these three faculties, Al-Fārābī added a fourth: "estimation" (وهم), later to play a prominent role in the psychology of the Latin Schoolmen, to whom it would be known as *aestimatio.*[47] Avicenna offered a number of different classifications of the internal senses, which alternately reproduced the two taxonomies of the tradition and exceeded them in their scope. In the medical treatise known to the Latin West as the *Canon,* Avicenna thus adopted a threefold classification at one point and suggested a fourfold one at another; and in the philosophical masterpiece of his maturity, the *Shifā'* as well as in its abridgment in the

Najāt, he went further, distinguishing five internal senses, which could also rise to seven depending on the principles by which one counts them.[48] At every point, however, Avicenna revised the classical definition of the first of the internal senses, the imagination: for from his earliest works to his last, he maintained that its activity necessarily implied that of common sense. The claim came to be canonical in the philosophy of the Latin Schools, and by the thirteenth century Thomas Aquinas could note simply and in passing in the first part of the *Summa Theologiae* that "in his book on the soul, Avicenna posits five inner sensitive powers, namely, common sense, imagination, the imaginative faculty, estimation, and memory [*sensum comunem, phantasiam, imaginativam, aestimativam, et memorativam*]."[49]

The "book on the soul" to which Thomas referred was the treatise on psychology of the *Shifā',* which, translated from Arabic into Latin in Toledo during the second half of the twelfth century, came to be known to the Christian West as Avicenna's *Liber de Anima* or *Sextus de Naturalibus.* It already contained a summary enumeration of the internal senses in the fifth chapter of its first book, which began with the faculty of "fantasy, which is common sense" (*bantāsīa, wal-hiss al-mushtarak, fantasia, quae est sensus communis fantasia, quae est sensus communis*).[50] But the work proposed a systematic account of the nature of the faculty only in the first chapter of Book Four, which considered all the internal powers of the soul as a whole. Avicenna began his discussion with common sense, and from the opening of the chapter he made it clear, with a characteristic gesture, that he believed at least some of his predecessors to have greatly misunderstood the true nature of the phenomenon. Against those who had invoked the power to explain common sensibles alone, he argued, in programmatic terms, that "common sense, on the contrary, is the faculty that receives all sensible things."[51] His proof was pellucid: were it not so, no animal, man or beast, could ever link a sensible object of one type to that of another. Were common sense not the sense of all things sensed, after eating something sweet, we would never know how to connect what we had tasted with something we could see, and after hearing the song of a certain man, we would not be able to recognize by vision the man who sang it. "The life of beasts" too, the philosopher commented, would then be harsh: had they no common sense, animals would not know to tie the sight of a wooden stick to the sense of pain, nor could they sense, from a certain smell, that they were close to the object of a certain taste.

Avicenna thus significantly extended the range and the significance of common sense even as he inscribed it, for posterity, as the most elementary term in the hierarchical ascent of the inner faculties of the soul. He argued that the capacity others had restricted to certain specific types of sensation was in truth no less than the "root (or principle) of all the external senses" (*principium sensuum exteriorum*), the single power which enabled the animal to be affected by various forms of sensitive reception that could be tied to, and separated from, each other. Common sense, with Avicenna, thus acquired a decisive and irreplaceable position within the systematic analysis of the powers of the soul. As the final faculty of sensation and the first internal sense, it articulated the transition from the bare externality of sense to the impassable interiority of thought; it bound the sensitive faculty to the intellectual in leading the five senses back to a nonsensuous principle without which they would have no sense. For in the end, Avicenna cast the inner power not only as the foundation of all the senses but also as their center, the point from which they all "emanated,"[52] engendered in the shared procession from a primary power. Common sense thus became more than the point toward which the five senses moved, the "king" of the Fārābīan parable to which the sensible advisors all brought their news; it now emerged as that from which the five senses originally departed, to which they then returned as to their source. The terms of the Persian philosopher's final characterization of the sense in his *Liber de Anima* are memorable not least for the distance they mark with respect to the source of the doctrine in the Aristotelian treatise on the soul. They were to return, as echoes, to be glossed and amplified, throughout the Arabic and Latin philosophy that followed them. "This power which is called the common sense," Avicenna wrote, "is the center from which the senses ramify, and to which the senses return, like rays; and it is in truth that which senses" (*Et haec virtus est quae vocatur sensus communis, que est centrum omnium sensuum et a qua derivantur rami et cui reddunt sensu, et ipsa est vere quae sentit*).[53]

Albert and the Mediality of Sensation

By the time Albert the Great composed his commentary on Aristotle's *De anima* in the middle of the thirteenth century, the Avicennian account of the soul was well established in the European universities: the philosophical production of such figures as Jean de La Rochelle, Alexander of Hales, and Roger Kilwardby, to say nothing of the various anonymous *Questiones in tres libros de Anima* published in the twentieth century, all bear witness to the depth and precision of the engagement of the thirteenth-century Schoolmen with the works of *Avicenna Latinus*.[54] But the thirteenth-century students of Aristotle benefited also from that monument of philosophical exegesis that is Averroës' *Long Commentary* on the Aristotelian treatise, which was translated sometime between 1220 and 1235 by Michael Scot (and which today survives in that form alone). It is clear that the argument of Albert's treatise on the *De anima* could not have been possible without either contribution to philosophical psychology. The master of Cologne continually departs, expressly and thoroughly, from a close reading of both Avicenna and Averroës, and he builds on the propositions of both *falāsifa* in offering an account of the nature of sensation that is in many respects unprecedented in the history of medieval thought.

Albert dedicates the fourth treatise of his commentary on the "second" book of the *De anima* to the nature of common sense. His method is that of the systematic and progressive interpretation of the Aristotelian text *ad litteram* practiced in the universities of the time, which he distributes in twelve chapters ordered by argument. Unlike Avicenna, his exposition of the theory of common sense therefore proceeds by means of the regular authoritative citation and exposition of the doctrine of the Stagirite. Recalling the setting of the original discussion of the "shared sense," Albert explains that this faculty alone can account for the five complex sensibles (*motus, status, figura, magnitude, numerus et unum*);[55] it alone can give rise to the self-reflexive perceptions expressed by such statements as "we feel ourselves to see and to hear" (*sentimus nos videre et audire:* the example is Avicennian);[56] and, finally, it alone allows for the composition and division of phenomena received by different forms of sense perception.[57] His conclusion unites in one stroke the doctrine of the Aristotelian text and the account of the foundation and source of the sensitive faculties proposed by Avicenna in the *Sextus de Naturalibus:* "We say," Albert writes, in the eleventh chapter of the treatise, "that common sense is the root of all the individual senses; it is the form from which sense flows into all the proper senses" (*dicimus sensum comunem esse principium omnioum sensuum particularium et esse formam, a qua est influentia sensus in omnibus propriis sensibus*).[58]

The next and final chapter of the treatise abandons the form of the commentary altogether. It is marked by the editors of the *Opera Omnia* as a "digression,"[59] but its argument, although novel, follows logically from the discussion of the common sense until this point. Here Albert, deepening his analysis of the status of the faculty as a single power that exercises itself in each of the five senses, reflects on the nature of its unity. He concludes that common sense can be defined as a "universal" form, not, to be sure, in the sense of the predicable, but rather in the sense that it is "a cause that formally preconceives that which emanates from it, just as the architectural plan preconceives the form of the house" (*est universalis non ut praedicabile, sed sicut causa formaliter praehabens ea quae oriuntur ex ipsa, sicut architectonica praehabet formam domus*).[60] The "universality" of common sense, Albert thus argues, consists in the specific causal relation in which it stands with respect to the individual senses: that of "pre-conception" (*praehabitio*). As Alain de Libera has shown, Albert here invokes a technical term of medieval Neoplatonism in his analysis of the Aristotelian faculty. *Praehabitio* hearkens back to Pseudo-Dionysius, who employs the Greek term *proekhein* in the *De divinis nominibus,* as well as to Eustatius of Nicea, who characterizes the Good as that which "preconceives" everything in itself, being at once *superhabens* and *praehabens* with respect to that which proceeds from it.[61]

In a manner that is both philosophically rigorous and conceptually original, Albert thus develops Avicenna's suggestion that the five senses "emanate" from common sense as the rays of a circle derive from its center. Common sense, we now read, constitutes the single power by which the entire sensorial faculty, with its many branches, comes into being. It is the *primum sentiens* which, in its formal universality, already contains the proper senses according to the mode of the Neoplatonic "preconception." Hence the new definition of common sense:

> the first sensing not in virtue of time, but in virtue of nature, that in which the entire sensitive capacity is originally founded—that is common sense, which is the origin of the individual senses, since the proper senses are derived from it, and since it cannot be constituted *e converso* from them, nor can anything of its being come from them.
>
> primum sentiens non quidem tempore, sed natura, hoc est in quo primitus salvatur tota virtus sensitive, est sensus communis, qui est origo sensuum propriorum ita, quo ab ipso derivantur sensu proprii, ita quod non e converso constituitur ab eis nec aliquid sui esse habet ab eis.[62]

Common sense comes close, at this point, to ceasing to be "a" sense at all. For unlike the other senses the "shared faculty" as Albert now defines it constitutes not a distinct form of receptivity but the one power in which "the entire sensitive capacity is originally founded" (*primitus salvatur totat virtus sensitive*). If, adopting a term of the medieval doctors, one gives the name *medium* to the spectrum in which the individual sense perceives its object, then one must conclude, like the editors of Albert's *Opera Omnia,* that common sense is the "medium of media," or, to employ the abstract noun of the medieval philosophers themselves, that common sense constitutes "mediality of all sensible things," *medietas omnium sensibilium.*[63] It is the ultimate element of sensation: the dimension in which, and from which, all sensation comes into being, preserving itself as long as it lasts.

Li fontaine et li sourgons

Translated from Greek to Arabic and from Arabic to Latin, common sense underwent a further transposition at the end of the thirteenth century: together with so much of the conceptual vocabulary of Scholasticism, it passed from Latin into the literary vernaculars of modern Europe. It was thus that Meister Eckhart, for instance, once set out to explain in the idiom of his audience that "the teachers say that there is one power that sees by means of the eye and there is another, that understands that it sees" (*daz in ander kraft ist, dâ von daz ouge sihet, und ein ander kraft, dâ ez bekennet, daz es sihet*).[64] And it was thus that it came to be discussed in the Middle French treatise known as *Li Ars d'Amours de vertu et de boneurté,* which was once attributed to Jean le Bel, later assigned to Jean d'Arkel, and more recently thought to have been the work of neither author. In the seventh chapter of the first part of this work, we find a short attempt, in the terms of the rubric, to "define common sense." The *Ars* offers us the following sketch of the philosophical concept:

> The common sense is a power that embraces all proper things which affect the proper senses. And the particular and single senses, which are external, descend from the common sense, which is internal. It is like the various rays of a circle, which move from the middle of the circle towards all the parts of the circle. And thus the semblances of things that are sensed by the individual senses are brought to the common sense; and this is how the common sense judges the properties of the individual senses, variously distinguishing between the different things by means of the senses that are sensed, just as we distinguish between white and sweet, for instance, in milk. We thus say that the common sense is the fountain and the source of all the individual senses, to which all sensible movement is brought back, as to its ultimate end. This faculty possesses a [particular] object insofar as it is a sense, and it possesses a [particular object] insofar as it is common. Insofar as it is a sense, it receives from things a semblance without matter and without the presence of any material form. Insofar as it is common, it has two activities. One is the judgment on the sensed thing, by which we are aware that we are sensing, as when we judge that we are seeing and hearing by means of

another sense. The second activity is to compare the different things that are sensed, and to imagine. Thus we say: this is sweet and this is even sweeter, this milk is white and it is sweet. And this is why all the aspects of sensed things are brought back to the common sense by each individual sense. Some locate this capacity in the back of the brain, where the nerves of the five senses meet; others place it in the heart, since it is the fountain and the source of life.

Li communs sens si est une puissance ki comprent toutes les propres choses, ki les sens particulars muevent. Et cil sens particuliers u singulars de dehors, si descendent dou commun sens ki est par en dedens; ensi con diverses lignes issent d'un cercle de c'un moïelon d'un cercle, issent à toutes parties de ce ciercle. Et ensi les sanlances des choses par les singulars sens senties, sunt au sens commun raportées; par lesqueles moïennes il juge des propriétés des singulars sens, et dessoivre et destinte entre les diverses choses diversement par les sens senties, si comme nos, entre blanc et douc, disons on lait. Dont disons-nous ke li sens communs est li fontaine et li sourgons de tous les sens singulars, ouquel tot li movement sensible sunt rapporté, si comme en fin derraine. Ceste possance a aucune chose en tant k'ele est sens, et aucune en tant k'ele est communs. En tant ke sens est, il rechoit des choses la sanlance sans matère et toutes voies de matère présente. En tant que communs est, il a deux choses: l'une si est li jugements de la chose sentie, par lequele nous connissons ke nous sommes sentant: ensi que quant nous nous jugoon véans et oïans a l'uevre d'aucun autre sens faisant; la seconde si est comparer les diverses choses senties ensanle, et deviser; ensi que dire: checi est douc et che plus douc. Ci lais est blans et si est dous. Et iche a-il pour ce k'a lui sunt raportées toutes les nuances des choses senties par cascun sens singular. Est cest virtue metent aucun en la derantraine partie de la cervel, là li nerf sentant de cink sens singulars s'asanlent. Li autre le metent ou cuer, pour çou k'il est fontaine et racine de vie.[65]

Each of the functions that define the medieval faculty of the soul appears here in an exemplary abbreviated form. The author has read his Aristotle, but also his Avicenna and his Averroës, and he is not far from Albert. For the French writer, whoever he (or she) may have been, defines common sense as an internal power (*en dedans*) that animates the external senses (*de dehors*) just as the "rays from the middle of the circle move towards all the parts of this circle"; and it is by means of this faculty, he specifies, that it is possible to "judge the properties of the individual senses, to variously distinguish between the different things by means of the senses that are senses," and "to know that we sense" (*ke nous connissons ke nous sommes sentant*). The author, however, does not only echo the *auctores.* He also finds his own expression for the power: it is, he writes, "the fountain and the source of all the individual senses, to which all sensible movements are brought back as to their ultimate end" (*li fontaine et li sourgons de tous les sens singulars, ouquel tot li movement sensible sunt rapporté, si comme en fin derraine*). But the fountain is in truth double. For common sense is not only *li fontaine de tous les sens singulars;* it is also, as we read at the end of the passage, "the fountain and the root of life" (*fontaine et racine de vie*). Perhaps this is because, for the sensitive animals that we are, to live is to know that we feel, and because, as Thomas once wrote, glossing Aristotle, "it is by common sense that we perceive that we are living" (*sensu enim communi percipimus nos vivere*).[66]

Notes

1. Réné Descartes, *Discours de la méthode* (1647), in *Œuvres,* ed. C. Adam and P. Tannery (Paris, 1896–1913), vol. 6, p. 2.

2. P. Chanet, *Traité de l'esprit de l'homme et de ses functions* (Paris, 1649), pp. 21ff.: "La première faculté interne où les Espèces sont portées par les Esprits, s'appelle dans les Escholes le sens commun: Elles n'entendent pas par ce terme, ce que vulgarement nous apppellons ainsi en nostre langue. Le sens commun en François n'est autre chose que la Raison qui est commune à tous les homes. . . . Quelquefois nous entendons par ce terme de sens commun, que ce quer nous nommons autrement les sentiments de la Nature, c'est à dire les lumières naturelles, qui sont restées à l'homme après le péché."

3. See F. de S. de la Mothe-Fénelon, *De l'existence de Dieu,* in *Œuvres* (Paris, 1787), vol. 2.

4. On the development of the terminology of the common sense, see the helpful entry in the *Historisches Wörterbuch der Philosophie,* ed. Joachim Ritter and Karlfriend Gründer, rev. Rudolf Eisler, vol. 9 (Basel: Schwabe & Co. AG, 1971–), "Sensus Communis," pp. 622–675, esp., for the modern period, pp. 639–662.

5. See ibid.

6. Immanuel Kant, *Kritik der Urteilskraft,* I, §40: "Vom Geschmack als eine Art von *sensus communis.*"

7. "Wir sind Ein denkendes *sensorium commune,* nur von verschiednen Seiten berührt," in J. G. Herder, "Über den Ursprung der Sprache" (1772), I, 3, in *Herders Sämmtliche Werke,* ed. B. Suphan et al. (Berlin: Weidmann, 1877–1913), vol. 5 (1891), p. 61.

8. Cicero, *Timaeus,* 12, 44.

9. Lucretius, *De rerum naturae,* I, 422–425.

10. Quintilian, *Institutio oratoria,* I, 2, 29; Seneca, Ep. I, 5, 4. See "Sensus Communis," in *Historisches Wörterbuch der Philosophie,* pp. 629–634.

11. See the helpful analysis in Jacques Brunschwig's "En quel sens le sens com-

mun est-il commun?" in *Corps et âme: Sur le "De Anima" d'Aristote,* ed. Gilbert Romeyer Dherbey and Cristina Viano (Paris: Vrin, 1996), pp. 189–218.

12. 414b; compare the list at 413b 13, which does not include the appetitive faculty.

13. 413b. Unless otherwise noted, all translations are my own.

14. 416b 30; cf. 424a: *to gar aisthanesthai paskhein ti estin.*

15. On the symmetries and asymmetries of the five senses and, in particular, the exceptional status of touch in Aristotle's doctrine, see Richard Sorabji, "Aristotle on Demarcating the Five Senses," in *Articles on Aristotle,* ed. Jonathan Barnes, Malcolm Schofield, and Richard Sorabji (London: Duckworth, 1975–1979), vol. 4: *Psychology and Aesthetics,* pp. 77–92.

16. 424a 2.

17. This is the basis of the so-called *logos* doctrine of *De anima* II, by which Aristotle has been said to elaborate on theories of several of his predecessors. See Deborah W. Modrak, *Aristotle: The Power of Perception* (Chicago: University of Chicago Press, 1987), pp. 56–62.

18. See, most explicitly, 424b, which opens Book Three in the modern edition: *hoti d' ouk estin aisthēsis hetera para tas pente (legō de tautas opsin, akoēn, osphrēsin, geusin, haphēn*). On this question, the later medieval writers were not so certain, as Jacqueline Cerquiglini-Toulet has demonstrated. See her essay, "Le Schéma des cinq sens, D'Une Théorie de la connaissance à la creation de formes littéraires," *Micrologus* 10 (2002): pp. 55–69.

19. 425a 15.

20. 426b 10.

21. 426b 10ff.

22. 425b 10ff.

23. 425b 15ff.

24. 425a 27.

25. Ibid.

26. 520a 12–14 and 451a 17.

27. 449a 18.

28. 455a.

29. There is a rich scholarly literature on the common sense in Aristotle. See, among others, D. W. Hamelyn, "Koiné Aisthesis," *The Monist* 52 (1968): pp. 195–209. For a convincing defense of the claim that the multiple terms are indeed designations of a single faculty, see D. W. Modrak, "An Aristotelian Theory of Consciousness?" in *Ancient Philosophy* 1, no. 2 (1981): pp. 160–170. Against "the doctrine of the 'common sense,'" see Wolfgang Welsch, *Aisthesis. Grundzüge und Perspektiven der Aristotelischen Sinneslehre* (Stuttgart: Klett-Cotta, 1987), pp. 307–380.

30. See 427a 17–429a 10 (citation from 427b 23–25).

31. On the relation between imagination and intellection—a subject that was to provoke the most heated debates in thirteenth-century Scholasticism, see, among other passages, 431a–431a20 and 449b 30: *noein ouk estin aneu phantasmatos.*

32. See *De memoria* and, on the relation of memory to the imagination, esp. 449b 24–450b 11.

33. The threefold classification of the postsensory faculties has for this reason often been called "Galenic": on this term and its appropriateness, see Harry Austryn Wolfson, "The Internal Senses in Latin, Arabic and Hebrew Philosophic Texts," *Harvard Theological Review* 28 (1935): pp. 69–133, rpt. in *Studies in the History of Philosophy and Religion,* vol. 1 (Cambridge: Harvard University Press, 1973), pp. 250–314, here pp. 253–254.

34. See Wolfson, "The Internal Senses," p. 250, who cites Averroës to support the explanation: "Et virtutes cerebri . . . quambis non habeant membra vel instrumenta, ipsa tamen habeant propria loca in cerebro" (Colliget II, 20, fol 30 F).

35. Aëtius Plac. IV 8, 7, *Stoicorum Veterum Fragmenta,* fragment 852, cited by Fazlur Rahman in his notes to *Avicenna's Psychology: An English Translation of Kitāb al-Najāt, Book II, Chapter IV, with Historico-Philosophical Notes and Textual Improvements on the Cairo Edition* (Oxford: Oxford University Press, 1952), pp. 77–78.

36. *Confessions,* I, 20, pp. 58–59.

37. Book 7, 17, pp. 384–387.

38. *De libero arbitrio,* II, 3–5, in Augustine, *La Felicità, La Libertà,* ed. Maria Teresa Fumagalli Beonio Brocchieri (Milan: Biblioteca Universale Rizzoli, 1995), pp. 168–185.

39. Wolfson, "The Internal Senses," p. 252.

40. Ibid.

41. Ibid., pp. 254–255.

42. Ibid.

43. For the Hebrew text cited here, see Salomon Fried, *Sefer ha-Yesodot, Buch der Elemente: Ein Beitrag zur jüdischen Religionsphilosophie des Mittelalters* (Frankfurt am Main: J. Kaufmann, 1900), p. 53. English in A. Altman and S. M. Stern, *Isaac Israeli: A Neo-Platonist of the Early Tenth Century* (Oxford: Oxford University Press, 1958), pp. 135–136. The Latin text can be found in part in Fried's notes: the passage cited is from Fried, p. 53, n. 3C.

44. See Wolfson, "The Internal Senses," pp. 274–275.

45. ةلضافلا ةنيدملا لها ءارآ باتك, ed. Albert Nasir Nadir (7th ed., Beirut: Dar al-Mashriq, 1987), pp. 88–89.

46. It has been argued that Al-Fārābī already considered common sense as an internal power of the soul: see A.-M. Goichon's annotated translation of Avicenna, *Le Livre des directives et remarques (Kitāb al-Išārāt wa l-tanbīhāt)* (Paris: Vrin, 1951), p. 318. No matter how one decides to understand the Fārābīan texts cited by Goichon, Avicenna remains the first thinker to inscribe common sense repeatedly and systematically within the set of the internal senses.

47. On Fārābī's classifications and the origin of the *virtus aestimativa,* see Wolfson, "The Inner Senses," pp. 267–276.

48. See ibid., pp. 271–281.

49. Thomas Aquinas, *Summa Theologiae,* 1, Q. 78, A. 4, section 6.

50. For the Arabic text, see Ján Bakoš, *Psychologie d'Ibn Sīnā (Avicenne) d'après son œuvre Aš-šifā'* (Prague: Nakladatelsví Čekoslovenské Akademie Véd, 1956), vol. 1, p. 44. The Latin text can be found in Gérard Verbeke, ed. with Simon van Riet *Avicenna latinus, Liber de Anima, seu Sextus de Naturalibus,* 2 vols. (Louvain: Peeters, 1968–1971), vol. 1, p. 87, 20.

51. IV, 1, Arabic in Bakoš, *Psychologie d'Ibn Sīnā,* vol. 1, p. 157 (P 182r).

52. *De anima* III 8, cited in Verbeke's Introduction to *Liber de Anima,* p. 50.

53. For the Arabic, see Bakoš, *Psychologie d'Ibn Sīnā,* vol. 1, p. 159 (B 153r); Latin in *Liber de Anima,* vol. 2, pp. 5, 57–59.

54. See, in particular, Jean de La Rochelle, *Tractus de divisione multiplici potentiarum animae* II, ed. P. Michaud Quentin (Paris: Vrin, 1964); Alexander of Hales, *Expositio super libros Aristotelis de anima* (Oxford: n.p., 1481); Roger Kilwardby, *De Spiritu phantasticu,* ed. P. Osborne Lewry, 2 vols. (Oxford: Oxford University Press, 1987–1993).

55. Albert the Great, *Opera Omnia,* ed. Bernhard Geyer (Westphalen: Aschendorff, 1951–), vol. 7, pt. 1: *De anima,* Lib. 2, Tract. 4, ch. 6, p. 155.

56. Ibid., Lib. 2, Tract. 4, ch. 8, pp. 158–159.

57. Ibid., Lib. 2, Tract. 4, ch. 10: *De Probatione sensus communis per hoc quod componit et dividiot inter sensato diversorum sensuum,* pp. 161–163.

58. Ibid., Lib. 2, Tract. 4, ch. 11, p. 164.

59. Ibid., Lib. 2, Tract. 4, ch. 12: *Et est digressio declarans, qualiter sensus communis est medietas omnium sensibilium,* pp. 164–165.

60. Ibid.

61. Pseudo-Areopagiticus, *De divinis nominibus* 13, n. 2; *Patrologia Graeca* 3, 977D; *sicut omnia in seipso praehabens et supermanens secundum unam impausabilem et eandem et superplenam et imminorabilem largitionem;* see Eustatius of Nicea, *In Primum Aristotelis Moralium ad Nicomachum,* 1096a 10–14; Alain de Libera, "Le Sens commun au XIIIe siècle, De Jean de La Rochelle à Albert le Grand," *Revue de Métaphysique et de Morale* 4 (1991): pp. 475–496, esp. p. 495.

62. Albert, *Opera Omnia,* vol. 7, pt. 1, p. 165.

63. See the title of ch. 12 in ibid.

64. Meister Eckhart, *Werke,* vol. 2, ed. Niklaus Largier (Frankfurt: Deutsche Klassiker Verlag, 1993), p. 328. See also *L'Œuvre latine de Maître Eckhart,* vol. 1: *Commentaire de la Genèse, précédé des Prologues,* ed. F. Brunner, A. de Libera, E. Wéber (Paris: Cerf, 1984), p. 487.

65. Jean d'Arkel, *Li Ars d'Amours de vertu et de boneurté, par Jehan le Bel,* ed. Jules Petit (Bruxelles: Victor Devaux, 1867), 2 vols., vol. 1, pt. 2, ch. 7 of sec. 1: "Cis capitles determine du sens commun," pp. 198–199.

66. S. Thomae Aquinatis, *Commentarium in Libros De Anima,* Lib. 2, lect. 13, in *Opera Omnia,* ed. Roberto Busa, vol. 4: *Commentaria in Aristotelem et alios* (Stuttgart-Bad Cannstatt: Fromann-Holzboog, 1980), p. 349.

3 Senses, Imagination, and Literature

Some Epistemological Considerations

Gregor Vogt-Spira

The starting point for the following considerations is the close connection between sensory perception and thought in Antiquity and the Middle Ages.[1] This link between the physico-physiologico-neurological dimension and the production of meaning has far-reaching consequences for all Antiquity and well beyond. It has its epistemological foundation in the model of the soul developed by Aristotle in *De anima,* and variously faceted in Stoa and Neoplatonism. Despite having been from that moment on, and particularly during Late Antiquity, the object of a rich commentary tradition, it remained basically unchanged and was passed down to the Middle Ages. The close connection between sensory perception and thought is actually to be understood here in two different ways: First, it implies the view that all thought is based on sensory perception—suffice it to think of the statement by Aristotle, influential for many centuries, that without sensory perception there is no thought.[2] Yet, at the same time, the contrary is also true, namely, since each sense partakes of the thought process, each sensory perception is already an act of cognition, even if only in a less-developed form.

In this chapter, I deal with some basic assumptions resulting from these epistemological presuppositions with regard to the literary field, focusing on the first few centuries AD of the Roman Empire as a link period in which ancient knowledge achieves a standard schoolroom form which is handed down to the Middle Ages. What is the position of literature in this fundamental nexus of perception and thought?

A first connection shows already in the characteristically twofold interpretation of the letter as *semantikos tis psophos,*[3] as something having a semantic as well as an acoustic side, as much a meaning as a sound. A standard definition of this fact is given by ancient and medieval grammarians: *littera est pars minima vocis articulatae.* This foundation in the physical and physiological dimension can be traced further into modern times with regard to the efforts to define the concept of "letter": it is only at the beginning of the nineteenth century that the systematic separation of sound and letter, and thus the separation of the sensory and the mental components, asserts itself, without actually proving to be entirely consistent.[4]

Yet, the connection between textuality and the sphere of sensory perception is not limited to the phonic aspect, but extends also to the complementary semantic side, or, in rhetorical terms, the relationship of *res* and *verba.* It is to this relationship in particular that we give attention in this chapter. In this way, a long-standing debate about a complex of problems that originated in ancient literary and art theory is taken up again, a debate that has continued to be productive through various metamorphoses until very recent times: the concept of *mimesis.* In view of the close connection of sensory perception and thought established by Aristotle, adopted by Hellenistic literary theory, and forming a part of the fundamental knowledge of later concepts of literature, a triadic structure results in which some of the *aporiai* of a binarily oriented post-Cartesian or post-Humian tradition are absent. In this context, a key role is taken by *phantasia,* the important introduction of a faculty halfway between (external) senses and (internal) powers of cognition in the Aristotelian model of the soul. Thus a field is opened that seems to touch with, for example, Wolfgang Iser's triad of the Real, the Fictive, and the Imaginary. Since, however, the epistemological preconditions and premises differ fundamentally—on the one hand a difference between, on the other a connection of, the sensorily perceptible and the cognitive world—it follows that, according to the historically specific epistemic conditions, the literary models based on them also diverge from each other in their fundamental aspects.

First of all I would like to discuss some characteristic features of the standard model that became basic knowledge in scholia, grammars, and anthologies of Late Antiquity and as such constituted a continuous line of development into the Middle Ages. The great role which is played by the element of sensory perception in observations about literary creation is striking. This becomes clear, for example, in the central postulate of *enargeia* that was developed for the first time within Hellenistic Homeric criticism, which was then fully formulated in the theory of rhetoric, and from there became basic knowledge for purposes of the production and reception of texts.

The postulated requirement is to represent things as if one could see them clearly in front of one's eyes.[5] This objective leads to an *ostendere* that is intended as an intensification surpassing a simple *dicere.* The process thus finds itself directly brought into contact with the sensory organs. It is stated explicitly that a speech fails its full effect and that it does not assert itself enough if its power appeals to the ears only; rather, its *summa virtus* is—in this passage paradigmatically with the reference to the case of judicial speech—that a judge should not simply feel that the bare facts on the basis of which he has to pass his decision are merely being narrated to him, but rather that they are displayed graphically and presented to the eyes of the mind.[6]

The mind's eye is exactly the capability of *phantasia,* or power of imagination, that became so commonly known in Late Antiquity, even by its Greek term, that it even occurs in schoolbooks about poetry written in Latin.[7] In a key passage, Quintilian puts the power of imagination into a formulation which has canonical status:[8]

> Quas φαντασίαν Graeci vocant (nos sane visiones appellemus), per quas imagines rerum absentium ita repraesentantur animo, ut eas cernere oculis ac praesentes habere videamur, [. . .]

This statement is based on the fundamental idea of a movement that goes in a direction that is opposite to the usual: Rather than from the organ of sense to the powers of imagination, the process runs in the contrary direction toward the *telos* of a connection back to the senses. Crucial is the expression *praesentes habere,* by which the rhetorical key competence of *pro ommaton poiein,*[9] to which *cernere oculis* corresponds in this passage, is put into more general terms.[10]

The aim of this becomes clear from the etymological interpretation of "presence" which Isidore of Seville gives in the section on the *sensus corporis* in his *Origines: unde et praesentia nuncupantur, quod sint prae sensibus*—which is explained in more detail with regard to the special case of the eyes: *sicut prae oculis, quae praesto sunt oculis.*[11] How physically concrete this is really meant is shown by the previous explanation concerning the senses: *Sensus dicti, quia per eos anima subtilissime totum corpus agitat vigore sentiendi.*[12]

Quintilian implies nothing less than the notion that words, by rendering present something that is absent, are putting it *prae sensibus.* That this is in fact the underlying idea can also be seen from the concept of the letter, the quintessence of which is encapsulated in a well-known definition by Isidore in which the same phenomenon is described not in visual but in acoustic terms:[13]

> Litterae autem sunt indices rerum, signa verborum, quibus tanta vis est, ut nobis dicta absentium sine voce loquantur.

The fundamental model according to which texts make our senses experience something absent, something not immediately available, and bring it *prae sensibus*—here, the senses of sight and taste are often mentioned *pars pro toto,* as in expressions like "bringing something before someone's eyes" and also "let something manifest itself"[14]—ultimately finds a programmatic formulation in the genre of *ekphrasis:* With the purpose of surpassing the visual by means of the linguistic medium, it claims to include potentially all the senses. It is precisely in this sense that Philostratus introduces the description of a painting with the remark that mere optical perception would not yet convey the fragrance of a garden, that through the use of words, however, even the smell of apples would reach the audience.[15] In another passage, he advances the claim that the hearer or reader can also smell the scent of roses, hear the noises of a scene, and taste the sweetness of some jam.[16]

In sum, the textual model to be recognized here is grounded on the fundamental idea that sensory perception brought about by the exterior world is not experienced as different from the one evoked through texts by way of *phantasia;* its objective and ideal is the elimination of the perception of difference—the model is not based on the concept of difference as such, but on its elimination and disregard. Many uncertainties can be traced back to the fact that our usual assumption of the impossibility of going beyond the concept of difference is projected back into premodern times.

This fundamental ideal of eliminating the perception of difference rests on several presuppositions: a central role in it is played by the fact that *phantasia* is capable of supplementation. This fact is described by Quintilian in connection with the techniques used to produce *enargeia,* one of which is located under the umbrella term of completion: *tota rerum imago quodam modo verbis depingitur.*[17] This refers to a passage in the concluding book of Cicero's *Second Verrines*—in other words, to the reaction of a reader, and expressly designated as such:[18]

> An quisquam tam procul a concipiendis imaginibus rerum abest ut non, cum illa in Verrem legit: "stetit soleatus praetor populi Romani cum pallio purpureo tunicaque talari muliercula nixus in litore," non solum ipsos

> intueri videatur et locum et habitum, sed quaedam etiam ex iis quae dicta non sunt sibi ipse adstruat.

We are fortunate in that Quintilian later introduces as an example also his own activity of supplementation:[19]

> Ego certe mihi cernere videor et vultum et oculos et deformes utriusque blanditias et eorum qui aderant tacitam aversationem ac timidam verecundiam.

One single sentence from Cicero has set in motion a lively process of supplementation resulting in a small scene in its own right that, depending on the individual's power of imagination, may have slightly different results each time. This is not to be confused with the concept of *logique supplémentaire* in the sense of a logic of difference.[20] Quite on the contrary, the elimination of difference with regard to sensory perception is stressed emphatically. The following example, Cicero's description of a sumptuous dinner party, shows this explicitly:[21]

> "videbar videre alios intrantis, alios autem exeuntis, quosdam ex vino vacillantis, quosdam hesterna ex potatione oscitantis. Humus erat inmunda, lutulenta vino, coronis languidulis et spinis cooperta piscium." Quid plus videret qui intrasset?

Thus verbal representation offers something which even a real observer could have seen. To appreciate better the guiding nature of such a reference, let me just adduce the judgment about Virgil's representation of the boxing-match between Dares and Entellus during the funeral games held for Anchises: the description would make the appearance of the boxers as they are getting ready for their fight visible to us, so visible indeed that it could not have been clearer to an onlooker.[22] This way of looking at the relationship of "fictional" and "real" world runs through the entire commentary on the *Aeneid* and confronts scholars nowadays with the striking absence of many familiar categories.

From the above examples it is clear that the underlying idea in this context is that literature can arouse something analogous to sensual perceptions, the ideal result of this process being that the induction by means of texts becomes undistinguishable from that which is brought about by means of the perception of the external world. This fundamental concept is further clarified by the cognitive model—or in Old European words: the model of the soul by means of which options for the description of the connection between the physico-physiological dimension and that of thought are generated. It is necessary to enquire into the importance of this epistemological basis for the entire system, especially since the important consequences for literary theory which derive from the assumptions discussed here are obvious.

To begin with, this can be explained by looking at the power to which, as we have just seen, a key role is attributed with regard to literature: *phantasia.* Its introduction into the model of the soul as a kind of link that should maintain the connection between sensual perception on the one hand and thought on the other, is a specific innovation introduced by Aristotle. In its later translations—just to mention *imaginatio, immaginazione, imagination, Imagination, fancy, Einbildungskraft*—*phantasia* has experienced an extraordinary reception in the history of philosophy—and beyond it—and has also remained a point of reference for literary theory. Yet, in the debate about the Aristotelian concept of *phantasia,* carried out intensively for roughly the last thirty years, its fundamental difference from all the interpretations advanced after Hume or even after Kant has been noted almost unanimously and with great vigor.[23] And rightly so, since "fantasy / imagination / power of imagination," however one may translate these terms,[24] have a completely different position when they are located within a continuum ranging from the sense organs to the highest noetic faculties, or alternatively, when they have been conceived of as a purely mental activity under the premise of the existence of a boundary which the sensory faculties cannot overstep.

The consequences for "premodern" literary theory have not been considered by scholars so far.[25] One of the main reasons for this is an overly strong adherence to the Aristotelian *Poetics,* where a link with the concept of *phantasia* is nowhere in sight—possibly already for chronological reasons. Rather, imagination finds itself developed from another starting point: *De anima,* the main text on this topic, deals with the differentiation of the capabilities of the soul with the aim of laying the ground for Aristotle's scientific and biological writings, and therefore without literature coming into view.[26] Anyway, the connection was established for the first time by Alexandrian literary criticism, especially in the context of the exegesis of Homer. From there, it permeated to rhetoric.[27] Thus it became basic knowledge without having developed the distinct contours of an all-encompassing literary theory.

Let us now turn our attention to ancient epistemology with its authoritative assumption that all knowledge derives from sensory perception. The foundations of the model of the cognitive process that was to become canonical had been laid by Plato and Aristotle; it was afterwards modified by the Stoics, and widened and refined in later debates, particularly in Neoplatonism, and in the process of compilation of commentaries on Aristotle's works. Yet its fundamentals remained unchanged.[28] A Latin summary dating from Late Antiquity and representing on its part a point of departure for the Middle Ages, is provided by Boethius. In the following, I will deal first with Aristotle, in whose writings the model of the soul was endowed with basic characteristics that retained their validity for a long time, and that, through the rich tradition of Aristotelian exegesis down to the time of Scholasticism, has proved to be particularly productive in the context of the formation of theoretical concepts in the Middle Ages.

The underlying tripartite structure leads to a division of the soul's cognitive capability into *aisthesis, phantasia,* and *noesis.* These three faculties are linked with each other insofar as the performance of each one of them is built each time upon the performance of the other two. Therefore, the indispensability of *aisthesis* for the generation of any kind of knowledge is stressed repeatedly. In *Analytica posteriora,* for example, it is stated:[29] "It is clear that in the absence of sensory perception knowledge necessarily is also absent." Similarly, in *De anima:*[30] "One could in no way recognize or understand something if one couldn't perceive anything." It is in this sense that we have to say that thought is based on sensory perception.

Nevertheless, we should ask how precise the link is which is established between the physico-corporeal dimension and *noesis.* This results, in the first place, from the concept of thought itself as the faculty whose main activity is defined as the making of distinctions. Insofar as distinctions can be made with varying degrees of precision and distinctiveness, the central disjunction is phrased as *confusum-distinctum,* a Latin translation of the Greek *synchorismenon-kechorismenon.* These two terms were introduced to philosophy by Plato; the examples adduced by him—like the one of the three fingers—have been the object of much debate and have been misunderstood many times, since they are diametrically opposed to the idea of the cognitive process familiar to us and of the capacity of sensory perception.[31]

In this context, the scale *confusum-distinctum* is conceived in a dynamic sense: something general and confused is at first perceived by the senses, and then an analytical process leading to the knowledge of the specific parts is initiated, taking the form of an upward motion. The interaction of the single parts of the soul is conveniently summarized in a representative fashion—here made explicit only for two faculties at the far ends of the scale, *aisthesis* and *noesis*—despite the Neoplatonic undercurrent of that work in Boethius's *De institutione musica:*[32]

> Sensus namque confusum quiddam ac proxime tale, quale est illud, quod sentit, advertit. Ratio vero diiudicat integritatem atque imas persequitur differentias. Itaque sensus invenit quidem confusa ac proxima veritati, accipit vero ratione integritatem. Ratio vero ipsa quidem invenit integritatem, accipit vero confusam ac proximam veri similitudinem. Namque sensus nihil concipit integritatis, sed usque ad proximum venit, ratio vero diiudicat.

A very important consequence of conceiving the act of thinking as an act of making distinctions, which has already been mentioned at the beginning, must be stressed once again. In fact, from this idea it also follows that the lowest capability of the soul, *aisthesis,* is already conceived as an act of thought. In a key passage in *Analytica posteriora, aisthesis* is described as "an innate capability of making distinctions": δύναμις σύμφυτος κριτική.[33]

Thus follows that there are only "cognitive senses": each sense takes part in the cognitive process as long as it makes distinctions—even if not as distinctly as the higher parts of the soul. The common view that sensory perceptions are exclusively passive and receptive is a projection of the modern model into the past. In the context of a grown interest in the study of *De anima* from different sides—Malcolm Schofield, Dorothea Frede, the school of Arbogast Schmitt and others—such a "Kantian conception" which reduces sensory perception to a purely passive influence and delimits cognitive acts to a narrowly confirmed space of "mental imagery," has been rejected as a basic misunderstanding.[34]

The idea that each sense is cognitive is to be carefully distinguished from the concept of the *sensus spirituales* and their later identification with the *sensus interiores* that begins to develop with Origen on the basis of a Neoplatonism transformed in a Christian sense, yet, despite being mentioned several times, never systematically becomes part of the Latin tradition. The Aristotelian model of the soul is systematically formulated for the first time by Avicenna, and thus a deep caesura is generated.[35]

Let us now turn to the concept of *phantasia* itself as it was located by Aristotle at the intersection of the senses and the cognitive act proper. With this a series of problems leading up to the question of whether or not it is a unitary concept manifests itself. In his incisive contribution of 1975, Malcolm Schofield had inimitably conceded the following points that were going to influence later controversies strongly:[36] "I shall suggest . . . that Aristotle can be fairly interpreted as adopting different but complementary vantage-points on a more or less coherent family of psychological phenomena. But it would be a triumph of generosity over justice to pretend that he manages to combine his different approaches to *phantasia* with an absolutely clear head." Nevertheless, the introduction of *phantasia* into the model of the soul has gained acceptance and, as the time of Greek and Latin literary and rhetorical theory from Hellenism to Late Antiquity shows, it went beyond its narrow philosophical framework and acquired the status of general knowledge.

Why such a link can be regarded as necessary becomes clear when one considers that the intellect as such can only conceive of the nonperceptible, the intelligible forms. Nevertheless, it needs images of something sensorily perceptible to decide whether or not something is desirable, and thus to be able to refer to concrete situations and objects.[37] According to the perspective adopted in each case, one can understand *phantasia* either as a necessary link or, as others do, as a diving line between the senses and the intellect. In any case, as Aristotle stresses frequently, it is characteristic that *phantasia* is neither identical with *aisthesis* nor with *dianoia,* yet that sensory perception is necessary for *phantasia,* and that the latter is necessary for thought.[38] *De anima* iii 3, the only focused and detailed discussion of this subject in the Aristotelian corpus, discussing the creation of a "conceptual room for an independent notion of *phantasia,* between thinking on the one side and sense-perception on the other,"[39] is written in an unusually cursory manner,[40] and this does not make things any easier.

Let me now turn to the connection of *phantasia* and *aisthesis.* In his *Rhetoric,* Aristotle defines *phantasia* at one point as *aisthesis tis asthenes,*[41] and this represents an earlier approach that was abandoned later. In fact, in *De anima* he stresses emphatically that the two do not coincide. An important difference is this: since *aisthesis* is basically a reception of perceptible *eide* without *hyle*—this is exemplified by means of the image of the impression of a signet ring in wax—it reveals itself as irresistibly attractive.[42] *Phantasia,* on the other hand, is based on the fact that sensations remain in the soul,[43] even after the objects of perception have been removed.[44] From this follows, to anticipate our conclusions, its specific capacity: to make present what is absent—to bring it *prae sensibus,* to take up Isidorus's etymological explanation.[45] This will offer the key to the idea that texts allow a sensory experience of "absent," of "nonpresent" things.

For our context, it is important that *phantasia,* even when designated as a form of *noein,* is, on the whole, brought very close to sensory perception and constitutes, together with it, the lowest part of the *psyche aisthetike.* Because of this it has even been argued recently that: "The faculty of *phantasia* is the same faculty as the perceptional faculty, although different in essence and definition."[46] The function that *phantasia* thus has for the act of thinking is decisive. Aristotle has proved influential throughout the centuries with the following statement:[47]

> τῇ δὲ διανοητικῇ ψυχῇ τὰ φαντάσματα οἷον αἰσθήματα ὑπάρχει. [. . .] οὐδέποτε νοεῖ ἄνευ φαντάσματος ἡ ψυχή

In a complementary fashion, one can look at it also from the opposite angle: consequently, from the perspective of what *phantasia* adds to the *aisthemata* in order to make sensory perceptions accessible to the dianoetic part of the soul. It is obvious that the very performance of semantization is assigned to *phantasia:*[48]

> δεῖ ἔμψοφόν τε εἶναι τὸ τύπτον καὶ μετὰ φαντασίας τινός (σημαντικὸς γὰρ δή τις ψόφος ἐστὶν ἡ φωνή).

Human vocal expression is also defined as a *semantikos psophos* which is produced physiologically and has at the same time a semantic side to it, while the creation of meaning as an activity of the soul is located especially within *phantasia.*[49] The background to this is the Aristotelian doctrine that each act of thinking implies visualization.[50] This even led to the explanation that the introduction of *phantasia* and *phantasmata* in *De anima* iii 3 is aimed at the specific faculty of visualization.[51]

The way in which *phantasmata* and *aisthemata* can be brought together more precisely so that "for the thinking soul the images generated by the faculty of imagination are like the images generated by the senses," is explained in a passage from *De memoria* in which *eikon* as an explanatory term establishes a relation between an image and a past event.[52] It shows how to understand this relation as one of similarity: "The image is able to represent the past event because the image is like the event," so that it can be formulated in Aristotelian terms "that a *phantasma* can function as a likeness that attaches the present mental state to an object in the world."[53]

We cannot pursue this idea further here, but I would like to emphasize in summary that *phantasia* is conceived as the key faculty of giving meaning to sounds, and that this semantization is represented as a kind of image-making procedure. By way of complement, the idea should be added that for *aisthemata* and *phantasmata* a relationship of similarity is assumed. In other words, if thought finds the former like the latter, it can dispense with their ontological difference. This leads to the consequence that the naturalistic question of whether something exists as a physical object or not becomes insignificant, and this in turn has immediate consequences for the objects of literature.

The rhetorico-poetical textual model broadly defined at the beginning, its main idea being that sensory perception induced from the outside is not experienced any differently from a perception stimulated by means of texts through *phantasia,* thus proves to be fully anchored in a common idea of how perception and thought operate. Out of this, new ways of describing more closely a concept of literature that antedates, even in a mere chronological sense, the "linguistic turn" may be found. For that reason, we would now like to address some of its consequences with a view to problems of categorization.

Let us take as an example Macrobius's *Saturnalia,* an implicit poetic treatise of Late Antiquity, which is a paradigm for a grammatical and rhetorical concept of the text, and which, in turn, had an authoritative effect on the Middle Ages and the beginning of the modern era. A characteristic definition of the relation between literature and reality in this work can be found: with reference to the *Aeneid,* it is said that the poet is not led by anyone else but the mother of all things herself, Nature—a standard formulation for the practice of *imitatio*—and that therefore it could be stated:[54]

> Quippe si mundum ipsum diligenter inspicias, magnam similitudinem divini illius et huius poetici operis invenies.

A relation of *imitatio* is claimed here and is further explained as a relationship of similarity—*similitudo*—between *res* and *verba,* between "World" and "Poetry." It is in continuation of the line of thought laid down here that Bernard Weinberg in his fundamental contribution to Renaissance poetics could emphasize that:[55] "the *Res* of poetry is indistinguishable from the *Res* of reality"—that is why *natura,* in turn, can be exemplified by means of texts, and the better the texts, the more effectively this happens.[56]

The *similitudo* claimed by Macrobius is nothing else but a shortened formula of the epistemological model developed above: the process by which the images of representation that are set in motion by means of the text are in a relation of similarity to those images which are triggered by the perception of nature. In fact, there is every reason to believe that the ancient model of *imitatio* is based completely upon such a relationship of similarity between *aisthemata* and *phantasmata.*[57] I must limit myself here to a few brief references and choose first of all a poetological treatise that provides a summary of the doctrine of *imitatio* and finds itself at the other end of the time span covered by the present volume: the *Poetices libri septem* of Julius Caesar Scaliger. Despite its rather unconventional philosophical reformulations, this work is essentially based upon assumptions about the theory of language and literature of the Roman imperial period, and at the same time belongs to a continuous tradition reaching back into the Middle Ages that used to be underestimated for a long time.

The dichotomy between *res* and *verba,* represented as a complete separation of the terms, is introduced in the preface to the third book dealing with the *res* under the very heading *Quid imitandum sit.*[58] In it, Scaliger boldly ventures to explain the various relations using the Aristotelian theory of the four causes. In the present context, the efficient *aitia* (*causa efficiens*) by means of which Scaliger outlines very clearly his own view of the relation between words and things is particularly important: words would receive their *forma* from objects of nature, but not in the sense of the Platonists, namely, that through the power of the objects words are created, but rather that it is we who would assimilate the nature and the scope of speech to the nature and the scope of the objects:[59]

> non idcirco quia cum Platonicis eo verser in errore, ut putem a rebus ipsis verba natura sua concreata esse, sed quia res ipsae quales quantaeque sunt talem tantamque non illae, sed nos efficimus orationem.

Consequently, *imitatio* is introduced into the framework of a triadic system of *res-verba-nos,* in which the decisive role is attributed to the faculty of perception and thought of either the producer or the audience of a text:[60] the object of this concept of *mimesis* is not so much the ontologically different status of *res* and *verba,* but the relation of reference of one to the other. Actually, between world and poetry a relation of similarity that requires an act of cognition is set up. The central point is constituted precisely by that model in which the thinking soul brings closely together the images of representation and perception:[61] τὰ γὰρ φαντάσματα ὥσπερ αἰσθήματά ἐστι, πλὴν ἄνευ ὕλης.

Thus one feature in particular that is well characteristic of the rhetorico-poetical concept of the text is clarified further: the combination of the model of *imitatio* and visuality. The frequency with which reference is made to the concept of the image is one of its most prominent characteristics: *sermo* is nothing but an *imago.*[62] With a certain exuberance, the idea of *pingere* is used for writing poetry or for the writing of any text in general—a semantic interference with *scribere* that can be traced right through the Middle Ages,[63] and the quality of the visualization is more and more regarded as one of the most important criteria for literary quality.[64]

In this context, a mutual connection concerning their very foundations is established within the relationship of imitation and image. On the one hand, imitation would be present in every text precisely because words would be images of things: *Denique imitationem esse in omni sermone, quia verba sint imagines rerum.*[65] On the other hand, one also comes across the opposite relation: since every speech would be *eidos, ennoia, mimesis,* quite like a painting, the words would be *rei effigies atque imago.*[66] In this rhetorico-poetical concept of the text, the relation of the image proves to be the nucleus of the concept of *imitatio.* The faculty that brings this about is no other than *phantasia.* Let us remember once more the result of the third section, where the ability of *phantasia* to carry out acts of semantization had proved to be a type of image-making under the presupposition that for the objects of images, and thus for the reference to *res,* there exists a relation of similarity between *phantasmata* and *aisthemata.*

Those *phantasmata* are, however, characterized by the fact that they are not directly identical with the *aisthemata;* rather, it is the matter of an act of identification carried out by the thinking soul: a mechanism that contains a "poetic" potential which is put to specific use in literature. In order to let it make its effects felt appropriately, one more aspect is connected with it in ancient debates. It is based on the view, characteristic as much of Greek as of Roman doctrine, that language undoubtedly reaches beyond the field of discourse: This is because it is taken for granted that, apart from the argument itself, the state of the soul of the speaker as well as of the person in front of him is of considerate importance. Within such double orientation, which, for instance, explicitly constitutes the starting point of and the central point around which rhetoric revolves, a key role is attributed to the sphere of the affects. It is for that reason that under the influence of rhetoric the sphere of the affects has found its place in literary theory—to the point that Pseudo-Longinus believes himself to be able to see the proper goal of the creation of effects of visualization in poetry in their influence on the stirs of emotion.[67]

Against this background, it is not accidental that Quintilian introduces the concept of *phantasia* right there in his chapter about affects. The reason is as follows: *Has* [*visiones*] *quisquis bene ceperit, is erit in adfectibus potentissimus.*[68] From such visual impressions in the mind, it is in a crucial way given rise to a disposition that makes the triggering of affects possible, as is clear from the words added to the definition of *enargeia: et adfectus non aliter, quam si rebus ipsis intersimus, sequentur.*[69] When stirs of emotion result in no other way but as if we were present ourselves, the present-tense framework that had proved to be a specific capacity of verbal description reaches out so far that it makes its influence felt beyond the sphere of imagination and actually reaches into the sphere of action: This model allows us to explain why the world of what can be perceived by the senses is immediately involved as a result of the action of *phantasia.* Let me now note in passing that such a focusing on the present ultimately produces a series of other peculiarities in ancient literary theory: in particular the standard mode of reading by identifying oneself and by "living through" what is read, a mode based on identification that is still present in the first poetological works of early modern times with their instructions for how poets should be read[70]—a phenomenon that seems to us like a peculiar blurring of the diving lines between the literary and the nonliterary.

To sum up, we maintain that the "poetic" capability of *phantasia,* namely, that of creating "presence," shows itself from various points of view to be crucial to the concept of literature as it was canonized in the grammatico-rhetorical tradition of the ancient world and its later transmission. At the same time, the doctrine that by interpreting *phantasmata* as *aisthemata* something merely imagined is experienced as "real" seems to reach its limit when it comes to objects that cannot be perceived by the external senses. Actually, this problem was already discussed in Late Antiquity, in particular with respect to the representation of mythological characters and gods. Still, we have to keep in mind that, even when the point of reference becomes uncertain, the effectiveness of the "assignment of fiction" is, as a rule, presupposed already as a given.[71]

This is made clear even in a particularly far-reaching case: in Philostratus's *Vita Apollonii,* the Olympian Zeus by Pheidias provides an occasion for the thought that a concept of imitation which merely refers to what is real is insufficient for the representation of the images of the gods.[72] As a possible solution, a singular and remarkable attempt at establishing a hierarchy among *mimesis* and *phantasia* is set up: *phantasia* would act as a better-informed demiurge than *mimesis,* because the latter would only create what it has seen; *phantasia,* by contrast, also what it has not seen, since *phantasia* would represent it by referring back to what exists. Despite the terminological fuzziness of the passage, pointing back to an origin with no connection to any philosophical school,[73] and rather to a use of concepts derived from common knowledge, it is significant that both *mimesis* and *phantasia* are here understood with reference to their constructive, "demiurgic" side: therefore, even if *phantasia* maintains its advantage, because it can represent also the invisible, this is also ensured by the fact that it operates in a formation by analogy to what is really available—and the causal "then" (γάρ) is meaningful. The terminological attempt to distinguish between *mimesis* and *phantasia* according to the criterion "real-possible" has not already affirmed itself because the formulation of the antithesis is not coherent: yet already in the popular use of this concept, the basic idea that *phantasia* proceeds according to the reference to reality independently from whether its objects can be perceived by the senses or not, shows itself even more clearly.

Let me amplify this by introducing a second example: Macrobius's treatment of the *paradeigma parabole eikon* with a specific example taken from Virgil. With reference to what he wants to prove, namely, that also in these cases affects would be triggered, he says about images:[74]

> Et imago [. . .] idonea est movendis affectibus. Ea fit cum aut forma corporis absentis describitur, aut omnino quae nulla est fingitur.

Insofar as, concerning *imago,* the alternative is opened up whether the absence of the body in question is to be regarded as merely accidental or as an absence in principle (as in the case of something which, like the Scylla, does not exist at all), it becomes apparent that the criterion for the mechanism of visualization is not constituted by an act of checking the reference; rather, this is presupposed as a given, quite like a rule in a game.

This view was commonly held for centuries. Let me demonstrate this by means of a passage taken from Cicero and later introduced by Quintilian as an example of a particularly virtuoso application of the technique of generating images.[75] It is taken from a speech, and thus from a text belonging to a genre which allows, due to the need of convincing a wider audience, an insight into commonly held beliefs. The listener is called upon to generate an image with the argument that the *cogitationes*—that is, in this passage, the concept of *phantasia* which had not yet been introduced into Latin[76]—were free and, at the same time, would allow us to see clearly what they want, just like one sees what is directly in front of one's eyes:[77]

> Fingite animis—liberae sunt enim nostrae cogitationes et quae volunt sic intuentur ut ea cernimus quae videmus.

It is obvious that the ability of making something up is not treated as the opposite of being truthful, imagined things not as being in contradiction to seen things, for Cicero would else undermine his own credibility. On the contrary, one of the self-evident faculties of thinking is to bring about the manifestation of things, just as if by means of sensory perception.

What has been said above has demonstrated the close interrelation between concepts of "text" and such models which describe sensory perception and its connection with cognition. This has consequences for the development of models in the area of literary studies. In fact, the perspective of historical epistemology proves to be indispensable for literary theory: each concept is based on presuppositions that find their foundation in models of cognition that are prevalent at the time.

This connection sheds light on numerous features of the ancient and, in addition to that, of the "premodern" concept of the text. It is, however, still largely unexplored. This is the case in spite of the fact that for the older model of cognition, whose key text is Aristotle's *De anima* and which is essentially founded on the tripartite model of the soul that is developed there, the huge difference that exists between it and all post-Humian, or even post-Kantian, models is actually part of its basic knowledge. This is explicitly stressed for the concept of imagination.[78] It is evident that considerable consequences for literary theory can be expected in this field. Perhaps the present phase of radical change sharpens our awareness of these interdependencies, not the least because neuroscience has begun to make the apparent certainties of the last centuries concerning the relationship of body and soul seem like a thing of the past.

Translated by Dr. Boris Dunsch and Monica Signoretti

Notes

1. The key categories of the concept of "text" and "literature" that was developed in premodern times have always provided a point of reference for literary theorists and continue to do so today. However, this concept shows a number of characteristics that are difficult to grasp when one considers them against the backdrop of the established practices and expectations formed as a result of the "linguistic turn." In many areas of research—orality, visuality, the concept of *mimesis,* ancient and medieval aesthetics—we witness the development of a lively debate to which this essay is intended to contribute. It adds to the range of the discussion by systematically introducing the perspective of historic epistemology. The reason for this is that the ancient and medieval model of cognition—a model that does not know of an unbridgeable difference between the sphere of the senses and the cognitive "construction" of texts and images (a difference familiar to us

moderns)—has enormously important consequences for literary theory today. This touches also on another discussion that has been extraordinarily stimulated by the studies of Hans Ulrich Gumbrecht, most recently in his book *Production of Presence: What Meaning Cannot Convey* (Stanford: Stanford University Press, 2004). In a way, our contribution is meant to complement this discussion from a historic point of view, demonstrating that "presence" is a core category by which the effects that texts may have on readers are defined in premodern times. My special thanks go to Sepp Gumbrecht, who has advanced the study of the stimulating question of the "Medieval Senses" over the years with his wonderful unflinching energy, and to Steve Nichols for his masterly organization of the conference in Florence. For the English translation my thanks go to Dr. Boris Dunsch and Monica Signoretti.

2. Arist. *Anal. post.* i 18, 81a 38f.; see below, nn. 29f.

3. Arist. *De an.* ii 8, 420b 32 (see also n. 49, below).

4. I have pursued this topic elsewhere: see G. Vogt-Spira, "Vox und littera. Der Buchstabe zwischen Mündlichkeit und Schriftlichkeit in der grammatischen Tradition," *Poetica* 23 (1991): 295–327.

5. Quint. *Inst.* 8, 3, 62.

6. Ibid.; the expression *oculi mentis* goes back to the Platonic τὸ τῆς ψυχῆς ὄμμα (*Resp.* 533d 2).

7. See G. Watson, *Phantasia in Classical Thought* (Galway, 1988), 134f. and idem, "The Concept of 'Phantasia' from the Late Hellenistic Period to Early Neoplatonism," in W. Haase, ed., *Aufstieg und Niedergang der römischen Welt* II 36.7 (Berlin and New York, 1994), 4765–4810, here 4801; see also the example in n. 8.

8. Quint. *Inst.* 6, 2, 29: "There are certain experiences which the Greeks call φαντασίαι, and the Romans visions, whereby things absent are presented to our imagination with such extreme vividness that they seem actually to be before our very eyes." (Here and in the following the translation is that of H. E. Butler.)

9. Arist. *Rhet.* iii 11, 1411b 23.

10. See its use in Servius's commentary to Virgil that testifies to a broad and self-evident diffusion in the fourth and fifth centuries and at the same time also plays a role in its further diffusion during the following millennium. In the case of *Ecl.* 2, 60, when the shepherd Corydon unhappily in love with Alexis addresses himself saying: *quem fugis, a! demens?* it is observed that *iterum per phantasiam quasi ad praesentem loquitur,* the idea that *phantasia* makes possible the presence of what is absent, is found again notably on the level of the schoolbook, and therefore as widespread basic knowledge.

11. Isid. *Etym.* 11, 1, 19.

12. Ibid.

13. Isid. *Etym.* 1, 3, 1: "Letters are indications of things, signs of the words, and in them is so much strength that they speak to us without a voice the words of those absent." Unless otherwise noted, all translations are my own.

14. Quint. *Inst.* 8, 3, 70.

15. Philostr. *Eik.* 1, 6, 1.

16. Philostr. *Eik.* 1, 2, 4; 1, 2, 5; 2, 26, 3.

17. Quint. *Inst.* 8, 3, 63.

18. Quint. *Inst.* 8, 3, 64: "Is there anybody so incapable of forming a mental picture of a scene that, when he reads the following passage from the Verrines [. . .], he does not seem not merely to see the actors in the scene, the place itself and their very dress, but even to imagine to himself other details that the orator does not describe? 'There on the shore stood the praetor, the representative of the Roman people, with slippered feet, robed in a purple cloak, a tunic streaming to his heels, and leaning on the arm of this worthless woman.'" The reference is to Cic. *Verr.* 2, 5, 86.

19. Quint. *Inst.* 8, 3, 65: "I seem to see before my eyes his face, his eyes, the unseemly blandishments of himself and his paramour, the silent loathing and frightened shame of those who viewed the scene."

20. It is not the question whether the "supplementary character" of word or writing is putative or not—as it is necessarily perceived under the influence of the opponent terms of *signifiant-signifié*—the way in which the issue is usually discussed. Derrida's distinctions may result in interesting ripples of thought. From the perspective of historical epistemology, however, all models built on Saussure's opposition show themselves to be only one of several conceivable options. First of all, it remains to be seen under which conditions which option has been realized in history. And at this point it should be maintained strongly that in Antiquity, until the time of Augustine, the theories of language and of signs are very much distinct from each other and that it is only from that time onward that they begin to coalesce gradually and over a long period of time. This means that ancient and imperial basic knowledge about the nature of literature which has been influential well into early modern times and with which we are concerned here, is not organized on the basis of a theory of signs. To admit such nonetheless constitutes an historically inadmissible anachronism.

21. Quint. *Inst.* 8, 3, 66–67: "'I seemed to see some entering, some leaving the room, some reeling under the influence of the wine, others yawning with yesterday's potations. The floor was foul with wine-smears, covered with wreaths half-withered and littered with fishbones.' What more would any man have seen who had actually entered the room?" The reference is to Cic. *fr. orat.* VI 1.

22. Quint. *Inst.* 8, 3, 63, with reference to Virg. *Aen.* 5, 426–460.

23. This has already been stated by M. Schofield in his contribution to the "Seventh Symposium Aristotelicum" 1975, a catalyst for the more recent discussion and reprinted more times, here quoted from "Aristotle on the Imagination," in M. C. Nussbaum and A. Oksenberg Rorty, eds., *Essays on Aristotle's "De Anima"* (Oxford, 1992), 249–277; see in particular 250f. The approach of Th. G. Rosenmeyer, "Φαντασία und Einbildungskraft. Zur Vorgeschichte eines Leitbegriffs

der europäischen Ästhetik," *Poetica* 18 (1986): 197–248, to deal with *phantasia* under the rubric of "prehistory," is to be considered with some caution—despite his, at times, excellent analysis of single issues.

24. There are some voices declaring themselves against translating the word *phantasia* with the term introduced through the Latin tradition *Imagination* or *imagination:* Schofield, "Aristotle on the Imagination," 250; J. Frère, "Fonction représentative et représentation. Φαντασία et φάντασμα selon Aristote," in G. Romeyer Dherbey and C. Viano, eds., *Corps et âme. Sur le "De anima" d'Aristote* (Paris, 1996), 331–348, here 337, et al. For the history of translation see Rosenmeyer, "Φαντασία und Einbildungskraft," 197–199; in particular for the development of the terminology in Latin, see P. Flury, "Phantasia und imaginatio im Bereich des antiken Lateins," in M. Fattori and M. Bianchi, eds., *Phantasia-Imaginatio. V° Colloquio Internazionale, Roma 9–11 gennaio 1986* (Roma, 1988), 69–79.

25. Frère ("Fonction représentative et representation") is justified in pointing to the lack of studies. He would like to distinguish between a *phantasia aisthetike* and a *phantasia logike,* however, and apart from those also a *phantasia mimetike* or *poietike,* nevertheless without carrying this through with sufficient conceptual clarity.

26. Faced with the well-known problems of relative chronology inherent in the Corpus Aristotelicum, nothing certain can be said about the chronological relationship of the two works, yet it is probable that the concept of *phantasia* was developed further only after the *Poetics* had been written. However, Frère ("Fonction représentative et représentation") tries to show that some observations in the *Poetics* are compatible with the concept of *phantasia,* and this is nonetheless also perfectly possible.

27. See the outline in P. H. Schryvers, "Invention, imagination et théorie des émotions chez Cicéron et Quintilien," in B. Vickers, ed., *Rhetorical Revalued* (Binghamton and New York, 1982), 47–57.

28. This line is drawn very clearly by A. Schmitt, "Zur Erkenntnistheorie bei Platon und Descartes," *Antike und Abendland* 35 (1989): 54–82; see now also the great synthesis in idem, *Die Moderne und Platon,* (Stuttgart, 2003).

29. *Anal. post.* i 18, 81a 38f.: Φανερόν δὲ καὶ ὅτι, εἴ τις αἴσθησις ἐκλέλοιπεν, ἀνάγκη καὶ ἐπιστήμην τινὰ ἐκλελοιπέναι.

30. *De an.* iii 8, 432a 7f.: καὶ διὰ οὔτε τοῦτο μὴ αἰσθανόμενος μηθὲν οὐθὲν ἄν μάθοι οὐδὲ ξυνείη, ὅταν τε θεωρῇ, ἀνάγκη ἅμα φάντασμά τι θεωρεῖν.

31. See on this point the lucid explanation by A. Schmitt which also sheds some light on the history of philosophy, "Das Schöne: Gegenstand von Anschauung oder Erkenntnis?" *FILOSOFIA* 17/18 (1987/1988): 272–296, here in particular 284–290.

32. Boeth. *De inst. mus.* 5, 2: "The sense perceives a thing as indistinct, yet approximate to that which it is; reason exercises judgment concerning the whole and searches out ultimate differences. So the sense discovers something confused, yet

close to the truth, but it receives the whole through reason. Reason itself comes to know the whole, even though it receives an indistinct and approximate likeness of truth. For sense brings nothing whole to itself, but arrives only at an approximation. Reason makes the judgment." (Translation by C. M. Bower.) This is later explained by means of the example of the circle: *Velut si quis manu circulum scribat; fortasse cum vere circulum oculus esse arbitretur, ratio vero nullo modo esse id quod simulatur intellegit.* On the position of this passage in the context of the history of philosophy, see Schmitt, "Das Schöne," 282f.

33. *Anal. post.* ii 19, 99b 35.

34. E.g., Schofield, "Aristotle on the Imagination," 250; Frère, "Fonction représentative et representation," 283; Schmitt, *Die Moderne,* passim, and with detailed references to previous scholarship W. Bernard, *Rezeptivität und Spontaneität der Wahrnehmung bei Aristoteles. Versuch einer Bestimmung der spontanen Erkenntnisleistung der Wahrnehmung bei Aristoteles in Abgrenzung gegen die rezeptive Auslegung der Sinnlichkeit bei Descartes und Kant* (Baden-Baden, 1988). See also H. Busche, "Hat Phantasie nach Aristoteles eine interpretierende Funktion in der Wahrnehmung?" *Zeitschrift für philosophische Forschung* 51 (1997): 565–589, particularly 572–575.

35. See H. Busche, "Die Aufgaben der phantasia nach Aristoteles," in Th. Dewender and Th. Welt, eds., *Imagination-Fiktion-Kreation. Das kulturschaffende Vermögen der Phantasie* (München-Leipzig, 2003), 23–43, here 27, and particularly Th. Dewender, "Zur Rezeption der aristotelischen Phantasialehre in der lateinischen Philosophie des Mittelalters," in ibid., 141–160.

36. Schofield, "Aristotle on the Imagination," 253.

37. See D. Frede, "The Cognitive Role of *Phantasia* in Aristotle," in Nussbaum and Rorty, *Essays on Aristotle's "De Anima,"* 279–295, here 289, but less stringently phrased.

38. See *De an.* iii 3, 427b 6–16 and passim.

39. Schofield, "Aristotle on the Imagination," 254.

40. To this, points specifically Frede, "The Cognitive Role of *Phantasia* in Aristotle," 281.

41. *Rhet.* i 11, 1370a 28–29.

42. *De an.* ii 12, 424a 17–24.

43. *De an.* iii 3, 429a 4–5.

44. *De an.* iii 2, 425b 24–25: διὸ καὶ ἀπελθόντων τῶν αἰσθητῶν ἔνεισιν αἱ αἰσθήσεις καὶ φαντασίαι ἐν τοῖς αἰσθητηρίοις.

45. See n. 11, above.

46. D. K. W. Modrak, *Aristotle's Theory of Language and Meaning* (Cambridge, 2001), 234.

47. *De an.* iii 7, 431a 14–17: "For the thinking soul images are like sensory perceptions. . . . For the soul never thinks without mental images."

48. *De an.* ii 8, 420b 31–33 with Ross's ἔμψοφόν instead of the ἔμψυχόν of the

direct transmission: "that which strikes should have sound and be accompanied by a certain kind of mental representation (for the voice is a sound endowed with a meaning)."

49. It becomes clear at once that, in the *Ars grammatica, littera* and *vox* are not connected at random, and thus textuality is established in the sphere of the sensorily perceptible; see also n. 3, above.

50. See, e.g., Arist. *De an.* iii 7, 431b 2, or *De int.* 1, 16a 3f. with Ammonios's commentary.

51. Schofield, "Aristotle on the Imagination," 255.

52. Arist. *De mem.* 451a 14–17: τί μὲν οὖν ἐστὶ μνήμη καὶ τὸ μνημονεὺειν, εἴρηται, ὅτι φαντάσματος, ὡς εἰκόνος ο φάντασμα, ἕχις, καὶ τίνος μορίου τῶν ἐν ἡμιν, ὅτι τοῦ πρώτου αἰσθητικοῦ, καὶ ᾧ χρόνου αἰσθανόμεθα.

53. Modrak, *Aristotle's Theory of Language and Meaning,* 234f. and 237.

54. Macr. *Sat.* 5, 1, 19: "For if you observe the world itself carefully, you will find a close similarity between that divine work and this work of poetry."

55. B. Weinberg, "Scaliger versus Aristotle on Poetics," *Modern Philology* 39 (1942): 337–360, here 348.

56. This applies mainly to Virgil's *Aeneid,* even in the sense that the nature to be imitated by the poet can be found in a more perfect form in poetry alone. To take up once more a pointed formulation of Weinberg, "Scaliger versus Aristotle on Poetics," 349: "Thus the norm of nature, represented only imperfectly by objects in the real world, is represented perfectly by Vergil's epic. Vergil *is* nature." This is directly evident from the perspective of the Platonic-Aristotelian scale *confusum-distinctum:* just think of the example of the circle (see above n. 32). In continuation of the passage quoted above Boethius gives a systematic explanation (*De inst. mus.* 5, 2): *Quare sensum quoque confusio sequitur, mentem vero atque rationem quoniam materia non moratur, species, quas pervidet, praeter subiecti communionem intuetur, atque ideo eam integritas comitatur ac veritas, potiusque, quod in sensu aut peccatur aut minus est, aut emendat aut conplet.*

57. Incidentally, this sheds light on the expansion of the field of the object, which is at the basis of rhetorical and poetic usage, against the Aristotelian concept of the limitation of *mimesis* to *pragmata;* through its more abstract and non-object-oriented approach such an expansion helps to avoid a number of problems.

58. Julius Caesar Scaliger, *Poetices libri septem. Sieben Bücher über die Dichtkunst,* unter Mitwirkung von M. Fuhrmann hrsg., übers., eingel. und erl. von L. Deitz und G. Vogt-Spira, 5 vols. (Stuttgart–Bad Cannstatt, 1994–2003), iii 1 (vol. 2, 60, 14–26).

59. Ibid. (vol. 2, 60, 21–25).

60. According to the principle: *omne enim quod cognoscitur non secundum sui vim sed secundum cognoscentium potius comprehenditur facultatem.* [. . .] *cum omne iudicium iudicantis actus existat, necesse est, ut suam quisque operam non ex aliena sed ex propria potestate perficiat* (Boeth. *Cons.* 5, 4, 71–74 and 113–115).

61. Arist. *De an.* iii 8, 432a 9–10: "In fact representations are like sensations, but without matter."

62. Scal. *Poet.* vii 2 (Bd. 5, 502, 10–11).

63. See H. Wenzel, *Hören und Sehen, Schrift und Bild. Kultur und Gedächtnis im Mittelalter* (München, 1995), 292–296.

64. A representative example is Macr. *Sat.* 5, 11, 11: *Hoc mire et velut coloribus Maro pinxit:* such judgment is sufficient in itself to justify why the passage of Virgil referred to here is superior to the corresponding Homeric passage.

65. Scal. *Poet.* vii 2 (Bd. 5, 508, 1–2).

66. Scal. *Poet.* iv 1 (Bd. 3, 256, 14–15).

67. Ps.-Long. *De subl.* 15, 2.

68. Quint. *Inst.* 6, 2, 30: "It is the man who is really sensitive to such impressions who will have the greatest power over the emotions."

69. Quint. *Inst.* 6, 2, 32: "our emotions will be no less actively stirred than if we were present at the actual occurrence."

70. Exemplary is the *Poetics* of M. H. Vida, which was reprinted more than forty times in the sixteenth century alone; see 1, 112–122 and passim.

71. In the present context, the focus is on literary and artistic theory. To be distinguished from it are theological questions. See the elegant solution of the problem in the Neoplatonic approach, namely, that the higher capability of knowledge would already subsume the lower ones, but that the opposite would not be true (Boeth. *Cons.* 5, 4, 71–115, particularly 88–90): *In quo illud maxime considerandum est: nam superior comprehendendi vis amplectitur inferiorem, inferior vero ad superiorem nullo modo consurgi*—here particularly with reference to the problem of how human freedom of will and divine providence could be reconciled.

72. Philostr. *Vita Apollon.* 6, 19; see Watson, "The Concept of 'Phantasia,'" 4766–4769, which gives a short summary of some problems raised by the passage; the suggestion to talk here of "creative imagination" is not a happy one, since in this context "creativity" barely displays any distinctive feature.

73. See the discussion in Rosenmeyer, "Φαντασία und Einbildungskraft," 236–240.

74. Macr. *Sat.* 4, 5, 9: "Also the image . . . is in the position of moving the affects. This happens when is described either the appearance of a body that is absent or when is evoked one that doesn't exist at all."

75. Quint. *Inst.* 9, 2, 41.

76. About its transmission, see Flury, "Phantasia und imaginatio im Bereich des antiken Lateins."

77. Cic. *Pro Mil.* 79.

78. See n. 34, above.

PART TWO
Fascinations

4 *The Critical Sense*

Some Spanish Examples

Marina Brownlee

The relationship between sensual perception and cognition, between cognition and thought, between the personal as well as social uses of the senses, is a contingent one. I realize that Aristotle's account of perception is considered to be "purely physiological"—and has often been juxtaposed with Cartesian "spirit" or "mindstuff." And yet, Aristotle demonstrates that perception and desire are really about external objects. When a man or beast judges an object to be food, and the perception causes a desire to eat it, the perception and desire are clearly directed at the external object. By such operations we see, as Terrell Bynum notes in his analysis of *De anima,* that Aristotle's theory of perception addresses "mental properties" like privacy and subjectivity.[1]

Not only is the ultimate number of senses open to interpretation (five according to some authorities, three or seven according to others),[2] but we must also acknowledge the complexities involved in the presence of both external/physical and internal/spiritual sense systems. In the case of extreme physical sensory deprivation motivated by religious fervor, we know, for example, that it can lead to extraordinary spiritual plenitude communicated through the senses: we can taste heavenly sweetness, see divine light, smell the pungent odor of sanctity through violets, and so on.[3] The senses are complex in yet another way as well, namely, they are polyvalent: writing is tactile, but also visual (and perhaps auditory); speech is not just auditory but kinesthetic (involving the olfaction of breath, perhaps even taste or touch). Sweat can be categorized according to sight (we see it), smell, taste (voluntary or involuntary), touch, conceivably it can even be heard (dripping or making other noises when in contact with friction).

In this chapter I seek to explore the cultural (as well as individual) relativism of the senses—their representation as dysfunctional in times of social disorder. That is to say, the senses in literature function not merely on biological and cognitive planes with relation to an individual agent, but in a broader, ideological framework as well, as an index of cultural plenitude or its opposite—cultural anxiety. To illustrate this phenomenon I consider examples drawn from the first half of the fourteenth century in Spain.

My focus is on the oral sense—taste (the most largely social sense)—the gustatory sense which is achieved through the lips and mouth, as is speech, lingua. As seemingly natural faculties of taste, not only eating and drinking, but also speech were occasionally classified as separate senses, and laughter (admittedly a difficult commodity to classify) was an equally serious topic of concern.[4]

The parameters of the senses involve not only sacred and secular considerations, but gender distinctions as well: historically, men were meant to speak about ideas, laws, and governance, while women were expected to be silent. With the exception of female religious, while women were ideally silent, when they did speak they were portrayed in unflattering ways, either as prolix in formal terms, semantically as inane, given to vain topics, and/or as positively sinister, as dangerously seductive. As we know, female seduction through speech originated with Eve's temptation of Adam with the proposition that he eat the forbidden fruit, which, in turn, led to the biblical injunction against women—disqualifying them from preaching and teaching.[5]

As we know, this view of the transgressive nature of female speech extends well beyond the Middle Ages, as, for example, the allegorical English play devoted to the senses (entitled *Lingua,* 1607), attests. Female speech, Lingua, announces her desire to be declared a sixth sense and for her presumption she is branded a "witch" and "whore," a sense she deploys for criticizing men in powerful places, and for providing wives with "weapons to fight against their husbands."[6]

My exploration of the oral sense draws examples from two texts from the first half of the fourteenth century: the anonymous *Libro del Caballero Zifar* (1300–1361?),[7] and Juan Manuel's *Libro de los enxiemplos del Conde Lucano et de Patronio* (1335).[8] Both texts were written during a time of political, economic, and social turmoil, and their exploitation of the senses is calculated to figure the instability of social and cultural relations treated by their respective authors.

Traditional categories of behavior and belief—the predictable pedagogical imperative—are seriously interrogated in these works. The two authors voice the desire to shape the interpretation of their readers—at times offering predictable depictions of people and events with their attendant transparent exegesis. At the same time, however, they clearly perceive the limitations of this pursuit, figuring, on several other occasions, unstable categories—generated by transgressive sensorial perceptions—and unexemplary actions in unpredictable ways that question the very notion of the pedagogical efficacy of exemplary discourse. Thus the circuit between perception and cognition is dramatically challenged. This essay explores some of this dark side that thematizes human complexity and unpredictability by considering some narratives in *Zifar* and *Lucanor* that offer problematic examples of behavior in society—all heavily based on manipulations of the oral sense.

Much work has been undertaken in recent years with respect to the body (in terms of pathology, sex and gender distinctions, trauma, the history of sexual practices, etc.),[9] and our work on the senses relates to it in important ways. In *Volatile Bodies,* Elizabeth Grosz rightly observes that: "Bodies have all the explanatory power of minds" (vii). And, although her study explores sex and gender relations in modern contexts of social constructivism, the semantic potential of bodily representation holds equally true for *Lucanor* and *Zifar,* and the same can be said for the representation of the role played by the *senses* in these texts.

The potential for (1) formulating social constructions of meaning through the body, along with (2) the articulation of the individual in bodily terms is as thorny and fascinating in the Middle Ages as it is for both earlier and later periods. And in this enterprise, poststructural criticism serves to nuance our thinking about these two corporeal functions. The influence of psychoanalysis in recent decades is now being rethought in meaningful ways. The Lacanian model that assumes the existence of a single body-image defined by the phallus—or its lack—with the privileging of the male embodied subject has sparked interesting critical responses. Butler, for example, writes about the undeniably distinct nature of the female body and its implications and, in a different light, thinkers such as Deleuze have challenged the totalizing corporeal ideology of the psychoanalytic model by reinstating the importance of the fragmented body.[10]

By way of exploring the unpredictable relationship of sensorial perception and cognition, I would like to consider first, the paratextual matter as well as several *exempla* of *Lucanor*. They will serve as a demonstration of the problem that Juan Manuel projects: namely, that the traditional medieval confidence in the ultimate viability of representing religious and social systems as being adequately figured by sensorial paradigms was losing its currency as the fascination with human agency and subjectivity and Nominalist skepticism were gaining in status.[11]

Juan Manuel offers a fascinating dialogue between the senses as cultural signifier and as unique event and identity, yielding a dynamic—and often unanticipated—array of relationships, of the senses as personal perception leading to personal cognition, and as icons of a symbolic cultural order. As we know, the links between sensorial and cognitive systems of organization work paradoxically: the relations between the two are encoded by the relation of a specific sense. Strivings for unity and psychic wholeness are produced and expressed—paradoxically—by the individual, sensorial fragment. (This would explain why we find in *Lucanor* so many representations not only of notable sensorial events, but of extreme events, of not only sensorial but corporeal violence.)

Like the regulation of the body, sensorial control was (and continues to be) an expression of cultural power—exploited in the Middle Ages by both Church and State for the articulation of official perspectives, for the imposition of homogeneity and dependence—whereas in modern times such "body language" tends to be exploited by the individual more often in the quest for uniqueness and autonomy.

Juan Manuel's fourteenth-century world was an era of disaffection and disenchantment regarding issues of caste and rank, where traditional wisdom and social hierarchies were no longer operative. It was a time that witnessed even Juan Manuel himself—as full of paradox and contradiction in an unstable world. Norman Schafter describes his *Libro del caballero y el escudero* (1326) as "a catalogue in outline form of the estates, and divisions within each estate, of Christian society,"[12] and one is tempted to view the relationship of this text to *Lucanor* as the difference between Spanish society in theory and praxis. Yet even the "ordered correspondences and similitudes" presented in the *Caballero y el escudero* register profound instabilities: notable among them, the conflict inherent in spending one's life either in pursuit of eternal salvation or of worldly fame and power (a subject dear to Juan Manuel himself).[13]

For a brief time—during the minority of Alfonso XI—he was all powerful: serving as regent of Castile and related by marriage to the throne of Aragón. A mere two years later, however, in 1325, rejected and humiliated by Alfonso (who held his daughter Constanza hostage), Juan Manuel took the radical step of renouncing his oath of fealty, thereafter seeking refuge with a Moorish king. Explicit legitimizing of the infidel monarchs (based on Christ's injunction: "Jesucristo nos mandó que por todas las tierras do fuesemos, obedeciésemos a los reyes et a los grandes señores" [Christ instructed us, wherever we went, to obey the kings and influential lords].[14] Also among the pages he offers us, we find that meditations on the true nature of honor (titular versus personal worth), on the questionable value of primogeniture as a meaningful category, on the paramount importance of dissembling, whether words instead of deeds are more reliable, and the power of magic are some of the most notable issues he raises.

Juan Manuel's reliance on lived experience rather than bookish authority (a feature which inclines many readers to view him as the first "modern" Spanish author) is, in part, a reflection of the influential Nominalist commitment to personal experience rather than bookish *auctoritas.* Models based on learned doctrine are not only questioned, they appear to be no longer relevant in conveying the instability of his time. Hence his reliance on empirical story-telling which as Louis Mink reminds us, "is the means we have of making sense of experience, of creating beginnings and ends, causes and effects, relations and dependencies."[15]

In fact, the text is full of mixed messages, with its dialogic exchange between Patronio and Lucanor functioning as a "juego de espejos enfrentados" [a game of mirrors that confront one another] as Marta Diz aptly remarks.[16] Its specular nature confronts the reader programmatically as both positive and negative *exemplum.* In those narratives where an unproblematic lesson is imparted positivistically, we cannot argue with the resultant pedagogical effect. The emperor's new clothes narrative (no. 32), and several Aesopic tales (nos. 5, 6, 9, 12, 19, 22, etc.), offer just such unproblematic exegesis for the reader. Yet the collection as a whole is consciously framed in paradox and obscurity, pointing to the deceptive nature of signs—a deception that is staged through the senses.

There are five—increasingly obscure—parts to the book, culminating in the alternation of clear and obscure *sententiae* in part IV and the transformation in part V of the Good-versus-Evil opposition into something relative. The General Prologue to the work instructs us that no two people in the world look identical in their facial features—just as no two men have the same intention. And yet, the last tale presents us with an exact look-alike to the king in the form of a madman. The theme of deception and dissimulation is crystallized at the work's structurally significant midpoint, where we are offered a typology of lies.

Whereas the adviser, Patronio, tells lies/fictions in order to teach truth throughout the collection of stories, at the midpoint we encounter an anatomy of lies, the "single," "double," and "triple lie" ("la mentira treble") that utters truth in order to deceive.[17] Even in its most basic discursive sense, this book is problematic—given that the Prologue asserts the impossibility of knowing one's intentions, yet Patronio can describe a situation or event as if he were an omniscient exception—since he always knows the intentions of all the many characters who populate the text. He paradoxically enjoys a kind of *entendimiento* that no other human has at his disposal.[18]

Deception, mendacity, and the proliferation of simulacra—sensorial as well as verbal—abound in Juan Manuel's world and in his text. Jean Baudrillard writes about the end of feudalism in Europe in a way that, I think, is pertinent to Juan Manuel's Spain. He speaks of the "disenchanted universe of the signified"[19] which resulted from the destruction of the feudal system—its hierarchies of caste and rank—and the substitution of open competition at the level of signs. Lamenting the "disappearance of syntax and semantics" (145), he explains: "There once existed a specific class of objects that were allegorical . . . such as mirrors, images, works of art (and concepts?); of course these too were simulacra, but they were transparent and manifest. . . . In these objects, pleasure consisted more in discovering something 'natural' in what was artificial and counterfeit" (146). It is for this reason that the second Prologue to the work deals with the sense of *taste,* and with the diseased patient-reader in need of aid, whom he will treat as a doctor does:

> Fiz este libro compuesto de las mas apuestas palabras que yo pude, et entre las palabras entremeti algunos exiemplos de que se podrían aprouechar los que los oyeron. Et esto fiz segund la manera que fazen los fisicos, que quando quieren fazer alguna melizina que aproueche al figado, por razon que naturalmente el figado se paga de las cosas dulçes, mezclan con aquella melezina que quieren melezinar el figado, açucar o miel o alguna cosa dulçe; et por el pagamiento que el figado a de la cosa dulçe, en tirando la para si, lieua con ella la melezina quel a de aprouechar. (28)

> [I wrote this book] in the fashion of doctors, who when they want to prepare a medicine that will minister to the liver, since naturally the liver likes sweet things, they mix with their medicine intended for the liver some sugar or

> honey or something sweet; and because of the pleasure that the liver gets from sweet things, as it takes them to itself, it takes along with them the medicine which is for its own good. (41)

Despite this professed, curative potential of his prose, indeterminacy invades the text as it reflects real life. Example no. 44 of *Lucanor* provides a clear case of the derailment of traditional forms of order and values, a derailment effected by the manipulation of normative forms of taste and speech.[20] This tale is recounted by Patronio in response to Lucanor's complaint that people whom he has treated generously have (most ungratefully) deserted him and even attempted to do him great harm. According to this narrative involving three historical figures, Count Rodrigo bore false witness against his virtuous wife, for which mendacity she asked God to perform a miracle to vindicate her.[21]

This is a text obsessed by lies, and the power of speech itself—the count's, his wife's, and that of all the other true and mendacious interlocutors—qualifies as a topic for our consideration since speech was often construed historically as a sense. As we know, there has not existed a consensus on the senses: Plato did not discriminate clearly between senses and feelings. In one cataloguing of the senses, he includes sight, hearing, and smell, but elects to exclude taste altogether. Rather than identifying touch as one of the senses, he speaks of the perceptions of hot and cold, adding to the list the sensations or emotions of pleasure, discomfort, desire, and fear. By contrast, Aristotle declares the intrinsic relationship between the senses and the elements (earth, air, fire, water, and the quintessence), therefore identifying five senses. A different accounting is offered by Philo, in the first century. Because he wanted the senses to total seven for allegorical purposes of biblical exegesis, he included the genitals and speech on the list.[22]

Philo, however, is not alone in construing speech as an organ, though it seems to elude such categorization as a rule, perhaps because we consider the senses to be passive receptors of data, while speech is an active producer of data, not a natural sense but a learned phenomenon. The ancients, by contrast, tended to conceive of the senses as media of communication, rather than as passive receptors of data. At the same time, speech has often been considered to be an innate ability shared by all humans. As Constance Classen observes, "So engrained was the notion [of speech as innate] that in the Middle Ages the Holy Roman Emperor Frederick II ordered that a group of babies be kept secluded from all language in order to find out which tongue would come naturally to them: Latin, Greek, Hebrew or the local language.

No conclusion was reached on the matter as, unfortunately, the babies died before they could speak."[23] Yet, not only has premodern Europe been tempted to construe speech as a sixth sense, so has Noam Chomsky.[24]

As soon as Count Rodrigo's wife prays to God, "as if by some miracle" her husband is stricken with leprosy, thus allowing her to abandon him. It is odd that her words of prayer elicit this effect, since, among other things, leprosy, while associated with sin, is especially identified with the poor.[25] This disease, which was most destructive in the late twelfth and thirteenth centuries, is associated with the *caritas* of religious men and women: for example, the unnamed bishop of the thirteenth-century *Dialogus Miraculorum* who "aided by God's grace . . . applied his tongue to the leper's diseased face, and miraculously received a precious gem from the nostrils of him who had seemed to be a leper but who was now revealed to be Christ, ascending into heaven in glory,"[26] or the similar example of St. Francis's kiss.[27]

As soon as the count and his wife are separated, the King of Navarre proposes marriage to her, and she accepts, becoming the Queen of Navarre in short order. Meanwhile the afflicted count decides to make a pilgrimage to the Holy Land in order to die there. Unfortunately, he and the three knights who accompany him run out of provisions during their stay in the Holy Land, becoming utterly destitute. The knights are reduced to extreme poverty, desperately hiring themselves out to toil for others as a means of survival. They demonstrate their allegiance to the count not only by this demeaning activity, but even by drinking pus from their lord's wounds to prove that they are not disgusted by having to care for him.[28] After his death, their degradation is still not ended, however, since they must beg for food in order to make the journey home to Spain, in order to deposit his remains in Castile. When they stop in Toulouse, they encounter a lady about to be burned at the stake because of an accusation of adultery made by her brother-in-law. It was proclaimed that if no knight comes forth to save her, she will die. Hearing this, one of the three knights, Pero Núñez, magnanimously steps forth to defend her if he can be assured of her innocence. In questioning her, she claims that she did not commit adultery—though she wished she had.

From this admission, Núñez realizes that harm will inevitably come to anyone who tries to save her, since she wished she had sinned. But because he took her *word* that she "had not committed the entire sin" at face value, he decides to save her. He enters the jousting ground after first informing the lady's relatives that some accident will, no doubt, befall him because of her adulterous thoughts. Sure enough, although he wins the battle and saves the lady, he loses an eye; "thereby," Patronio adds, "what he had said before came to pass."[29]

Upon their arrival in Castile, the king greets his loyal knights, offering a worthy burial for the count, whereupon the knights return to their homes: Ruy González is greeted by his wife, who has fasted in his absence, refraining from eating meat or drinking wine. But rather than being appreciative of her fortitude and selfless devotion, he is saddened to hear of her fasting, saying that he had told her to live well and eat well. Because she had not eaten anything but bread and water, he considers her to be disobedient.

Likewise, Pero Núñez is dismayed by his wife. Because she begins to *laugh* (prompted by the sheer delight she experiences at his return alive), he is convinced that she is instead laughing *at* him.[30] To dispel this misinterpretation by a dramatic gesture, the lady "[runs] a needle into her own eye and [puts] it out," telling her husband that "if she ever laughed again, he would never think that she was laughing to shame him."[31]

From this story, Patronio derives three lessons: (1) that although some people whom you have treated generously will treat you badly, others will serve you well; (2) do not expect to be served well by all whom you have supported; and, (3) the epigraph of the story (which departs somewhat from the diegetic lesson): "If by men you have been ensnared / Do not therefore go unprepared" [Maguer que algunos te ayan errado, / nunca dexes de fazer aguisado] (222). So ends the tale.

Yet this tale is, in fact, a bold series of departures—or violations—of religious, social, political, and literary systems, offering the reader a series of dysfunctional simulacra. The first is the "miracle" by which God answers the lady's prayer, causing her husband to contract leprosy, so that she can abandon him to trade up and marry the King of Navarre. Whereas his false witness is reprehensible, her abandonment of him is unsavory as well. The contraction of leprosy is also atypical of miracles involving marital disputes. These anomalous events in the teleology of miracles are striking. The chivalric and courtly episodes offered by the knights with the dying count and with the woman accused of adultery and with their wives are equally strange. The drinking of the count's pus by the knights is bizarre—the type of activity associated with (usually female) saints: their abject poverty and need to do hard labor for hire is similarly and strikingly uncanonical behavior. Knights are supposed to work for their lord, who provides for them.

Pero Núñez vows that he will defend the accused woman "if he [can] be certain of her innocence," but how could he be? He takes her word against her brother-in-law's (thereby defying not only him but the judicial system as well). She is problematic in saying that while she didn't commit adultery she wished that she had. (This desire itself—even if unfulfilled—is a sin, as the Bible reminds us—e.g., in Matthew 5:28.) Don Pero is aware, therefore, that she is tainted in part. (The complexity of her case exposes the untenably totalizing nature of the judicial system, as well as the complications of the religious and chivalric perspective in terms of human subjectivity.) Núñez's realization that he will suffer misfortune given the lady's problematic vindication attempt is followed by his almost immediate ocular mutilation. The swiftness of this divine retribution seems mechanical, as does the king's misguided honoring of the dishonorable (mendacious) count, affording him full burial honors. Thus the justice system itself, as represented by the king's decree, functions as an empty simulacrum of the truth.

The domestic relations of the two knights and their wives are equally problematic, generating upsetting simulacra that take the form of dire misreadings: Ruy González is affronted by his wife's fasting, motivated by her mourning of his absence. Yet, why does he not construe her abstinence as a mark of uxorial devotion instead? The final—and most graphic misunderstanding—is Pero Núñez's misreading of his wife's laughter: her joy at his return leading to laughter, is interpreted by him as mockery due to his lost eye.[32] Not only does he obviously not understand the depth of her devotion, he leads her to mutilate herself by putting out her own eye. This last misreading resulting in self-mutilation, hence permanent physical disfigurement, is troubling indeed, for in the world of literature (as in life itself) it is particularly unacceptable—and in a noble woman no less—given the standards of beauty and physiognomy that were operative at the time.

In this way, Juan Manuel figures the instability at issue in the most hallowed social institutions of his day—in the political, religious, and amatory spheres—through the senses, primarily the oral sense of speech (its truly perilous nature), and its effects: the contraction of leprosy as a divine punishment for the count's mendacity—a direct result of his wife's words of prayer, the resultant lack of food and drink to and from the Holy Land for the count's vassals, the gustatorial sense of pus (imbibed not for its taste but for its *dépassement* of revulsion by the three loyal knights, as proof of devotion to their lord). The would-be adulteress, however, goes free, while Pero Núñez saves this tainted woman (who had sinned in thought). And while he demonstrates great generosity in rescuing this woman, he treats his own wife cruelly, leading to her violence against herself. Likewise, another of the three knights, the generous Ruy González, who has also made significant sacrifices for his mendacious lord, mistreats his long-suffering wife.

In other words, the senses are unreliable in terms of cognition—people can and do act very unpredictably. Indeed, even such putatively sane individuals can act irrationally.

Looking now to *Zifar,* a text that is contemporary in its production to *Lucanor,* we find a wealth of sensorial depictions which, again, short-circuit our expectations in terms of cognition and agency—here, specifically in terms of eating and laughter, an oral/aural product that, as we have seen in *Lucanor,* can pose a terrible threat. *Zifar* in Arabic means "errant" or "wandering," and it is appropriate to the eponymous protagonist, who faces innumerable adversities as a result of an evil ancestor's malediction (leading to Zifar's perpetual poverty and exile, and to the ten-day life span of his horses). The tale begins in an ambiguously defined land known as "las Indias," and it has been viewed as deriving from Eastern and Western versions of the legend of St. Eustache, the *Thousand and One Nights*' tale of "The King Who Lost His Kingdom and Wife and Wealth and Allah Restored Them to Him," and/or the French *Chanson de Floovant,* which is related to the legend of Octavian.[33] Contained within this romance (which claims to be translated from Chaldean—normally denoting Syriac, a dialect of Aramaic, though some Hispanists assume that it was written in Arabic), is also a sizeable didactic section in which Zifar instructs his two sons with lessons on life, the universe, and everything. This treatise draws material from the Arabic *Flores de filosofía,* but is also related to other Semitic-based didactic texts, for example, the *Bocados de oro, Poridat de las poridades,* the *Siete partidas* of Alfonso X, and the *Castigos e documentos del rey don Sancho.*

I would like now to briefly consider two episodes devoted to *taste as eating* in *Zifar* to reflect on the representation of this sense and its surprising possibilities for meaning-production. The first is a tale designed to explore the parameters of friendship, with variations found in the *Disciplina clericalis,* the *Scala coeli,* the *Libro de los exemplos,* the *Speculum laicorum,* as well as *Lucanor.*[34] The *Lucanor* version (no. 48, "A Man Who Tested His Friends") has a father tell his son to kill a pig, put it in a sack, and tell one of his friends that it is the corpse of a man whom he has murdered—hence the need to get protection from the friend, and to destroy the corporeal evidence. Each of the putative friends refuses to provide refuge, until the father's one and only true friend finally offers protection to the son. When it becomes known in the town that a murder has been committed, the sack-wielding youth is logically incarcerated and sentenced to death. The true friend, in order to comply with his bond of undying friendship, swears to the youth's innocence, implicating his own (innocent) son instead, who is summarily executed. While this tale proves that a good friend is hard to find, it is perverse in that a father sacrifices his wholly blameless son to comply with a simulated crime devised by another man in order to illustrate the meaning of friendship to his own son.

In *Zifar*, by contrast, a variant of this *exemplum* leads to cannibalism. The "Parable of the Half-Friend" once again is intended by a father to prove to his son that a good friend is hard to find. After going from door to door of friend after friend, receiving no help, the youth finally goes to the father's so-called half-friend, who receives him and *laughs* when the youth tells him that his father has instructed the friend to slice up the corpse and eat it—realizing that the father wanted to test his son, noting, at the same time, the son's transgressive gullability.

The man cooked the flesh and the father invited the son to eat it, "since," he claims, "the flesh of an enemy had the same flavor as that of pork" (14) [que atal era la carne del ome como la carne del puerco (67)]. The son loved the taste of the roasted meat, so much that he said to his father, "[T]he other enemy of mine who was with this one when he insulted me cannot escape my killing and eating him with great pleasure; because never have I eaten meat that tastes so good as this" (14) [non puede escaper el otro mio enemigo que era con éste quando me dixo la sobervia, que le non mate e que le non coma muy de grado, ca nunca comí carne que tan bien me sopiese como ésta (68)]. Upon hearing these words, the father and friend become understandably concerned at the son's appetite for human flesh, their *exemplum* having generated a truly perverse sense of taste. Intellection and morality should provoke revulsion at the thought of eating a human corpse, yet this text wants to signal the unpredictability of cognition generated from perception.[35]

Another example—this time of literal cannibalism—involves a mother and her son. The story explains how a lady was happily married to a knight, who died an untimely death, leaving her widowed with a young son, whom she loved, and upon whom she doted. As the son grew, he became a monstrous murderer and rapist, a repeat offender in these and other heinous crimes. When the emperor learns of this grotesque behavior he logically sentences the offender to death. For her part, the devoted mother is disconsolate, begging the king to embrace and kiss her son one last time. At this request, the son speaks in a loud voice, saying:

> Let my mother be welcome for she wishes to make me see that justice is carried out as it should be. I well believe that God would not want anyone else except the person who deserves it to suffer punishment. (171)
>
> Bien venga la mi madre, ca ayudarme quiere a que la justiçia se cunpla segunt deve, e bien creo que Dios non querrá al sinon que sofriese la pena quien la meresçe. (253)

The assembled masses are amazed at the son's words of wisdom.

> Friends, said the [condemned man] . . . I will not run away, for I desire, and am pleased, that justice be carried out. I consider myself a terrible sinner for doing so much evil as I did, and I want justice to begin with the one who deserves it. (171)
>
> Amigos—dixo [el condenado] non creades que me yo vaya; antes quiero e me plaze que se cunpla la justiçia e me tengo por muy pecador en fazer tanto mal como fis; e yo lo quiero començar en aquel que lo mereçe. (253–254)

While all present marvel at these wise and ethical words, his actions soon betray them, revealing, in fact, an inhuman impulse:

> he took [his mother] by the ears beneath her hair with his hands, and he placed his mouth against hers, and began to gnaw and eat away her lips so that he did not leave her anything up to her nose, nor of her lower lip to the point of her chin, and all her teeth were exposed and she remained very ugly and disfigured. (171)
>
> tomóla con amas a dos las manos por las orejas a buelta de los cabellos e fue poner la su boca con la suya e començóla a roer e la comer todos los labros, de guisa que non dexó ninguna cosa fasta en las narizes, nin del labor deyuso fasta en la barbiella; e fincaron todos los dientes descobiertos, e ella fincó muy fea e muy desfaçada. (254)

The disfigured mother has lost the power of speech, given her barbaric injury, and is reduced to the minimal pathetic signs she can make with her hands. We are shocked not only at the son's savage cannibalism, at the action's contrast with his words,[36] but equally at the emperor's response. For rather than executing him on the spot, the son is exonerated and his mother condemned—for overly permissive parenting(!). While this story exists in earlier sources, Jacques de Vitry, Philippe de Navarre, Vincent de Beauvais, Eude de Cherington, and others, in them it is the father who is punished.[37] Nowhere except in *Zifar* is the mother condemned. Her punishment strikes us as unfair not only because her flaw was excessive love, it seems particularly incongruous because philosophical speech is male gendered—it is the male who is the lawgiver and transmitter of ethical doctrine.

The potential chasm separating perception and cognition is dramatized in fourteenth-cenury Spain—given that people all too frequently eschew Aristotle's description of a reasonable "critical mean."[38] And the oral phenomenon of laughter (what Descartes defines as "this inarticulate and explosive voice that we call laughter" is one of those complex sense-productions, like sweat, for example, that cut across several sense-categories, and also several social situations. French fabliaux, Italian *novelle,* and Chaucer's tales, but also serious texts, can surprise us with laughter—its salutary potential as well as its perceived threat. Is it good or evil? Who is authorized to laugh? Should clerics indulge in it? In short, as Del Kolve avers in his work on the Corpus Christi plays, the Middle Ages considered "its peril, its necessity, its potential usefulness."[39]

The *Zifar*-author considers laughter in several places, but one of the most curious is the encounter between Zifar's son Roboán and the Emperor of Tigridia, in the Fertile Crescent. The newly arrived young knight distinguishes himself so impressively that several of the emperor's vassals soon become insanely jealous and determine to destroy this competitor. Knowing that the emperor never laughs and beheads anyone who asks him why, the knights urge Roboán to ask him the fatal question. Yet, the emperor—surprisingly—does not kill him. Instead, and with no explanation, he puts him in a boat that transports him to the Blessed Isles (Yslas Dotadas), where he marries the Queen (Nobleza/Nobility), since they experience love at first sight. Having spent a year of bliss, the devil (disguised as a lovely lady) tempts him to ask for a horse that swiftly returns him to the emperor, with no hope of seeing his beloved again. He now realizes that the emperor had undergone the same sad experience.

We are prompted to wonder why the emperor did not explain his sad news, the reason why he never laughs, and also the extreme penalty he imposes on people who ask him why. The reason why he spares Roboán is also not divulged. Does he not explain his sadness because he feels that words cannot convey it adequately? Does he realize that Roboán must experience this profoundly sad event for himself—that words need a particular experiential context in order to be meaningful? Does he spare Roboán because he sees him as a version of his earlier self? In any case, Roboán becomes the emperor's best friend, until the latter dies, bequeathing the empire to him. For his part, Roboán *does* overcome his sad experience, thus offering us a meditation both on the power and constraints of language as a meaning-producing system, of perception, of its polysemously possible relationship to thought, and of the unpredictable nature of human subjectivity and agency.

In closing, and by way of relating the oral sense—taste, drinking, speech, and laughter to perception and cognition—I would conclude by saying that the "critical sense" (of my title) signifies the inscrutable, unpredictable judgment formulated by the fourteenth-century perceiving subject in a world of indeterminacy, lies, and simulacra.

Notes

1. Terrell Ward Bynum, "A New Look at Aristotle's Theory of Perception," in *Aristotle's "De anima" In Focus,* ed. Michael Durrant (London: Routledge, 1993), 106–107.

2. Constance Classen, *Worlds of Sense: Exploring the Senses in History and across Cultures* (London: Routledge, 1993), 1–5.

3. See Caroline Walker Bynum, *Holy Feast and Holy Fast: The Religious Significance of Food to Medieval Women* (Berkeley: University of California Press, 1987), and also, e.g., Béatrice Caseau, "Christian Bodies: The Senses and Early Byzantine Christianity," in *Desire and Denial in Byzantium: Papers from the Thirty-first Spring Symposium of Byzantine Studies, University of Sussex, 1977,* ed. Liz James (Aldershot: Ashgate Variorum, 1998), 101–109.

4. See *The Philosophy of Laughter and Humor,* ed. John Morreall (Albany: State University of New York Press, 1987).

5. E.g., 1 Timothy 2:11–12.

6. Thomas Tomkis has Common Sense decree that a court of law will rule on whether Lingua can be considered as one of the senses. Common Sense decrees that "as the senses must number five in order to correspond with the four elements and 'the pure substance of the heavens,' speech cannot be counted as a sense. An exception is made in the case of women, however, who may deem Lingua to be 'the last and feminine sense' (an interesting instance of the engenderment of perception)." Constance Classen, *The Color of Angels: Cosmology, Gender and the Aesthetic Imagination* (London: Routledge, 1998), 75.

7. All citations to the anonymous *Zifar* will refer to the edition by Joaquín González Muela, *Libro del Caballero Zifar* (Madrid: Clásicos Castalia, 1982). Translations refer to *Book of the Knight Zifar,* ed. Charles L. Nelson (Lexington: University Press of Kentucky, 1983).

8. All citations from *El Conde Lucanor* will refer to volume 1 of the two-volume *Obras completas* edition by José Manuel Blecua, (Madrid: Gredos, 1982). Translations refer to *The Book of Count Lucanor and Patronio,* trans. John E. Keller and L. Clark Keating (Lexington: University Press of Kentucky, 1977).

9. Judith Butler, *Gender Trouble* (New York: Routledge, 1990); Thomas Laqueur, *Making Sex* (Cambridge: Harvard University Press, 1990); Elizabeth Grosz, *Volatile Bodies* (Bloomington: Indiana University Press, 1994).

10. Gilles Deleuze, *Foucault* (Paris: Minuit, 1986).

11. G. L. Bursill-Hall, *Speculative Grammars of the Middle Ages* (The Hague: Mouton, 1971).

12. Norman Schafter, "Don Juan Manuel and the Changing Structure of Society: A Conflict," *Kentucky Romance Quarterly* 26 (1979): 181–187.

13. José Antonio Maravall, "La sociedad estamental en las obras de Don Juan Manuel," *Nueva Revista de Filología Hispánica* 16 (1962): 329–354.

14. Celestino del Arenal, "Don Juan Manuel y su visión de la sociedad internacional del siglo XIV," *Cuadernos Hispanoamericanos* 38 (1976): 104.

15. Louis O. Mink, *Historical Understanding* (Ithaca: Cornell University Press, 1987), 239.

16. Marta Ana Diz, *Patronio y Lucanor: La lectura inteligente "en el tiempo que es turbio"* (Potomac, MD: Scripta Humanistica, 1984), p. 37.

17. "Et deuedes saber que la mentira senziella es quando vn omne dice a otro: 'Don Fulano, yo fare tal cosa por vos,' et el miente de aquello quell dize. Et la mentira doble es quando faze iuras et omenages et rehenes et da otros por si que fagan todos aquellos pleitos, et en faziendo estos seguramientos, ha el ya pensado et sabe manera commo todo esto tornara en mentira et en enganno. Mas la mentira treble, que es mortal mente engañosa, es la quel miente et le enganna diziendo verdat" (211).

18. Another example of Don Juan Manuel's attraction to paradox is his observation that no two faces are identical, as he observes in the Prologue, while he thereafter discusses the case of a madman who is identical in features to the king.

19. Jean Baudrillard, *Jean Baudrillard: Selected Writings,* ed. Mark Poster (Stanford: Stanford University Press, 1988), 136.

20. "De lo que conteşçio a don Pero Núñez el leal et a don Roy Gonzalez de Çauallos et a don Gutier Royz de Blaguiello con el conde don Rodrigo el Franco." In his edition of this work for Castalia (Madrid, 1969), 217, Blecua gives the following biographical information about the three knights: "Pedro Núñez de Fuente Almejir mereció el sobrenombre de 'Leal' por haber salvado a Alfonso VIII, niño aún, huyendo conél a Atienza desde Soria; Ruy González era señor de Cevallos, primo de Rodrigo el Franco; Gutierre Royz de Blaguiello estaba también emparentado con el anterior y Rodrigo González de Lara, el Franco, fue conde de las Asturias de Santillana en tiempo de Alfonso VII. Hacia 1141 estuvo en Jerusalén." Hermann Knust's edition of the work, *"El Libro de los Enxiemplos del Conde Lucanor et de Patronio." Text und Anmeruingen aus dem Nachlasse* (Leipzig: Adolf Birch-Hirschfeld, 1900), 399ff., gives more historical details on these figures.

21. "[E]lla, quexando se desto, fizo su oración a Dios que si ella era culpada,

que Dios mostrasse su miraglo en ella; et si el marido le assacara falso testimonio, que lo mostrasse en el" (356).

22. Classen, *Worlds of Sense,* 2.

23. Ibid., 2–3.

24. *Language and Mind* (New York: Harcourt Brace, 1968), 79.

25. Catherine Peyroux, "The Leper's Kiss," in *Monks and Nuns, Saints and Outcasts: Religion in Medieval Society: Essays in Honor of Lester K. Little,* ed. Sharon Farmer and Barbara H. Rosenwein (Ithaca: Cornell University Press, 2000), 174.

26. Ibid., 184–185.

27. Thomas of Celano offers details in his *Life of St. Francis* regarding Francis's attitude toward the ministry to lepers that "emphasized the foulness and corruption of the disease, and by appending Francis's own account of having once so loathed the sight of lepers that seeing a leprosarium two miles away would cause him to hold his nostrils. And then one day, as Thomas recounted it, by God's grace prompted to thoughts of holy things, Francis met a leper and, having been made stronger than himself, he kissed him. . . . Some sixteen years later, Thomas was commanded to write a further, expanded version of his biography of Francis. In it he reinterpreted Francis's embrace of the leper in two important ways. As we have seen, in this second *Life* the mysterious disappearance of the leper hinted that the diseased beggar was in fact an agent of the divine or perhaps Christ himself." Peyroux, "The Leper's Kiss," 186–187.

28. "Et por que el conde entendiesse que non avian asco de la su dolençia, tomaron con las manos daquella agua que estaua llena de podre et de aquellas pustuellas que salian de las llagas de la gafedat que el conde avia, et bebieron della muy grand pieça" (357).

29. "[A]ssi se cunplio todo lo que don Pero Núñez dixiera ante que entrasse en el canpo" (358).

30. "[L]a buena dueña et sus parientes ovieron con el tan grand plazer, que ally començaron a reyr" (359).

31. "[S]i alguna vez riesse, que nunca el cuydasse que reya por le fazer escarnio" (359).

32. Freud's theory of laughter (found in his *Jokes and Their Relationship to the Unconscious*) is interesting in this regard. As John Morreall explains, "the core of the theory is that in all laughter situations we save a certain quantity of psychic energy, energy that is usually employed for some psychic purpose but which turns out not to be needed. The discharge of this superfluous energy is laughter." John Morreall, "A New Theory of Laughter," in *The Philosophy of Humor and Laughter,* ed. John Morreall (Albany: State University of New York Press, 1987), 131.

33. Charles P. Wagner, "The Sources of *El Cavallero Zifar,*" *Revue Hispanique* 10 (1903): p. 103.

34. Reinaldo Ayerbe-Chaux, *El Conde Lucanor. Materia tradicional y originalidad creadora* (Madrid: Porrúa, 1975), 367–370.

35. As Kenneth Scholberg observes, in this case, "La raíz de la comicidad se basa al principio en la candidez del joven, pero el episodio se hace aún más cómico con la inversión de la relación entre inventor de la trama y víctima. Si era risible el desconcierto del hijo, lo es aún en mayor grado el embarazo de los viejos." "La comicidad del *Caballero Zifar,*" in *Homenaje a Rodríguez Moñino,* vol. 2 (Madrid: Castalia, 1962), 160.

36. "Bien venga la mi madre, ca ayudarme quiere a que la justicia se cumpla segunt debe, e bien creo que Dios non querrá al sinon que sofriese la pena quien la merece" (253).

37. Wagner, "The Sources of *El Cavallero Zifar,*" 86.

38. Aristotle, *De anima,* trans. Hugh Lawson-Tancred (London: Penguin, 1986), 169.

39. V. A. Kolve, *The Play Called "Corpus Christi"* (Stanford: Stanford University Press, 1966), 131.

5 The Place of the Senses

MICHEL ZINK

The *locus amoenus* is a place of pleasure, a place where time is suspended and the senses, saturated. While feeling only exists in the *present:* in other words, paradoxically, in what we might explain as the awareness of an ungraspable moment of perception known as the present moment, this place of fusion between subject and Nature (fusion and immersion being the only conceivable relationships between man and Nature during the Middle Ages, apart from a relationship of distancing) is nevertheless a place of change. Nature is change as the etymologies of the words *natura* in Latin and *physis* in Greek remind us. Related to the movement of the stars, the *locus amoenus* is the product of one of Nature's alterations: the changing seasons. Periodic and cyclical, the origin of the seasons may be traced to Chaos and the first separation of the four elements.

This chain, like the one Jean de Meun describes as the *chaîne dorée* with which Nature holds together the four elements, seems at once too long and serious to reach the sensual euphoria of the *locus amoenus* and the lightheartedness of its poetic form. Yet, as I will demonstrate in the following instances, this metaphorical distance is often traversed.

For example, Boethius follows this chain from one end to the other in poems I, 5 and I, 6 of *The Consolation of Philosophy,* where each poem opens with a description of the four elements and ends by inviting man to live and experience, in the present moment, the fruits of each season. Poem I, 2 ("Heu quam praecipiti mersa profundo") uses Beauty to show the order, harmony, and regularity of Nature's movement, and to imply that it is subject to the laws of the

Creator. The opposition between the harmony of a world governed by the Creator and an uncontrolled, unjust randomness to which Fortune subjects men is developed in I, 5 in the famous poem "O stelliferi conditor orbis":

O stelliferi conditor orbis
Qui perpetuo nixus solio
Rapido caelum turbine versas
Legemque pati sidera cogis,
Ut nunc pleno lucida cornu
Totis fratris obvia flammis
Condat stella luna minores,
Nunc obscuro pallida cornu
Phoebo propior lumina perdat,
Et qui prima tempore noctis
Agit algentes Hespero ortus,
Solitas item mutet habenas
Phoebi pallens Lucifer ortu.
Tu frondifluae frigore brumae
Stringis lucem breviore mora:
Tu, cum fervida venerit aestas,
Agiles nocti dividis horas.
Tu vis varium temperat annum
Ut quas Boreae spiritus aufert
Revehat mites Zephyrus frondes
Quaeque Arcturus semina vidit
Sirius altas urat segetes.
Nihil antiqua lege solutum
Linquit propriae stationis opus.

O Maker of the circle of the stars,
Seated on your eternal throne,
Spinner of the whirling heavens,
Binding the constellations by
your law—
As at one time the shining moon
with crescent full,
Reflecting all the sun her brother's
fire.
Hides all the lesser stars,
And at another closer to Phoebus
pales,
And loses all her light, her
crescent dark;
Or when, at fall of night,
Venus, as evening star, arises cold,
And then, as morning star, paling
at sunrise,
Changes again her long-
accustomed role;—
You with the winter's cold when
leaves pour down
Draw in the short day's light;
You when the summer comes
aflame,
Hasten the passing of the night's
swift hours.
The changing year is ordered by
your power,
So that the leaves the north wind
strips away,
The west wind brings again in
gentleness,
And what Arcturus saw as
sleeping seed
As tall crops under Sirius burn dry.
Nothing escapes your ancient
ordering
Or fails its proper office to fulfil.[1]

Why, the poem inquires, always addressing the Creator, do you not extend into the world of man where, on the contrary, the randomness of Fortune and injustice reigns? The last lines of the poem take up the evocation of natural phenomena to paint Fortune's storms, this time in a metaphorical way:

Operis tanti pars non vilis	Of that great work far from the meanest part,
Homines quatimur fortunae salo.	We men are buffeted by fortune's seas.
Rapidos rector comprime fluctus	Ruler, restrain their rushing waves and make the earth
Et quo caelum regis immensum	Steady with that stability of law
Firma stabiles foedere terras.	By which you rule the vastness of the heavens.[2]

Philosophie responds to this with the same type of comparisons and metaphors. To construct her argument, she relies upon every consideration that poetry transforms into as many figurations of Beauty: the order of Nature, natural phenomena, man's perception and the effects they produce on him, related sensations, and so on. Philosophie says we must bow to the order of things in the same way that man must conform to Nature and live in the rhythm of the seasons:

Cum Phoebi radiis grave	When heavy Cancer burns
Cancri sidus inaestuat,	Under the rays of the sun,
Tum qui larga negantibus	He who then sows his seed
Sulcis semina credidit,	In unreceiving furrows,
Elusus Cereris fide	must, cheated of grain, go look,
Quernas pergat ad arbores.	For acorns under oak trees.
Numquam purpureum nemus	Never would you seek in reddening woods
Lecturus violas petas	To gather violets,
Cum saevis aquilonibus	When grasses shake their rustling spears
Stridens campus inhorruit,	Under the fierce north winds.
. . . .	. . . .
Signat tempora propriis	God marks out the seasons
Aptans officiis deus	Each for its proper duty;
Nec quas ipse coercuit	Nor does he suffer the order he has fixed
Misceri patitur vices.	To be disturbed.
Sic quod praecipiti via	So, whatever deserts that order

Certum deserit ordinem	Rushing headlong
Laetos non habet exitus.	Comes to no happy ending.[3]

Philosophie's teaching comes from a perception of feeling in Nature. And, what the senses teach us is that we are subject to the laws of Nature, which are ultimately laws of change.

On the other end of the chain, which goes from the Cosmos to the *locus amoenus,* one can observe that the privileged lyrical expression, that is the spring song (*la strophe printanière*), is characterized more by mentioning the changing seasons than it is by evoking spring. Once again, sensual pleasure draws its justification from change itself.

Outside the traditional fields of philosophy and theology, we find the two qualities of Nature—while remaining inseparable and interdependent—which, as we underlined above, hold together the very notion of change and, in their duality, nourished poetic imagination and gave shape to forms of medieval poetry: mutation or metamorphosis on the one hand, generation and love on the other. Poetry of love, poetry of mutation: the changing seasons, from the weather (*le temps qu'il fait*) to the passing of time (*le temps qui passe*), from feelings, and from the formation of our state of being. This is the lesson Arnoul d'Orléans draws from the inherent change of Nature (*mutatio*) as we read in Ovid's *Metamorphoses.* The change of weather marks the storm, another privileged term in poetry, less for its picturesque qualities than for its significance.

In this way, there is not only a meeting point between the generative nature of cosmographic poetry and the *Natureingang* of lyric love poetry. Indeed, if we look closely, within the very framework of lyricism, the elements of Nature in themselves are brought to light along with—first, perhaps—the nature of their changes. Moreover, the *Natureingang,* the winter or spring song, and the *chanson de reverdie* are characterized not only by emphasizing the appearance of Nature and the phenomena that mark certain times in the year, but also by their being placed at the moment where the season changes, where the weather changes, that they point out such change: "Quand la douce saison fine / Et que froid hiver revient," "Quant lo rius de la fontana / S'esclarzis, si cum far sol."

From one end to the other during the Middle Ages, from the ambrosian hymn "Jam lucis orto sidere" to Bernard de Ventadour's "Lo tem vai e ven e vire," from Charles d'Orléans's spring songs ("Le temps a laissé son manteau," but also "Je fus en fleur au temps passé d'enfance"), Latin rhythmic poetry, as in vernacular poetry about Nature, depends first on the "when" of time passing ("Lancan li jorn son lonc en mai," and Châtelain de Coucy transposes this into French as the "*Lancan* Occitan"), the "when" of the change in time that brings the weather (*le temps qu'il fait*), on the quaking weather, on contrast. The weather is a palpable manifestation of time passing ("Hiver, vous n'êtes qu'un villain"), and that is why we feel the weather at the moment when it makes its turn, when the seasons are changing, just like Rutebeuf in the *Griesche d'hiver:* "Au temps que li arbre defueille."

Perhaps—though this would be another topic—we could bring together this change, enclosed within the cycle of the seasons, with the sort of exaltation constructed around youth. Youth was less conceived of as an age of life or a physiological state than it was a quality of regeneration: like the choice of the lover (*amant*) and *vivant* where Nature's transformations are valued only for their movement which brings back spring each year. In this way, associating love and spring would not be in order to attain a certain perfection in love, as certain *trouvères* soon believed, but on the contrary, in order to affirm its splendid and courageous permanence in the face of time's passing.

The *locus amoenus,* which reunites the perfections and delights of spring, is, then, a place of pleasure for the senses and a place forever reminding us that we are subject to the laws of Nature. This is why we have been able to suggest a direct link between the *locus amoenus* and the four elements. When the lyrics engage the five senses, it is the spring songs which, to portray the singer's fusion with Nature, frequently manage to convey a systematic desire to take account of the elements.

For example, Simonetta Bianchini tried to make this relationship clear using the example of a song by Guillaume IX in an article with a significant title: "Guglielmo IX, *Pos vezem de novel florir* (BdT 183, 11): esordio stagionale o invocazione alla natura?"[4] Her argument is that the famous song from the first troubadour not only manifests itself in spring-like exordium, that is to say a harmony between Nature and the poet's feelings, it also constitutes an invocation to Nature and to the four elements, an approach inspired by ancient literature up to the time of Lucretius. While we cannot be certain that Lucretius was much read at the end of the eleventh century, the author creates a link between Guillaume's implied Epicureanism and the opinion he borrows from Guillaume de Malmesbury, that events are governed by chance and not by providence. Following is the strophe in question:

Pos vezem de novel florir Pratz, e vergiers reverdezir,	Since we see again blooming the prairies, and the orchards growing green,

Rius e fontanas esclarzir,	brooks and springs flow clearer,
Auras e vens,	and breezes and winds,
Ben deu cascus lo joi jauzir	each must revel in the joy
Don es jauzens.	Which is pleasure [jouissance].[5]

Simonetta Bianchini thus comments on verses 2–4 :

> Sono dedicati ciascuno ad un elemento "descritto" attraverso le sue manifestazioni più caratteristiche, già elencate da Isidoro nelle sue *Etymologiae:* della terra vengono presi in considerazione prati [« Pratum est cuius feni copia armenta tuentur », XV, xiii, 17] e giardini, come dire l'utile e il dilettevole [. . .]; sempre seguendo le *Etymologiae* isidoriane [XIII, xxi, 4–6] nelle descrizione dell'elemento acqua *rivus* e *fons* sono vicini [« Rivi dicti quod deriventur ad inrigandum [. . .]. Gurges [. . .]. Puteus [. . .]. Fons caput est aquae nascentis »] e, rispetto alla tradizione del *topos,* vengono a sostituire i *maria* in una connotazione più "domestica" e bucolica di quest'elemento. Ancora più strettamente collegati *aer* e *ventus,* descritti come conseguenza l'una dell'altra [XIII, vii, 1]: « aer [. . .] commotus ventos facit », come, poco dopo [XIII, xi, 1], « Ventus [est] aer commotus et agitatus ».
>
> Anche l'ordine nel quale vengono elencati gli elementi ripete quello divenuto ormai "classico": terra [*pratz* e *vergiers,* v. 2], acqua [*rius* e *fontanas,* v. 3], aria [*auras* e *vens,* v. 4], per cui si può rivolgere, ancora una volta ad Isidoro, il grande collettore di conoscenze scientifiche [*Etymologiae,* XIII, iii, 2]: « terra diluatur in aquam, aqua rarescat in aera, aer in ignem extenuetur ».[6]

This is all quite scholarly and convincing to a certain point. But, the author must admit that immediately following, in the same spring song, there is a rather exceptional example of a meeting of the four elements. Even in the one she comments on, it takes a trick to introduce the fire instead of quoting Isidore. In Guillaume IX's poem, the least we can say is that his presence is discreet—their reunion is so frequent that it is hardly significant. Perhaps, however, it might be possible to imagine the considerations made above on the changing of the seasons in the spring songs in order to make a connection between Bianchini's hypothesis on Guillaume IX and the analysis of Jörn Gruber on the *trobar naturau* "natural" love in Marcabru and later in Alphonse le Savant. In such a connection, it may be possible to argue that the spring songs imply a certain natural order: They appear as elements and seasonal cycles which harmonize with a kind of "morale de l'amour."[7] But this takes us away from the five senses.

The most bothersome aspect of Simonetta Bianchini's analysis—and again, I would like to emphasize its suggestiveness—is that, despite everything, the weight of the scholarly apparatus is set in motion in reference to a lighthearted strophe. Once again, we get the impression that the scholarly reading is plastered, somewhat artificially, onto verses where rather than gaining access, she forces her way in. Such a reading renders Simonetta Bianchini like the disciple of Matthieu de Vendôme, to whom she does not forget to refer.

Already in the twelfth century, Matthieu de Vendôme in his *Ars versificatoria* unites the four elements and the five senses as the culminating point and conclusion of his bravery piece on the *locus amoenus.* In a lengthy, sixty-two-verse *descriptio loci,* he illustrates the poetry and amorous resonances of the *locus amoenus* by presenting it, as soon as the opening lines, as a product of the arrival of spring and Nature's zeal: "Naturae studium locus est, quo veris abundant / Deliciae, veris gratia, veris opes." In the last part of the poem, the constituent elements of the *locus amoenus* are related to the five senses. Moreover, they are associated with the four elements, thus bridging the gap between cosmographic and spring-like poetry:

Flos sapit, herba viret, parit arbor, fructus abundat,	The flowers give fragrance, the grass grows, the trees bear,
Garrit avis, rivus murmurat, aura . tepet	Fruit overflows, the birds chatter, the river murmurs, the air is cool.
Voce placent volucres, umbra nemus, aura tepore,	Birds please by voice, the grove by shade, the air by coolness
Fons potu, rivus murmure, flore solum.	The fountain by drinking-water, by its murmur the stream, by its flowers the ground.
Gratum murmur aquae, volucrum vox consona, florum	The murmur of water is charming, the voices of birds are harmonious
Suavis odor, rivus frigidus, aura[8] tepens.	The smell of the flowers fragrant, the stream cool, the shade warm.
Sensus quinque loci praedicti gratia pascit,	The beauty of the mentioned place feeds the five senses,
Si collative quaeque notata notes.	were you to note all the marked points together
Unda juvat tactum, gustum sapor, auris amica	The water delights the touch, flavor the taste, the bird is
Est volucris, visus gratia, naris odor.	The friend to the ear, and grace to sight, scent to the nose.
Non elementa vacant, quia tellus concipit, aer	The elements are not absent: the earth conceives, the air
Blanditur, fervor suscitat, humor alit.[9]	Caresses, heat awakens, moisture nourishes.

It is important to avoid exaggerating the significance of Matthieu de Vendôme's Treaty. Unlike Geoffroy de Vinsauf's *Poetria nova,* for which Jean-Yves Tilliette was able to show to what extent the title is profoundly justified, *l'Ars versificatoria* appear as nothing more than a compilation of recipes by an author who knows Cicero, Horace, Ovid, and Lucien. However, in the treaty, Matthieu de Vendôme reveals the way he reads poetry of his time. All the elements he finds figure in the spring songs (but, gratefully, without systematic heaviness or didactic pedantism). At the expense of a heavy commentary, his reading of the spring songs puts them spontaneously in relation to cosmographic poetry, describing the universe through its four elements. This was indeed what the student of Bernard Silvestre, the colleague and enemy of Arnoul d'Orléans, knew so well. In other words, he attempts to establish the same relationship that we do between Nature as beauty and Nature as creator: *les cuistres se rencontrent.* Yet, he is not completely erroneous.

We might be brought to the point where we ask ourselves about the place Génius describes at the end of *Roman de la Rose:* Beau Parc, where a perpetual springtime and daytime reigns. On the one hand, Beau Parc seems to want to resolve the contradiction between the suspension of temporal progress or the dilation of the moment of perception in the pleasure (*jouissance*) of the senses. On the other hand, he is confronted with the perpetual change that the laws of Nature implement as a condition for those who want to perceive the senses of the *locus amoenus,* this place of this pleasure.

Translated by Alison Calhoun

Notes

1. Edition H. F. Stewart, E. K. Rand, and S. J. Tester, *Boethius: The Theological Tractates; The Consolation of Philosophy* (Cambridge: Harvard University Press, 1973 [1918]), pp. 159–161.

2. Ibid., p. 161.

3. Ibid., pp. 165–167.

4. S. Bianchini, "Guglielmo IX, *Pos vezem de novel florir* (BdT 183, 11): esordio stagionale o invocazione alla natura?" *Annali dell'Istituto Universitario Orientale-Sezione Romanza* 41, no. 1 (1999): pp. 113–120. (CR Cinzia Licoccia, dans *Critica del Testo* III/3 [2000]: p. 1146).

5. Mario Eusebi, ed., *Guglielmo IX. Vers* (Parme: Pratiche, 1995), p. 62.

6. Bianchini, "Guglielmo IX," pp. 115–116.

7. Jörn Gruber, "*Porque trobar é cousa en que jaz entendimento.* Zur Bedeutung von *trobar natural* bei Marcabru und Alfons dem Weisen," in *Homenagem a Joseph*

M. Piel por ocasião do seu 85° aniversário, ed. Dieter Kremer (Tübingen: Niemeyer, 1988), pp. 569–579.

8. Variant indicated by Faral, who prefers the lesson *umbra.*

9. Matthieu de Vendôme, *Ars versificatoria* I, 111, *Descriptio loci,* vv. 49–60, ed. Edmond Faral, *Les Arts poétiques du XIIe et du XIIIe siècle. Recherches et documents sur la technique littéraire au Moyen Age* (Paris: Champion, 1924), p. 149.

6 Seeing and Hearing in Ancient and Medieval Epiphany

Rainer Warning

In Plato's *Republic* ideas are thought but not seen (507b). He points out in this way the difference between sensory perception and spiritual sight, seeing with the "eye of the Soul" (533d). Of course, sight is the sharpest of all senses (*Phaedr.* 250d), but to the extent that Plato does not attribute a value to the senses according to their physical function but according to their contribution to knowledge, sight is not in principle more valuable than hearing. We "observe the revolutions of reason in heaven" and we attribute to them the "convolutions of our own thought," just as the harmony we hear "brings the soul in unison with itself" (*Tim.* 47 a–d). The hierarchy of the senses passed down to us—with sight in the highest position—goes back to Aristotle and implies two variations vis-à-vis Plato. On the one hand, with his concept of entelechy, he brings into the dimension of the visible the transcendental ideas of Plato; on the other, he ascribes to the senses a physical function. In this process, sight moves clearly into the first position, as hearing is more important only for its contribution to knowledge. In fact, sight, and only sight, perceives nature in its entirety and divinity as *theoria.* Philosophy is as much a theoretical as a theological science.

As theory, visual contemplation belongs as much to cult as to play in the context of religious festivals. The emissaries of the polis to religious festivals and oracles were called *theoroi,* and *theorós* was derived etymologically from *theós,* the god. When this god or his divine messengers appear, they present what they have to say in shimmering beauty, they bring transcendence to momentary evidence, as Athena does at the beginning of the *Iliad* to placate

Achilles' wrath (194ff.) and to induce Odysseus not to abandon Troy inconsiderately (166ff.). Sight is given unquestioned priority. This can be expanded with dramatic effects as Euripides does in the central scene of the *Bacchai,* when Dionysos's voice can be heard from the depths of the palace, and he then walks out and is beheld by the chorus in his splendor (574ff.). This priority of sight is still valid in the case of verbal epiphanies. Likewise, in connection with the oracle of Delphi, it is ultimately Apollo himself who becomes visible in the person of the Pythia, and talks through her (Pax 1955, 35).

The epiphanies of the Old Testament are to be associated with the appearance of fire as well: the burning bush (Exod. 3:2ff.), the nocturnal pillar of fire showing the way out of Egypt to the people of Israel (Exod. 13:21), the Sinai enveloped by smoke (Exod. 19:18). And yet, the examples already show that Jahve does not manifest himself here in the splendor of light, but that, at the same time as he shows himself, he also surrounds himself with fire. While he can be heard, he is not seen. Under cover of lightning and thunder, he moves all the way up the Sinai giving out smoke like a furnace, in order to manifest himself by means of words to his people. The epiphany of Jahve is hearing, not sight. It realizes itself in the duplication of concealment and manifestation: "non poteris videre faciem meam non enim videbit me homo et vivet" (Exod. 33:20).

Of course, the prophetic books, first among them Isaiah, know the pure epiphany of light: "surge inluminare quia venit lumen tuum et gloria Domini super te orta est" (Isa. 60:1). In this case, theology takes care to distinguish between historical and eschatological epiphany and makes clear that even in the latter case what we are dealing with is something basically different from that which antedates the spread of Christianity. The momentary evidence is replaced by temporality: the history of the people of Israel to whom Jahve reveals himself at first only while hidden, and to whom he will appear one day in the pure fullness of light.

The New Testament brings an end to this distinction between historical and eschatological epiphany. In doing so, in the case of historical epiphany it distances itself from the ancient law even more clearly than from the rest of the Old Testament. Jesus's appearances after his resurrection have the goal of giving proof. These are self-manifestations in which God-made-man gives himself to be recognized as such through a sign—as in the case of the disciples of Emmaus, whose eyes he opens by breaking the bread (Luke 24:30f.), and in the case of the disbelieving Thomas, who lets himself be convinced by tasting the embodied God. The development into an episodic event does not lead to questioning of the concept of epiphany itself, only its structural course. God is not present as God directly and manifestly, but he must offer himself for recognition, with the consequence that the appearance reaches its climax precisely at the moment of his disappearance—not at the beginning, but at the end, as in the episode of Emmaus. Understandably the appearances of Christ are marked at the beginning, as they start with a clear reference to the speaker himself or with greetings. They are mostly the occasion for an announcement and for the entrustment of a task, such as with the order of mission and baptism in Matthew 28:16ff., or with the assignment of the office of shepherd in John 21:15ff.

Both types of historical epiphany often transform themselves into each other. What is more important is something else: the evident reserve of the synoptic Gospels about the motif of the shimmering luminosity, the splendor of light as a key element of ancient epiphany. It appears in the epiphanies of angels, in the miracle of the Pentecost and, of course, in the Apocalypse of John (Apoc. 21:23), in the manifestations of Christ, but only on the occasion of his transfigurations (Matt. 17:1–5; Mark 9:2–7; Luke 9:28–36), as well as in the appearances with eschatological connotations. In the Resurrection, the light motif is completely absent, replaced by the jubilant "Resurrexit" of the angels at the empty grave, and even the transfigurations have their *telos* not in the luminous clothes of Jesus, but in the cloud darkening the scenery from which the voice of God resonates, announcing that Christ is his son so that everyone could hear him.

The fact that this transfiguration is completely missing in John corresponds well to the late canonization of this fourth Gospel, explaining the history of the dogma with the postponement of the *parusia:* the "consistent-eschatological interpretation of primitive Christianity" (Werner 1957, 9) is substituted as early as the Gospel of John with a Christology of the *logos* valorizing even more strongly the word and, with it, the hearing in opposition to the other senses. For this reason, even according to the miscreant Thomas, what is decisive is not the reevaluation of touch, but the reappraisal of this instrument of authentification offered immediately afterwards from the word of Jesus: blessed are they that have not seen and yet believe (John 20:29).

The same strategy can be seen at work in the episode of the "hortulanus" which is transmitted only by John. John 20:14–16 says that Mary Magdalen saw Jesus suddenly standing in front of her ("vidit Jesum stantem") and took him for a gardener ("illa existimans quia hortulanus esset") which leads to the initial misunderstanding: "Domine, si tu sustulisti eum, dicito mihi ubi posuisti eum." Most significantly, we do not learn from John whether this mistaken assumption is reached by Mary on the basis of the vision itself, or only on the basis of the place in which it appeared: the garden of Joseph of Arimathia. The appearance is not of interest, since the recognition is not brought about by sight but rather through the word: "Dicit ei Jesu: Maria. Conversa illa dicit ei: Rabboni (quod dicitur, Magister)." The word, the *logos,* is not only given priority over what is seen but is played precisely against what is seen.

One could easily attempt the opposite reading, and not let the "hortulanus" go as a simple mistake on the part of Mary but take it as an authentic appearance by a gardener—and this time it would no longer be Mary's mistake but a metamorphosis and, as such, a trick that shortly after his resurrection Jesus plays on Mary. In fact, the scene was read exactly in this way by no other than the authors of popular Easter plays in the thirteenth and fourteenth centuries. They seized the potential of metamorphosis for play and exploited it when they had Jesus appear in the clothes of a gardener playing tricks on Mary, trying to chase her away from his garden, even suspecting her of a *rendez-vous.* I have expounded this idea in detail elsewhere (Warning 2001, 74f.) and am limiting myself here to the observation that the play in the vernacular adheres to the epiphany in the word heard but not to the hierarchy implied by the Bible of a subordination of sight to hearing.

It is as if the theological exegesis had perceived such problems in advance, since we have a homily to be dated to the twelfth century and wrongly attributed to Anselm of Canterbury which strives to explain why the misunderstanding brings blame upon Mary alone. Mary had not sought Jesus in the right way, that is, with the "oculi cordis." She had tried to find with her physical eyes the one who was about to enter her heart, "per aures corporis" and thus the mistake happened: "Ecce Jesus venit ad te, et tu hortulanum eum existimas!" Thus the reason of the misunderstanding is sought in Mary alone and not in connection with the appearance of the resurrected. The "hortulanus" is a product of the act of seeing with the wrong eyes, and at no point is the question raised of whether the bodily appearance of a gardener might perhaps have been at the origin of this episode. Of course, Jesus is also a gardener, but an allegorical gardener, who lays the good seed in the heart of the believer; he manifests himself in word, he is identical with the "Jesus qui tem loquitur" (further details again in Warning 2001, 83f.). What the homily presupposes is not only the superiority of hearing over sight already given by the Bible, but a spiritual understanding of both senses. As is well known, this theory about the *sensus spirituales* was established by Origen and spans the entire Middle Ages, because with it is resolved the antithesis between divine transcendence and personal, concrete, bodily experience of God, the latter assigned to the spiritual senses.

For my example, even more important is the destruction of the unity of the biblical experience of the epiphany. The miracle play seizes a potentially mythical element in order to develop it in this dimension, namely, in the sensory dimension of the mythical evidence, as metamorphosis. "Metamorphosis," in the words of H. Blumenberg, "is present already in the genesis of myth itself, as anthropomorphosis: the gods lose their terror by changing their appearance. In the process, for the most part, they become poetic. Jacob Burckhardt premised a section on 'The Metamorphosis' to his discussion of the Greek gods. However, he did not reflect on the reasons why this staple of divine stories 'strikes' us so much: everything that comes after can be explained from the effort not to be understood as metamorphosis or not to accept anything like that in the world" (Blumenberg 1971, 38f.). The episode of the "hortulanus" in John occupies here an indeterminate place and the homily immediately reacts to it without clearly being able to prevent the miracle play from later representing precisely what should not be.

The miracle play, however, is only a relatively late example of the reception of an antiquity propounding a deferment of the *parusia* on the part of the Christian Middle Ages, a reception that appropriates in equal measure philosophical, theological, and poetical norms and leads to the creation of ever less transparent hybrids. Of course, this applies also to the conception and hierarchy of the senses that is the object of our interest here and, furthermore, to the relationship of sight and hearing constituting theophany. This history of reception is not only extremely complex in itself but its reelaboration has also continued to be controversial to this day every time preliminary hermeneutic decisions have come into play, particularly with the theologians. Here, I shall limit myself to some key terms before going back to concrete textual examples.

If the aforementioned Origen establishes a parallel between the senses of the body and the *sensus spirituales,* he still remains within the ancient tradition when he establishes a hierarchy among the latter: the word heard is subordinated to the wordless sight of God. The ancient premises were not adjusted one-sidedly to a biblical Christianity, but, on the contrary, a constant attempt was made to harmonize this biblical Christianity with antiquity. In the process, at times one pole, at times the other, is more strongly accentuated. But, overall, sight has the preference even when in the case of the *visio Dei* an eschatological connotation is still presupposed. However, the tensions are not eliminated with it, as is shown by the most carefully and well-documented contribution to the history of this concept and its development written by F. K. Mayr in the *Realenzyklopädie für Antike und Christentum* (1991). So, according to Athanasius, the hearing yields to the sight by referring to the mirror through which God can be recognized, a solution of which Dante will often make use. On the other hand, Cyril of Alexandria defends the priority of hearing in faith against the Hellenism of Origen, followed on this point by John Chrysostomos. A different position is defended by Pseudo-Dionysius Areopagita, where, next to the *sensus spirituales,* the eye is attributed higher symbolic value than the ear, as by Origen. Yet, a different position is defended by Ambrosius, who made an impression on St. Augustine with the "suavitas" of his sermons (*Conf.* 5, 13). However, Ambrosius himself later turned Augustine into a critic who ended up dedicating a certain amount of reflection to this seducing "suavitas."

In reality, St. Augustine gives back priority to sight over hearing, as has been convincingly demonstrated by M. Duchrow (1965). His often quoted critique of the pleasure of sight, the "concupiscentia oculorum" (*Conf.* 10, 30) should not make us forget that Augustine criticizes here only an exercise of sight fallen to the state of "curiositas" and, thus, losing itself in the visible world without a sufficient memory of its creator. This world offering itself to the external perception is to be recognized as simple "vestigia rationis" (*De ordine* II, 35), an invitation to the ascent "a corporeis ad incorporea" (*De musica* VI, 2). This noncorporeal, spiritual perception has the intrinsic character of a *visio* to which the hearing is also subordinated. Therefore, Augustine conceptualizes music not in connection with the tones heard with the senses but in relationship to a numerical order contemplated by the mind: a music whose harmony achieves its perfection in the number one, "unum." With this joy for the "unum," which corresponds also to the sight of the only God, an eschatological foundation is preserved. Yet, nothing is changed in the subordination of the word itself to the imagery of sight and light which reaches into the trinitary speculation of the Verbum. The "verbum cordis" is not heard, but can be seen as inner light: "verbum quod foris sonat, signum est verbi quod intus lucet, cui magis verbi competit nomen" (*De trinitate* 15, 20). We must take into consideration these positions of Patricism to which even Scholasticism does not introduce important modifications now that we turn ourselves to our real subject, the role of seeing and hearing in postantique and postbiblical theophany.

As is well known, the vernacular lyric of the Middle Ages is not derived from the—more recent—church poetry on Mary. Yet, as I have already demonstrated in detail elsewhere, the troubadours also reelaborated key lexemes with a feudal or Christian connotation in order to be accepted and, even more, in view of their self-legitimization, to demonstrate the compatibility of courtly love and *caritas* (Warning 1979). The stilnovists have embraced, continued, and narrowed this reelaboration down to the quote of the epiphany: they stylize the meeting with the beloved into a transcendental experience. For this reason, from the perspective of theology, a critical point is reached and it requires an explanation. Dante's *Vita Nuova,* in its quality of prosimetrum, highlights this point by presenting lyrical texts, turning Beatrice's entrance into the appearance of an angel, in parallel with a narrative commentary generally given the status of allegory. Already with the final perspective on the *revocatio* of the stilnovistic theology of Amore in the *Divina commedia,* the young man's love was given a moral direction—of course, not explicitly, but in such subtle cipher that the allegorical commentary ends up adding to its own ambiguity, something that has continually engaged the Italianists interested in allegorical consistency. For the questions I am asking I can avoid going into these controversies and move at once to one of the best-known poems from Chap. XXVI:

Tanto gentile e tanto onesta pare
la donna mia quand'ella altrui saluta,
ch'ogne lingua deven tremando muta,
e li occhi no l'ardiscon di guardare.
Ella si va, sentendosi laudare,
benignamente d'umiltà vestuta;
e par che sia una cosa venuta
da cielo in terra a miracol mostrare.
Mostrasi sì piacente a chi la mira,
che dà per li occhi una dolcezza al core,
che 'ntender no la può chi no la prova:
e par che de la sua labbia si mova
un spirito soave pien d'amore,
che va dicendo a l'anima: Sospira.

"Pare" (1) has the connotation of "apparire," that is, of appearing; "saluta" (2) has the connotation of "salute," as well as of salvation, in the same way as the eyes of the observer, as they close, suggest the fear of the sight of the divine, the *tremendum.* The second quatrain makes explicit, again with "par" (7), the appearance of an angel. Finally, the sestet goes beyond sight by means of the word, which, again connected to a "par" (12), is given the aura of a "spirito soave"(13)—with the invitation to a sigh of yearning: "Sospira"(14).

With all this, an ultimately Christian and nonancient dominance of word over sight seems to be realized. On the other hand, with the "gentilezza" of the "fedeli d'Amore" is imposed a norm that enters in competition with the Christian *caritas.* Dante's commentary suggests such a reading (particularly Chap. III) but does not clearly mention the point that is really critical, namely, not the inner norm, but the word that sings it. It is never the question of the speaker's speech but of the words of Beatrice to whom the speaker gives the aura of a "spirito soave pien d'amore" (13). But this "suavitas," as we have learned in the meantime, is not harmless even if it is inspired by God, for the god is no other than Amore and Dante is his servant with a practice of poetry that produces in the form of fictive speech the "suavitas" previously heard. Officially, in the mystic discourse of the appearance, the speaker makes himself disappear. But, this removal of the self is an effect of the text, of the discourse of the speaker himself. What is decisive is not the epiphany represented, but the dependence of what is represented from the means of representation, the dependence of what is seen and heard from the fictive speech of the speaker. The epiphany finds its *telos* not so much in Beatrice's speech but in the seducing *melos* of the "stilo de la loda." And this latter is not only read, but heard, when read aloud in the circle of the "fedeli d'Amore." It is at this point, then, that presence manifests itself, but a presence that is the effect of the rhetorical *ars* and not of the irruption of transcendence.

Thus, not only the apparent priority of what is heard over what is seen is deconstructed, but language as a means of deconstruction remains within the limits of this world. It covers the way "a corporeis ad incorporea" only according to the theology of Amore, its seducing "suavitas" remains under the domination of the false god. In the *Vita Nuova,* the allegorical commentary points out this error. The *Divina commedia* makes it explicit from the moment that Beatrice's words lead here to the vision of Christ. Yet, as we will see in a moment, Petrarch will refuse to follow Dante with his own choice of thematizing the very deconstruction of the hierarchy of eye and ear. Thus fictionality's attempt to draw attention to itself brings to light a theologically heretical, but aesthetically sanctioned, potential.

The verb "parere" or "apparire" together with the religious connotation of an angelic appearance is as frequent in the *Vita Nuova,* both in the poems and the prose, as it is rare in Petrarch. One of these texts is *Canzoniere* III, a sonnet of greeting:

La donna che 'l mio cor nel viso porta,
Là dove sol fra bei pensier d'amore
Sedea, m'apparve; et io per farle onore
Mossi con fronte reverente e smorta.
Tosto che del mio stato fussi accorta,
A me si volse in sí novo colore
Ch' avrebbe a Giove nel maggior furore
Tolto l'arme di mano e l'ira morta.
I' mi riscossi; et ella oltra, parlando,
Passò, che la parola i' non soffersi
Né 'l dolce sfavillar de gli occhi suoi.
Or mi ritrovo pien di sí diversi
Piaceri, in quel saluto ripensando,
Che duol non sento né senti' ma' poi.

The intertextual reference to the *Vita Nuova* cannot be missed. The same applies to the "Tanto gentile" (Chap. XXVI), just introduced, as well as to the sonnet in Chap. XXI:

Ne li occhì porta la mia donna Amore,
per che si fa gentil ciò ch'ella mira;
ov'ella passa, ogn'om ver lei si gira,
e cui saluta fa tremar lo core,
sì che, bassando il viso, tutto smore,
e d'ogni suo difetto allor sospira:
fugge dinanzi a lei superbia ed ira.
Aiutatemi, donne, farle onore.
Ogne dolcezza, ogne pensero umile
nasce nel core a chi parlar la sente,
ond'è laudato chi prima la vide.
Quel ch'ella par quando un poco sorride,
non si pò dicer né tenere a mente,
sì è novo miracolo e gentile.

Precisely as in "Tanto gentile," the woman passing by is stylized across pragmatic and semantic planes into a superpersonal dimension and is invested with the aura of a transcendental appearance. The lyrical ego is hardly to be perceived: the circumstances of the speech are as unspecific as the circumstances spoken of, the temporal gap between them is abolished, the verbal tense is, as a rule, the present, creating general and typified situations. Again it is Beatrice who speaks, so that in the represented "parlare" (10) of the mistress the speaker makes himself disappear; his role is implicitly generated by the voice of the mistress through whose mouth Amore speaks.

All of this is purposefully modified in Petrarch with a deconstructive effect in regard to the epiphany (on this point, see Warning 1983). "M'apparve" (3) has the connotation of the image of a dream, the vision, but it does not refer to transcendence by the fact that the appearance is stylized as a product of the "pensier d'amore" (2). The encounter is psychologically isolated. Contextual details given and thematized each time by Dante are not excluded here but rather dissolved. The lover could be in a public square; Laura could, just like Beatrice for the most part, be in the company of other women. But we never hear of this, precisely because the ego brings the appearance into his own space of meditation.

To the reduced reference to transcendence corresponds the connotative evocation of sensory commotion both on the speaker's and Laura's part. For Dante, "la mia donna" (1) meant the recognition of the mistress's right of possession over her servant. Petrarch eliminates this possessive and adds it to "cor," whereby he refers to the most intimate, most secret thoughts of the speaker. And this "mio cor" (1) is not by chance in the middle of the verse where it is surrounded by the glance of the beloved: "La donna che 'l mio cor nel viso porta" (1). Also, "porta" is a quote, but in Dante it has the god Amore as object, while in Petrarch the object of "porta" is only "il mio cor," whereby the *topos* of Amore's arrows is desemanticized to the knowing and benevolent, if not full of desire, glance not only of the lover, but also of his beloved. In the second verse, the god Amore is deprived of divinity in the "bei pensier d'amore" (2), the courtly love thoughts of the speaker, away from which the appearance suddenly robs him and makes him turn pale.

This transformation of the epiphany into a more subjective experience, its psychologizing, continues in the second quatrain with what would have been an unthinkable turn in Dante, Laura's address to the pale lover, and even more with her own change of color, her "novo colore" (6), that could have been read as pitifulness's paleness, had the following comparison not followed. Carducci and Ferrari identified it as a quote from Ovid, *Amores* II, where a restless Corinna, whose kisses of reconciliation would have disarmed even Jupiter, is introduced. The sensory excitement applies to both the lover and Laura, at least as the lover's projection. Similarly, with the visual anacrusis of the octave, the closeness to the topic of epiphany is maintained at the same time as it is secretly deconstructed, and this opposed movement extends, as it was to be expected, to the sestet as well.

The tripartite narrative structure of the appearance is realized: "m'apparve" (3), "a me si volse" (6), and now the final "passò" (10). And precisely as expected, the crescendo culminating in this conclusion brings into play hearing after sight. Just as in Dante, we do not learn what is said by the woman passing by, nor to whom she is talking, and nothing suggests that she is even addressing the lover himself. At any rate, the aura of speech is marked by a shock of dismay, and all this in the verbal understanding of the symbolism of language. It begins with the "oltra" (9), elegantly anticipated within the verse and only fully taken advantage of in connection with the "passò" (10), marked by means of a parenthetic insert. In between we have "parlando" (9), in the last part of the enjambment, temporarily suspended. Walking past and speaking are connected, and hardly has the beloved announced her greeting when she has already disappeared again.

From the point of view of the figures of sound, this important moment is marked by the vocalism in "a" and "o" and, more immediately, by the use of the phonetic closeness of "passare" and "parlare" as well as by the repetition of "parlando" in the etymological figure "parlando"/"parola" (9, 10). This vocalism of "a" and "o," along with the reappearance of the motif of the glance in v. 11, is framed at the beginning of v. 9 by all the other vowels, in particular the prominent "i," so that this becomes some sort of self-display of verbal "suavitas." In Dante, as we have seen, the verbal aura is evoked almost discursively:

9 Ogne dolcezza, ogne pensero umile
10 nasce nel core a chi parlar la sente

In the represented "parlare" of the beloved, the "parlare" of the mise-en-scène itself is made to disappear. Petrarch takes just the other way, and this is alluded to in the context of "passò" (10). The connection between "parlare" and "passare" allows a specific temporal moment to break into the language with the fugacity of an appearance. Petrarch marks the difference through repetition, particularly at the level of vocalism.

Of course this phenomenon is not limited to the language. The connection between passing by and speaking fixes the appearance also in its visual component. Thus in the last verse of the first tercet the initial "viso" (1) of the beloved returns, elaborated into "dolce sfavillar de gli occhi suoi" (11). From this, it becomes clear that, in the Middle Ages, the biblical hierarchy of the senses is not coherently preserved. As we have already seen, in a philosophical context, under the influence of the reception of antiquity, the ancient order of hearing and sight could be restored. The same applies to poetry under the ancient constraints or under the sought-after effects of the structure of the text. For this reason, in the *Canzoniere,* the sequence sight/hearing is much more frequent, but the opposite is also equally possible (see as examples, *Canzoniere* 133, 158, 167, 253, 273). In our text, the eyes in v. 11 must be mentioned once again only because the main caesura of the entire text falls between the two tercets. The remembered, and past, appearance comes to an end here, only to be euphorically reevoked in the last tercet by looking back from the very moment in which the locutionary act takes place. But how could this presence be even more closely characterized?

If, in the first part, the temporal sequence already gave a specific nuance to semantics, syntax, meter, and phonetics, with the last tercet it also extends to pragmatics. If the *passato remoto* of the epiphany alternates with the present moment of remembrance ("Or mi ritrovo," 12), the appearance itself is expressly subordinated to the opposition of then and now. This temporal structure of remembrance is the defining moment in Petrarch's deconstruction of Dante. The *Vita Nuova* is part of the "libro de la mia memoria," and this "memoria" is, as Augustine decisively defined it, a timeless repository of images acquired by means of the senses, in which the "I" meets himself spiritually (*Conf.* 10, 8). Measured against St. Augustine's, Dante's encounters with himself in the *Vita Nuova* are morally wrong in their renewed sensuality. In their celebration of the object of sight, they are the expression of the "voluptas oculorum" (*Conf.* 34, 51), and, in their inebriation with the object of hearing, they are the expression of the "voluptates aurium" (*Conf.* 33, 49). But, by exploring the possibilities of the present tense, they retain the *nunc stans* of "memoria."

Petrarch knows that Augustine casts a judgment upon these "voluptates" but this does not keep him from implicitly appreciating them with the formula of the "dolendi voluptas" (*De remediis* II, 93). This "voluptas" coincides in part with sensual desire, nostalgia for the beloved in her wordly corporeity, the "desio," that is unacceptable from a theological point of view, and yet which the poetic imagination cannot forego. Laura's appearances are not recalled from the "memoria," but they are the product of a "curiositas" that can crystallize in units of memory. This "curiositas" generates appearances whose fugacity is not based upon the fugacity of the transcendental appearance, but upon the momentary quality of interiority's discontinuity.

This fugacity is not only represented by language, but has its real place in the medium of this representation, that is, in language itself. This is the metapoetic effect of the described connection between "parlare" and "passare." The "dolendi voluptas" not only aims at the bodily dimension of the beloved, but also at the bodily dimension of the medium, namely, of a writing that when followed with the eyes is at the service of the "voluptas oculorum" and when read aloud of the "voluptas aurium." Petrarch's epiphanies are known and experienced as a product of desire—fleeting, momentary, and differential. They are unthinkable without Augustine, whom they obey and against whom, at the same time, they are opposed. It is precisely in this double juxtaposition that they mark the beginning of a genealogy in which, centuries later, another passerby will emerge.

La rue assourdissante autour de moi hurlait.
Longue, mince, en grand deuil, douleur majestueuse,
Une femme passa, d'une main fastueuse
Soulevant, balançant le feston et l'ourlet;
Agile et noble, avec sa jambe de statue.
Moi, je buvais, crispé comme un extravagant,
Dans son œil, ciel livide où germe l'ouragan,
La douceur qui fascine et le plaisir qui tue.
Un éclair . . . puis la nuit!—Fugitive beauté
Dont le regard m'a fait soudainement renaître,
Ne te verrai-je plus que dans l'éternité?
Ailleurs, bien loin d'ici! trop tard! jamais peut-être!
Car j'ignore où tu fuis, tu ne sais où je vais,
Ô toi que j'eusse aimé, ô toi qui le savais!

—Baudelaire, *Les Fleurs du mal*

I have already analyzed in detail this sonnet with regard to its intertextual reference to the sonnets of greetings by Dante and Petrarch elsewhere (again Warning 1983). I will only quote it here in conclusion as perhaps the most pregnant example of differential epiphany under the conditions of modernity. Once more, it is the matter of eye and ear. Yet, what the speaker hears is still only the deafening noise of the street of the great town, no longer the seducing words of the person encountered. She is alone just as he is. What he notices about her could lead him to imagine the elevated sorrow of a widow just as well as a coquette. And, when their glances crossed, it is unclear whether eye contact was ever made. The speaker can only assume it, without any prospect of ever finding confirmation.

Jorge Luis Borges once tried to define the aesthetic as the imminence of a revelation out of his reach: "esta inminencia de una revelación, que no se produce, es, quizá, el hecho estético" (Borges 1980, 133). We could say that the sonnet by Baudelaire offers the image of such an epiphany, but not only its own. Borges understands the formula cited as suprahistorical and, given the historical differences, it applies to Dante's Beatrice and Petrarch's Laura as well as to Baudelaire's anonymous passerby. They all are, as merely assumed epiphanies, flowers of evil. Dante tells us precisely this with his allegorical commentary, Petrarch in the opposition between a history of conversion and the euphoric passion for earthly charms, and Baudelaire with the sorrow of deprivation, that in *Le peintre de la vie moderne,* he once clearly refers to Augustine's "amabam amare" (II, 691). Yet, the crowd of the great town that causes him this sorrow with its outpouring of stimuli, visual as well as auditory, is pursued and approved. He explicitly allegorizes this curiosity into a "Curiosité" (I, 130), and, for the essays on poetry devoted to it, he chose already during his lifetime the title of *Curiosités esthétiques.*

Translated by Monica Signoretti

Bibliography

Primary Sources

Augustine. *Confessionum libri XIII, Corpus Christianorum, Series Latina.* 27 vols. Turnholt, 1981.

Baudelaire. *Œuvres complètes.* Cl. Pichois, ed. 2 vols. Paris, 1975.

Biblia sacra. *Biblia sacra iuxta Vulgatam versionem.* R. Weber, ed. 2 vols. Stuttgart, 1975. (Orig. publ. 1969.)

Borges, J. L. *La muralla y los libros,* in *Prosa completa.* 2 vols. Barcelona, 1980, 2:131–133.

Dante Alighieri. *La Vita Nuova* M. Barbi, ed. Firenze, 1960.

Petrarca. *Le Rime.* G. Carducci and S. Ferrari, eds. Firenze, 1956. (Orig. publ. 1899.)

Platon. *Werke.* G. Eigler, ed. 8 vols. Darmstadt, 1970–1983.

Secondary Sources

Blumenberg, H. "Wirklichkeitsbegriff und Wirkungspotential des Mythos," in *Terror und Spiel.* M. Fuhrmann. ed. München, 1971, 11–66.

Duchrow, M. *Sprachverständnis und biblisches Hören bei Augustin.* Tübingen, 1965.

Jeremias, J. *Theophanie. Die Geschichte einer alttestamentlichen Gattung.* Neukirchen-Vluyn, 1965.

Mayr, F. K. *Realenzyklopädie für Antike und Christentum,* s.v. "Hören," 119/20 (1991): 1023–1111.

Pax, E. *Epiphaneia. Ein religionsgeschichtlicher Beitrag zur biblischen Theologie.* München, 1955.

Warning, R. *Funktion und Struktur. Die Ambivalenzen des geistlichen Spiels.* München, 1974. Quoted in the English translation *The Ambivalences of Medieval Religious Drama.* Stanford, 2001.

———. "Lyrisches Ich und Öffentlichkeit bei den Trobadors" (1979), in *Lektüren romanischer Lyrik.* Freiburg/Br., 1997, 45–84.

———. "Imitatio und Intertextualität. Zur Geschichte lyrischer Dekonstruktion der Amortheologie: Dante, Petrarca, Baudelaire" (1983), in *Lektüren romanischer Lyrik,* Freiburg/Br., 1997, 105–141.

Werner, M. *Die Entstehung des christlichen Dogmas.* Stuttgart, 1959. Quoted in the English translation *The Formation of the Christian Dogma: An Historical Study of Its Problem.* New York, 1957.

PART THREE
Hidden Energies

7 *Perception, Cognition, and Volition in the* Arcipreste de Talavera

Joachim Küpper

It is a widely accepted view that during the Middle Ages the split between the body and the senses on the one hand and the mind on the other was less strict than what we are used to from times that are marked by the Cartesian dichotomy of *res cogitans* and *res extensa.* I have consciously chosen the wording "less strict" although it might seem a little vague. The reason for this is that during the long period which we call the Middle Ages, there were various theories on the connection between sensory perception and cognition which cannot be reduced to a sharply defined standard model. This said, one can state the following concerning the dominant tendencies:

1. The model derived from Plato according to which the senses play only a minor part in the cognitive process was known during the Middle Ages, but was less relevant. It becomes more important again during the fifteenth century, and one can even consider Descartes's model of cognition, which he bases on "innate ideas," as a secularized Christian variant ("catholic" in the etymological sense of the word) of the Platonic model of cognition.[1]

2. During the period of interest to me, the dominant model is the Aristotelian one as advocated by Avicenna, Averroës, Albert the Great, and Thomas Aquinas. According to this model, cognition always starts with sensory perception. As to the further steps of gaining knowledge, there is great variation. It ranges from a basically materialistic anthropology[2] to the reformulation of the Aristotelian concepts of *nous pathetikos* and *nous*

poietikos[3] as the dichotomy of *intellectus possiblis* and *intellectus agens:* The "passive" *intellectus possiblis* is responsible for those parts of the process of cognition that are connected to objects of perception and thereby to the senses. All "higher" achievements of the intellect, however, necessitate an "illumination" of the consciousness by the immaterial *intellectus agens.* Depending on which authority one follows, this category is understood as a transpersonal or as an individual one, in any case as one that supplies the model of cognition with the idea of an instance which is *not* bound to sensory perception.[4]

3. In all variants of the model outlined above, the acts of cognition that are bound to sensory perception always refer to the material world (including man).[5] Philosophically speaking, what is at stake is cognition on the level of natural history on the one hand and on the level of moral philosophy on the other. What shall be of interest to me in the following is only this latter field, the connection between perception, volition, and action.

Aristotle's moral philosophical concept is strictly purpose orientated. It sees "well being" (*eudaimonia,* "true happiness" [literal sense: having a good guardian spirit]) as the aim of all action. *Eudaimonia* is the term for a state which one would call "self-sufficiency" (*autarkeia*); trying to avoid too evaluative a terminology, one might also call it a successful *conservatio sui.* Although most people do not seize the opportunity but dedicate themselves to the base aims of "pleasure" (*hēdonē*) or "honor" (*timē*), "the good" (*agathon*), or rather the "good life" (*euzōia*), is available to "all that are not mutilated regarding virtue" (*tois mē pepērōmenois pros aretēn*)[6] via "teaching" (*mathēsis*) and "solicitude" (*epimeleia*). The senses ("sensation" [*aisthēsis*]) take in all data of the world, which finds itself in constant transformation and which, in the end, cannot be fully systematized. From this data, they abstract possibilities of action that all seem to be capable of guaranteeing the *conservatio sui.*

"Intellect" (*nous*) chooses from these possibilities of action the most useful ones and establishes "volition" (*prohairesis*), which in this respect is either "thought brought by desire" (*orektikos nous*) or "desire guided by thought" (*orexis dianoētikē*). Useful are the nonextreme variants of the possibilities of action. This, in turn, arises from the data on the surrounding world which is perceivable by the senses: What we call moderate is the behavior that keeps within the bounds of the main strand of what can be perceived, and we call extreme or excessive all kinds of behavior that deviate from successful behavior as can be observed. It is useful to let oneself be guided by the principle of "moderation" (*mesotes*), and this insight in turn is a manifestation of "reason" (*logos*) as a specific human quality. "Virtues" (*aretai*), that is, the patterns of action that allow for bliss, are, in this way, neither automatic promptings of the soul ("passions"/ *pathē*) nor "capacities/ potentialities" (*dynameis*), that is, a kind of naturally innate opportunity that only needs to be taken. Rather, they are *hexeis,* patterns of action that have to be acquired and *can* in principle be acquired by all humans via reason and then become qualities by habitualization.

Aristotle's model of the interplay between cognition, volition, and action could be criticized for being schematic. His answer to this reproach can, in the final analysis, be found, not in the *Nicomachean Ethics,* but in the *Poetics,* his theory of tragedy: Reason, which is based on the perception of the senses, is not able to completely eliminate the possibility of an "error" (*hamartia*), not even with "good" people. And the connection of such an error with a contingent second event—likewise not influenced by reason (when the old man that the young man has beaten thus to death, disregarding the rule of moderation, is the father of the young man)—can lead to something we call "tragedy." But it is important to note that from the point of view of Aristotle's theory of action, tragic catastrophe is an absolute exception.

When Christianity becomes dominant, it removes the basis of this pragmatic theory of action. Monotheism is not even the crucial problem, as the comparison of Christian and Jewish moral philosophy could show us. Of course, the ideal of the *conservatio sui* being substituted by the sovereign commandment of the one God changes the frame for "right action." But the God of the Decalogue is not a God of despotism. In the end, he does not ask for anything opposed to the *conservatio sui.* The reason why the relation between the perception of the senses and reasonable action becomes problematic is to be found at the core of Christian dogma: The sacrificial death of the Son of God can only make sense if there is no other way of restoring the possibilities of "right action." The idea of a universal need for redemption requires the idea of universal sinfulness, that is, the categorical exclusion of the possibility that even one solitary human being is capable of doing what is morally required out of his own cognition and his own power.

The paradoxical concept of the "original sin" has for various different reasons that cannot be discussed here been connected to a reevaluation of the senses since early Christian theology.[7] In ancient pagan, Aristotelian anthropology, the senses are first of all means of cognition. They mediate between world and mind. Apart from that, they are the means of the irrational faculty of desire, of the "passions" (*pathē*). They convey to the faculty of desire the perception of possible objects of desire and themselves become the instances of the fulfilment of desire.[8] Yet, from an Aristotelian point of view, reason is always capable of "restraining" the faculty of desire (*sōphrosynē*). Thereby, virtue is based on "decision" (*prohairesis*), virtue is "in our power" (*eph' hēmin*), "it is up to us to be decent or mean" (*eph' hēmin ara to epieikesi kai phaulois einai*), virtues and wickedness are "voluntary" (*hekōn*), the possibility of a life guided by reason is therefore not to be assigned to "chance" (*tychē*). At most, a "lack of self-control" (*akrasia*) can set aside reason momentarily.

Christianity continues to conceive of the senses as means of the cognition of the world and at the same time of the faculty of desire. But the crucial point is that from a Christian perspective, the faculty of desire finds itself in a constant conflict with *ratio,* a conflict whose outcome is never decided beforehand. According to Paul and Augustine, original sin is nothing but the permanent rebellion of desire against *ratio,* but most of all *ratio*'s systematic inability to control the faculty of desire by itself.[9] It is the latter that distinguishes Christian from ancient pagan moral philosophy.

Both *ratio* and its antagonist, the faculty of desire, can only interact with the world via the means of the senses. This was already true for ancient pagan (i.e., Aristotelian) thought. But only when the relation between *ratio* and the faculty of desire ceases to be hierarchical, when the two instances are in a state of permanent conflict which, in the final analysis, is undecided until the hour of death, are the senses both a means of cognition of the world and of a successful *conservatio sui,* and a means of the failure to recognize truth and thereby of (metaphysical) self-destruction.[10]

Therefore, we could say that the Christian Middle Ages have a hysterical relation to the senses.[11] The presence of the senses is stronger than in Modernity (this is what connects medieval with ancient culture),[12] but the repudiation of the senses is also a stronger one (this is what distinguishes medieval culture both from ancient times and from Modernity, although the respective reasons differ from one another). On the level of the given texts, this contradictoriness produces an obsessive preoccupation with the topic of the senses which comes close to repetition compulsion. This attitude toward the senses, which is rather glaring at times and which experiences its final peak during the European Baroque, ends with Cartesianism. In Cartesian thought, the senses are of little relevance. Because they are less relevant, they do not have to be staged as emphatically as in the premodern phase in literature (and other arts). And because they do not have to be staged as emphatically as before, in turn they do not have to be anathematized as emphatically as they were in those times.[13]

I will demonstrate what I called the "hysterical" relation to the senses in the following with the help of a text from late medieval times, the *Arcipreste de Talavera,*[14] which was finished in 1438 and which the author deliberately left without a title of its own. Since it was printed, it has also been known as *Corbacho,* in following the corresponding text by Boccaccio, and it has always been assigned the subheading of "Reprobación del loco amor."[15] As far as the overall structure is concerned, it is a text, mutatis mutandis, like the *Roman de la rose, De amore* by Andreas Capellanus, and the *Arcipreste de Hita:* The emphatic praise of the senses and sensual pleasures is accompanied by a harsh denunciation of the senses.[16]

In modern receptions the texts mentioned above are frequently classified as "subversive"[17]: It is claimed that repudiation of the senses and the sensual pleasures was, in a certain way, the tribute that those texts pay (more precisely: have to pay) to Christian orthodoxy, and that the praise of the senses and of sensual pleasures was their real intention which fought for its access to articulation in the disguise of a pretended denunciation. The price that this dominant thesis has to pay normally remains unnoticed. It regards as a matter of course the very attitude toward religion which was developed during the Age of Enlightenment and which reached its peak with Marx and his proselytes: religion, especially the Christian one, is an ideological system which distorts the nature of things with the intention of securing power. Not only could this assessment quite possibly be an historical one, bound to a certain epoch and its established ways of seeing. With regard to the texts mentioned above, it also implies the additional dilemma in that it requires the idea of a revolt of the caste of priests against the basis of its own authority. It is possible that not everyone who is entrusted ex officio with the divulgence of an ideology sticks to the maxims that he preaches in his personal life. But to live by double standards is completely different from undermining or even destroying the ideological basis of one's own authority in recorded texts. And concerning M. M. Bakhtin's theses, one might add that all of the quoted texts are too early to assign them to Renaissance culture, to the generalization of the carnivalesque.

The line of argumentation followed here would relieve the evaluation of the texts mentioned above and of the corresponding structure in many other important medieval texts of all of these pressures, and moreover, it would avoid suggesting a coherence that the texts obviously do not have. The "incoherence" of the modeling of the senses would in the first place be an expression of a basic incoherence of the medieval attitude toward the world: connecting an epistemology which, in the end, is based on the senses with a metaphysical truth whose indispensable basis is the denunciation of the senses. It is only when epistemology becomes detached from sensory perception that this incoherence comes to an end,[18] and with it the production of literary texts like the one that I will turn to in the following.

If the "Reprobación del loco amor" was nothing but a warning about *luxuria* written by a priest, it would suffice to state the official Christian moral doctrine and maybe emphasize the First Commandment by giving a vivid description of the torments of hell. And indeed, the Arcipreste starts his text with this declaration:

> Él ansý lo mandó en el primero mandamiento suyo de la ley: "Amarás a tu Dios, tu criador e señor, sobre todas las cosas." Por ende—pues por Él nos es mandado—conviene a Él sólo amar e las mundanas cosas y transytorias del todo dexar e olvidar, e, por quanto verdaderamente a Él amando, verdaderamente la su ynfinida gloria no es dubda que alcançaremos para sienpre jamás. Enpero, sy, su amor olvidado, las vanas cosas queremos e amamos, dexado el ynfinido Criador por la finida criatura e syerva, dubda non es quel tal aya condepnación, donde infinidos tormentos para sienpre avrá.

> He has commanded so in the First Commandment of His law: "You shall love God, your creator and lord, above all things." Therefore—because He has commanded us so—it is necessary to love Him alone and to give up completely all worldly and transient things and forget about them, the more because if we honestly love Him, we shall truly and without any doubt achieve His endless glory, for ever and ever. But if we, not being aware of His love, like and love vain things, if we give up the infinite creator in favor of the finite and dependent creature, there is no doubt that He will punish us with damnation in which there will be eternal torments forever. (p. 42)

But it does not seem to suffice—in those times and probably at any point in time—to base the "truth" and the whole knowledge about the world on the preterrational belief alone, on the hope for paradise ("ynfinida gloria") and the fear of "infinidos tormentos." It does not suffice because one cannot perceive with the senses the consequences of obeying or violating the First Commandment. If one were able to do so—and this is where the materialistic, senses-based epistemology of the epoch becomes tangible—there would not be so many violations against the divine law: "Sy el triste del onbre o muger *syntiese derechamente* qué cosa es perdurable, o para sienpre jamás, o por ynfinita secula seculorum aver en el otro mundo gloria o pena, sy sola una ora en el día en esto pensase, *dubdo sy pudiera faser mal*" / "If the pitiful man or the woman *felt directly* what is long-lasting, for ever and ever, or for what there will be punishment or glory for all eternity in the other world, if he thought of that for only one hour per day *I doubt that he could do any wrong*" (p. 43).[19]

The Arcipreste is eager to support faith by "knowledge." Again and again he refers to the senses-based epistemology of his time: What he gives in the following is a picture of the world gained via perception ("*veyendo* tanto mal e daño" / "*seeing* so much evil and so much damage" [p. 44]), that is, a multiplicity of sensory perceptions which have hardened into "experience" ("*esperiencia,* [. . .] la[s] qual[es] por prátyca puede cada uno *ver* oy de cada día" / "an *experience* that anyone can *see* every day for himself" [p. 44]).[20] And the reason why he writes it down is none other than saving the reader from having to make the detour of his own experience:

> [P]ropuse de fazer un conpendio breve en romance para ynformación algund tanto de aquellos que les pluguiere leerlo, e leýdo retenerlo, e retenido por obra ponerlo; e specialmente para algunos que non han follado el mundo, nin han bevido de sus amargos bevrages, nin han gustado de sus viandas amargas, *que para los que saben e an visto, sentydo y hoydo non lo escrivo nin digo,* que *su saber* les abasta para se defender de las cosas contrarias.

> [T]his is why I have decided to draw up a small piece of writing in the people's language in order to inform all those who would be pleased to read it and to keep it and once kept to put it into effect; and especially for those who do not know the world, who have neither drunk from its bitter beverages nor tried its bitter meat, *because for those who know and who have seen, and felt/smelt and heard I do not write and speak,* because *their knowledge* suffices to protect them from harmful things. (p. 41)

As we see here, the sense of seeing and the sense of hearing are understood as means to access knowledge ("saber"), that is, the level of cognitive condensing. It is this very level, the systematized transformation of sensory data into "experience," that Martínez's book which is based on hearing, seeing, and feeling places itself on.

The last part of the sentence just quoted which describes the purpose cognition serves ("para se defender de las cosas contrarias" / "to protect oneself from harmful things") opens up the conflict that I have mentioned above: The "cosas contrarias" are nothing but the promptings of the senses that moral theology calls *concupiscentia.* But the knowledge about the harmfulness of those promptings is mediated by those very senses that are themselves the site of the adverse. There is no escape from this contradiction (apart from basing all knowledge about the right behavior on faith), and while the fact that there is none accounts for the nature of the whole text, for its permanent, obvious inconsistency, it also accounts for the stagnancy or circularity of its argument, which is no less obvious and which is a quality completely unknown to Modernity.

The text continuously repeats itself, each new attempt of expressing its message varying only marginally from the previous one: The world, which we can perceive (only) by the senses, teaches us that the senses are something harmful. He who has experienced ("padesce") the pains/discomforts ("penas") caused by the promptings of the senses will not claim that he had not known about the consequences: "quien en esto pensase [. . .] como que *vee aquellas penas e las padesce,* e ya en esta vida ge las dan, ¿faría tanto mal como de cada día faze? [. . .] Por ende, non alegue ninguno: '*non lo sope, nin lo sentí*'" / "he who thought of this . . . , *as he sees those pains and suffers them,* and as they are caused him already in this world—would he do so much evil as he does every day? Therefore, no one shall say: '*I did not know anything about it, or rather I did not perceive it*'" (p. 118). But this does not change the fact that the "defrenado apetyto" / "the unrestrained desire" (p. 47) stirs again and again, and correspondingly one sees and hears the consequences every day: "O quánto dolor de coraçon, quánta amargura para las ánimas, de lo que de cada día *oýmos, sabemos, leemos, veemos* por fechos viles, torpes, orribles, de luxuria que de cada día por guisas diversas se cometen!" / "O how much heartache, how much bitterness is there for the souls, of which we daily *hear, learn, read, see,* created by base, disgraceful, terrible deeds caused by lust, that are committed every day in different ways" (p. 47).

A great part of the text, in fact the whole of the *primera parte,* is dedicated to the display of the whole range of what concupiscence of the senses causes, that is, to what is perceptible of those results ("segund de cada día *enxienplo muestra*" / "as the daily *example shows*" [p. 49]): Sensuality ruins families, undermines friendships, destroys honor (in the sense of reputation), indeed, if the persons involved belong to a certain social level, sensuality is even fit to cause wars and thereby bring death and misery to countless others (I, 2). The archpriest asks his readers chapter by chapter to look at what damage the sensual desire causes: "*Mira,* pues, desordenado amor quántos e quáles dapños procura e trae" / "Therefore *see* how much and what kind of suffering the unrestrained love causes and brings with it" (p. 50). The reader may widely open both his "inner" and the bodily/outer eyes in order to understand the nature of the "amor loco": "Pues, amigo, *abre los ojos espirituales e corporales; mira e vee* quántos daños de locamente amar provienen" / "Therefore, my friend, *open the mind's and the body's eyes; look and see* how much suffering is caused by the mad loving" (p. 117). Every day, he could see all of this, and he may just make sure for himself and in this manner gain experience which then will help to master all problems in life: "E de cada día tú lo puedes *ver* sy quisyeres; [. . .] *mucha prática e espirencia de todo es maestra*" / "And you can *see* this every day, if you want; . . . *a lot of practice and experience are the master of all action*" (p. 119). But after this and many similar statements, the author still continues his panorama of "dapños" caused by the senses which evidences that the senses as a means of cognition and the senses as a means of desire find themselves in an unsolvable conflict.

The content of what Martínez de Toledo intends to communicate from his experience in the following is this: "las malas mugeres, sus menguas, vicios, e tachas [. . .]; eso mesmo digo de los malos, perversos, e malditos onbres, dignos de ynfernal fuego en el solo ynonesto amar de las mugeres con locura e *poco seso* e bestialidad" / "the wicked women, their imperfections, their vices, their faults . . . ; I say the same about the wicked, perverted and damnable men who deserve to roast in hell-fire, if only because of their indecent love of women, their madness, their *poor sense* and their bestiality" (p. 44). The "deseo," the "delectación carnal" reduce the human to a beast ("vestia [bestia] salvaje" [p. 48]). Someone who has at least a little sense/reason ("juycio") should realize that one should better keep away from a seductive woman "como de bruto animal [. . .] como de bestia venenosa e de perro ravioso, que mordiendo poçoña todos los que muerde e comunican con él" / "as from a wild beast . . . as from a poisonous animal and from a rabid dog who poisons by his biting everyone whom he bites or who has contact with him" (p. 51);[21] "non es crimen fallado más grave que la fornicación" / "there is no greater sin than fornication" (p. 52); "amor deve ser aborrescido" / "love has to be despised" (p. 65). The archpriest's book gains its justification solely from the fact that what the senses perceive day by day and what the *virtus aestimativa* as one of the *sensus interiores* condenses into a clear instruction ("fuyr e se apartar" / "flee and getting away" [p. 51]) is turned into the opposite, "por conplyr un poco de vano apetyto" / "to follow a little the vain desire" (p. 52), by another prompting of the senses.

The whole paradox of the activity of the senses—also when understood as purely worldly, leaving aside the question of the salvation of the soul—is put in a nutshell in a passage in which the archpriest describes what is caused by the demand of the senses for a fulfilment of desire ("apetyto"), the self-destruction of the senses, and the self-destruction of the *virtutes* of the mind which turn the sensory perceptions into cognition:

> E como los otros pecados de su naturalesa maten el alma, *éste, enpero, mata el cuerpo* e condepna el ánima por do *el cuerpo luxuriando padesce en todos sus naturales cinco sentydos:* primeramente [faze] *la vista* perder, e menguar *el olor* de las narizes natural, qu'el onbre apenas huele como solýa; *el gusto* de la boca pierde e aun el comer del todo; casy *el oyr* fallesce, que parésce le como que oye abejones en el oreja; las manos e todo el cuerpo pierden todo su exersycio que tenían e comiençan de tenblar [tactus]. Pues, *las potencias del ánima tres, todas son turbadas;* que apenas tyene *entendimiento* [*virtus aestimativa*], *memoria,* nin *reminiciencia;* [. . .] *pierde el seso, e juyzio natural.*
>
> And as the other sins kill the soul due to their nature, *this however kills the body* and condemns the soul which is why *the body that gives itself to lust comes to harm in all of its five natural senses:* Firstly, it [the sin of lust] causes the loss of the *eyesight* and reduces the natural *sense of smell* of the nose, so that man can hardly smell anything as he used to before; he loses the *sense of taste* of the mouth and even his appetite completely; his *sense of hearing* nearly abandons him, so that it seems to him that he hears bees in his ear; the hands and the entire body lose the control that they had before and start to shake. And ultimately, *the three faculties of the soul are completely disturbed;* so that he has hardly any *reason/understanding, memory* and *remembrance* anymore; . . . *he loses his mind, and the natural faculty of judgment.* (p. 52)

What becomes clear in this passage in the most concise manner is the impasse of medieval anthropology as characterized at the beginning of this essay: If the senses have an inherent irrational tendency to effect their own ruin, how can they be a means of cognition to *avoid* this very way into ruin at the same time? Thereby, man[22] is not only an inconsistent being, but also a being that finds itself in permanent struggle with itself ("e lydia consygo mesmo" [p. 53]). At first sight, this sounds like a reference to the pattern of psychomachy. I will not deny that this pattern is of great importance for the whole of the epoch as described above, that is, for the times up to Descartes. But the quoted passages of the *Arcipreste de Talavera* are *not* concerned with the traditional struggle between virtues and vices;[23] rather, they are concerned with the struggle between the senses as means of perception and cognition and as means of the fulfilment of desire. What is at stake is not a dualistic moral philosophy, or rather theology, but an anthropology that is contradictory in itself.

How much this is true and how much the whole undertaking of the *Arcipreste de Talavera* deconstructs itself in the light of this contradiction perhaps becomes nowhere as clear as it does in the passage where he admonishes his reader not to think that he was immune against the supremacy of sensual desire: Even "Adam, Sansón, Davyd, Golyas, Salamón, Virgilio, Aristótiles, e otros dignos de memoria *en saber y natural juyzio*" / "Adam, Samson, David, Goliath, Solomon, Virgil, Aristotle, and others who are worthy of commemoration *due to their knowledge and their natural faculty of judgement*" (p. 55) had fallen victim to the concupiscence of their senses with grave, even dreadful consequences. But if "saber" and "natural juyzio" are based on sensory perception and experience, how can the reader of the book defend himself against something that not even the paragons of "saber" and "juyzio" that the author mentions were able to control? The archpriest comes back to this thought a few chapters later, adding further poignance:

> Pues, faser dioses estraños e ydolatrar, byen es cabsa [causa] el amor; que Salamón non se pudo dello abstener que por su coamante non ydolatrase. Mira en onbre tan sabio, e pues, ¿qué será, mesquino de tý, sy éste, *que Dios lo fiso el más sabio de los sabios,* pecó en tal pecado por amar? Pues, *¿quién nos defenderá a nosotros,* dignos de non ser, en su esguarde nin respecto, onbres llamados? E como te dixe de Salamón, asý de otros muy sabios e valyentes varones.
>
> Because the reason for making up other gods and worshipping them is love; for Salomon could not abstain from becoming an idolater for the sake of his lover. Look upon this man so wise, and then, what becomes of you, good-for-nothing, *if he whom God made into the wisest of the wise,* became guilty of such a sin for love? For *who will defend us,* we who are not worthy of being called humans compared to him? And what I have told you about Salomon, this is also true for other very wise and brave men. (p. 62)

The questions which Martínez uses to rhetorize his argument point to the dead end that was mentioned already: If wisdom as the peak of experience which can be reached only in very rare exceptions is not enough to control sensual desire, how can one expect that the degree of experience available to the average person ("nosotros") would provide enough orientation in the world? And in a chapter which is especially dedicated to the wise and the learned (I, 17), Martínez emphasizes this thought, referring again to the authorities mentioned, even up to the final claim of an inverted relation between wisdom and abstinence: "los que más cientýficos son, [. . .] menos se saben desenbolver dello [del uso, sc. del amor loco] que los sinples ynorantes" / "those who are the most learned, . . . are less resourceful concerning those matters [sc. refraining from lust] than the simple ignorants" (p. 76).

In an intellectual sense, the passage quoted above is the hinge joint with which the archpriest prepares for the transition to the third and fourth part of his treatise. In those later parts, he draws the conclusions from that passage: If the experience which is mediated by the senses does not accomplish much against the supremacy of sensual desire, then the only alternative left (unthinkable for contemporaries) is the general dismissal of the senses as a means of cognition, or otherwise the assumption of external powers which can prevent the consciously cognized from having an effect on volition. Those latter parts of the book, as we will see, deal with the problem of determinism.

However, before these two parts at the end there is the *segunda parte,* which is the part of the text that the modern reception, which starts in the nineteenth century, deals with most. At least on the Iberian Peninsula, but possibly in the whole of Europe, the *segunda parte* has been seen as the origin of literary "realism" ever since Ferdinand Wolf characterized the respective chapters as a "portrayal of the customs of that time" and as a witness to the fact that Martínez de Toledo knew how to "draw directly from life,"[24] and even more since Marcelino Menéndez Pelayos's famous description in the first part of the *Orígenes de la novela.*[25] The *segunda parte* starts with a formula that connects what is to be read in the following with the topic of the *primera parte,* at first addressing the male readers: "visto el efecto que loco amor procura, quántos dapños trahe, *veamos,* pues, por quién nos condenamos: nin qué cosa son mugeres" / "in view of the effect that the mad love has on us and how much suffering it causes let us *look* at those for whom we condemn ourselves: and what kind of thing women are" (p. 120). The reason the author gives for elaborating on what follows and which applies to the female readers adds to the stages of "perception" and "evaluation" the aspect of action: "*Vea,* pues, cada qual en sý, si es culpada, *e fiera su conciencia con verdadera corrección*" / "Each [woman] should *look* in herself whether she is burdened with guilt and *put her conscience in order with the aim of true improvement*" (p. 120). In fact, what is at stake in the *segunda parte* is a representation of the female world as perceived quite passionately by the senses of a moderately misogynous, though in the end a rather amused, male observer.

The first chapter deals with the women's material avarice ("avaricia" [II, 1]), in the sense that they are willing to sell their virtue at any time to a man who presents them with a gift big enough: "por dones library[ía] su cuerpo" / "she would give her body for presents" (p. 122). At the very beginning of the chapter, Martínez de Toledo tells an "authentic" story ("un exienplo que contesció en Barcelona" / "an example that took place in Barcelona" [p. 121]) which is of interest because, as a kind of mise en abyme, it anticipates the essence of the whole of the *segunda parte:* Once there had lived a queen in Barcelona who had prided herself so much on her virtue that one could only call her self-image the result of *superbia,* the worst of all sins: "Un[a] reyna [. . .] muy honesta con ynfingimiento de vanagloria, que pensava aver más firmeza que otra, diziendo que quál era la vil muger que ha onbre su cuerpo librava por todo el aver que fuese al mundo" / "A queen . . . , very honorable, of absolutely unfeigned vanity/self-confidence, who thought that she had more steadfastness than any other, and who wondered of what low kind the woman was who gave her body to a man for all the wealth in the world" (pp. 121–122). The lady also articulates this claim in public, which makes a knight who hears about it demonstrate to her that not even she is immune against temptation.

First, he asks her if she might not give herself to a man who gave her a diamond ten times worth the one that adorned her ring. Self-confident, the lady contradicts: "Non le amaría aunque me diese uno que valiese más que ciento" / "I would not love him, even if he gave me one that is more than a hundred times worth" (p. 122). The knight mentions other gifts, and a few more questions and replies later, things get to a point where the lady says that not even for the "reyno de Castilla" would she sacrifice her virtue. But then, the knight goes for broke: "Señora, quien vos fiziese del mundo enperadora e que todos los onbres e mugeres vos besasen las manos por señora, señora, ¿amarle ýedes?" / "Madam, he who would make you the ruler of the world and who would make all men and women kiss the hands of you as sovereign, Madam, would you not love him?" Already, the queen wants to give her usual, self-assured answer but then stops in the middle of the sentence, "E non dixo más" / "And said nothing more" (p. 122), because at this very moment she realizes her own desire: "E la reyna pensó en sý e vido que avía mal dicho, e conosció entonce a dádyvas non ay azero que resysta, quanto más persona que es de carne e naturalmente trahe consygo la desordenada cobdicia" / "And the queen started to think and saw that she had spoken wrongly, and then realized that there is no kind of steel that could resist gifts, let alone a person who is made out of flesh and by nature bears unrestrained avarice/desire for material wealth."

The subtext to the knight's last question is, of course, the scene of the temptation of Christ by the devil,[26] and the queen's gain in self-knowledge is nothing but the recognition of herself and any ordinary man being in the state of original sin. In order to make absolutely clear what he refers to, the author extends the lesson that the story teaches to all humans, from the king to the emperor and even the pope ("Por dádyvas farás venir a tu voluntad al papa a te otorgar lo que quisyeres" / "With the help of gifts you will even get the pope to meet your will and to grant you whatever you ask for" [p. 123]): By nature ("naturalmente"), man has a tendency toward sin and thereby toward disorder ("desordenada").[27]

This at first sight inconspicuous story at the beginning of the *Arcipreste de Talavera*'s *segunda parte* refers to a sore point in Christian anthropology that led to a divide of Western Christianity into two denominations a little less than a century after this text was written: If sinfulness is the inevitable quality of the human, then the attempt to restrain sensual desire by means of experience-based rationality becomes useless. In the end, this attempt is always doomed to fail. In the final analysis, Christian dogma implies a reverse of the hierarchy that the function of the senses had adopted in ancient times: It is not the cognitive faculty that governs the faculty of desire, but rather the faculty of desire that governs the cognitive faculty; "todo a su voluntad lo trastorna" / "everything has to comply to its will" (p. 123), as the Arcipreste puts it, or "reason is a whore," as Luther will later put it.[28]

Basically, Martínez de Toledo would have had to stop his text at this point and destroy what he had already written as his whole undertaking is based on an appeal to the readers' cognition. This appeal, in turn, is based on cognitive data which—as one would have to state in view of this *exemplum*—always carry ("trahen consygo") the natural tendency of the human consciousness to take its subjective wishes for the objectively true.[29]

In that epoch, there is no way out of the contradiction between an epistemology which is based on the senses and a dogma that anathematizes the senses. Therefore, in spite of its inconsistency, the way that the Arcipreste takes in the following is the only alternative at hand if he does not want to fall silent: He continues to relate what he perceives of the world with his senses and continues to draw abstractions from what he perceives, to value them according to "good" and "evil" and to inform his readers of the result of his insights for the purpose of application. And he draws another conclusion from the story on the queen in Barcelona which is as pragmatic as the first, pragmatic in the sense of unsatisfactory from a systematic point of view: If the disorder ("desorden") caused by the function of desire is an inevitable part of human nature, and if human nature is nevertheless something that its creator loved so well that he gave his own life for the overcoming of the metaphysical consequences, then the representation of the "desorden" cannot be completely inadmissible. What develops under the pressure of a rigorous doctrine of original sin is a kind of license for *representing* the sinful.

The author extensively uses this license obtained for himself in the beginning of the second part.[30] And it is obvious that the representation—although it might be impartial in substance—of something that everyone is subjected to, including everyone who reads this representation, leads to an affirmation of the portrayed. The pleasure that the reader finds in recognizing the whole range of the inevitable human (here the female) weaknesses sets the tone for his role implied in this part of the text. The amusement, which is diametrically opposed to a moralizing condemnation, is evoked by the fact that in large passages of the *segunda parte,* Martínez reports on things that can potentially be perceived, or of which he claims he perceived just the way he reports them. The abstractive performance of the "inner senses" only reaches the level of typification. The evaluation that is the *virtus aestimativa*'s task is left out, which is nothing but consistent after the introductory *exemplum* about the queen in Barcelona. And from the perspective of the perceivable, leaving aside all "higher" rational components of the conscience, the archsin of "cobdicia," which metonymically stands for the faculty of desire (*concupiscentia*) as such,[31] is reduced to a range of scenes of harmless everyday life[32] that are only too well known in their almost mimetic immediacy and that could also be taken from Petrus Alphonsus's *Disciplina clericalis* or Boccaccio's *Decameron.*[33]

It is not until the last, the fourteenth, chapter that the archpriest tries to reintegrate the whole range into the didactic intention of the text stuck in front of it with the help of an *argumentum e contrario:* "Por ende, amigo, sy considerases cómo sólo amar a Dios es sabyeza [. . .]; e que amar cosas mundanales—riquezas, mugeres, e estados—es loco e vano amor e vicio contra virtud, por el qual tantos dapños, como susodicho he, se syguen e provienen [. . .]" / "Therefore, my friend, if you now thought of the fact that only loving God means wisdom . . . ; and to love worldly things—wealth, women, privileges that are connected to status—is a mad and vain kind of love and a vice against virtue, and from which follows and stems, as I said above, so much suffering [. . .]" (pp. 175–176).

I would like to make a few closing remarks on the realism-thesis to which I referred at the beginning. It is true that the text of Martínez de Toledo shows some structures that are characteristic of both theory and practice of the realist novel of the nineteenth century, such as the revaluation of the trivial, of the particular, of the contingent detail and mimicry of "the people's" oral speech beyond any kind of rhetoric. However, these parallels might only extend to the surface. The novel of the nineteenth century, too, is determined by the depiction of what can be perceived immediately; Stendhal's famous mirror-metaphor is only the most convincing example. But one need not bring in Foucault's description of the episteme of the nineteenth century as a system of "profondeur" in order to see that the literary realism of Modernity decidedly does not consist in a depiction of the perceivable. The novels of Balzac, Flaubert, Stendhal, and Zola (with all their differences), show that what is immediately perceived does *not* grasp the real essence of the world. What is always needed is a narrator that either implicitly or explicitly articulates and reveals to the reader the true being of the things beyond the surface of the perceivable. The realist novel's obsession with perceivable details stems from the intention to create *illusion.*[34] The *cognition* of the world, however, needs "higher" registers than simply that of perception.[35] With Martínez de Toledo's treatise, things are completely different. Its conceptual substratum is Aristotelian epistemology: What the senses perceive is the "real essence" of the world. Knowledge, as represented by the *virtus imaginativa,* is evaluated by the *virtus aestimativa* according to usefulness and harmfulness, and it is this evaluation that paves the way for right action.

One could therefore say that while Martínez de Toledo presents the whole range of contradictions that are inherent in the senses in the *primera parte,* he concentrates in a nearly scholastic way on basing the *segunda parte* upon the idea of a cognitive efficacy. Therefore, the very question which arose already in the first part gets more pressing at the end of the second part: If the senses are capable of cognition of the world, then why do people not act according to what they cognize?

The superficial connection between the *tercera parte* and the *segunda parte* is that the third part is concerned with a characterization of male human beings, of men.[36] But the viewpoint of the presentation has shifted; what is at stake are not men in general, but a typology of the male half of humanity.[37] First, the author presents the pseudo-Aristotelian theory of the temperaments.[38] The four types (the sanguine, the choleric, the phlegmatic, and the melancholic type) are portrayed as such and then in their respective relation to sensual desire. In turn, the temperaments are explained with the help of astrology: The constellation of the stars at the time of birth determines to which type the person belongs, and it is the belonging to a respective type that determines the range of how well the person manages to cope with sensual desire. For example, the archpriest characterizes the sanguine man on the level of general qualities as the best type, because he is the most sociable, just, and sympathetic of them all (III, 2). Nevertheless, these good qualities, especially the first one, are accompanied by a very strong tendency toward the "amor loco": "que, comoquier que es alegre e plazentero, es mucho enamorado e su coraçon arde como fuego, e ama a dyestro e a syniestro" / "he, as anyone who is cheerful and sociable, is susceptible to love and his heart burns like fire, and he loves without caution" (p. 187).

The respective passages from the text could be seen as an expression of materialistic determinism. The archpriest tries to limit the tendency toward legitimizing sin that accompanies such an approach. He claims to inform about the weaknesses of sanguine persons, firstly, for them to be able to prepare themselves better against their own inclinations, and secondly, for the women to know which men they should be careful of in order to protect their virtue. But already in the chapter on the love qualities of the phlegmatic persons (III, 9), the evaluation according to moral aspects is withdrawn in favor of the aspect of suitability for love: "Asý que los tales non son buenos para amar, nin aun para ser amados; que nin tyenen lo que amor requiere, nin han lo que la fenbra quiere" / "So that those are not suited for love, neither for being loved; as they neither have what love requires nor what the woman wants" (p. 198). And the *tercera parte* ends with a seemingly value-free typologizing, but in substance unconcealed hedonistic, description of possible couplings according to age groups:[39] Young man and old woman, old man and young woman, old man and old woman, finally young man and young woman. Only the last of those variants is approved of by the archpriest ("aprovado"), the other three are rejected ("reprobado"),[40] and this classification is by no means carried out from a moralistic point of view, that is, the point of view whose aim is to avoid *luxuria*'s temptations in the best possible way. Neither is it the theologically appropriate one, that is, that of the best possible conditions for procreation. Rather, it is the one that has consistently been denounced as the road to doom in the other parts of the book, the pleasure of the senses.[41]

It is obvious that as a Christian priest, Martínez de Toledo cannot confine himself to this presentation of materialistic determinism. Nevertheless, it is striking[42] that he expands so much on this concept before denouncing it as heretic. The derogation is based on the fundamental principle of monotheism: If there is only one God, it is He alone who decides on what happens in the world. Martínez manages to weaken the materialistic determinism only by postulating a metaphysical determinism which he foregrounds as rigidly as monotheism demands.[43] The fourth book (*media parte*)[44] consists of an attempt to put the whole of the discussion back on the orthodox track—with foreseeable consequences. The problem of divine omnipotence and human freedom has never been discussed without opening up an abyss.

The questions discussed in the *media parte* take up the belief in fate, or more precisely the belief in the stars resulting from the *tercera parte.*[45] The archpriest specifies this problem in the middle of the first chapter of the *media parte:* "sy el malo nasció en mal sygno [. . .] ¿qué justicia sería ésta aver dapñación, pues él non procuró de nascer en aquel mal sygno, planeta, o fado?" / "if the bad person was born under a bad sign of the zodiac . . . and thereby be condemned, what kind of justice would that be, as he did not ask to be born under a bad sign of the zodiac, planet, or fate?" He who is predestined for condemnation in such a way would rightly accuse God: "-¡O Señor!, pues de nescesario me tengo de dañar, ¿por qué quesiste que nasciese, pues a Ty era notorio, en tu paresciencia [praesciencia] eternalmente dispuesta, que yo me avía nasciendo de dañar?" / "Oh Lord, as I have to bring about my own damnation out of necessity, why did you want me to be born although you knew before, preordained in your eternal knowledge, that I was born to be condemned?" (p. 212). Martínez says what the church would, after all, have said whenever this question arose: The problem is precarious and those who are not especially experienced theologians should rather refrain from discussing it.[46] But whether or not he thinks of himself as one of those experts, the very question is already implicit in his text so that he cannot but elaborate on it. Indeed, the alternative would have been an annihilation of what he had written so far.

The pained argumentation that has very good reason not to become too concise deals with the logical circle of monotheism. The popular belief in stars and fate which results in freeing man from responsibility is rejected with the help of the basic dogma that God is omnipotent, that He alone is mighty.[47] However, thereby the real problem has only been shifted. Because if one takes monotheism seriously, that is, the exclusive power of disposal of the one God, then there is as little human freedom as there is in the belief in fate.[48] Confession, moralizing, and rites all lose their meaning.[49] Since the belief in the hereafter prevails, or rather because without it, talking of faith could only be metaphorical, the question of divine justice is raised, a question considerably more dangerous.

Sooner or later, the inevitable result of what the archpriest discusses here is modern posttheism. But it suggests itself that this text from the late Middle Ages tries to cover up the explosive force of the questions raised by means of the familiar maneuvers: The problem of justice belongs to the realm of the *arcana Dei.*[50] Evil does not come from God, God only permits it.[51] Its purpose is to punish man for his sins.[52] The archpriest is only able to answer one of the two new questions that this solution raises, and even this answer remains dubious: If the fact of a violent death finds its reason in the past sins of the murdered, what about his murderer? According to Martínez, the murderer, too, is punished for his sins by his becoming a murderer. These sins necessarily have to be less grave,[53] which opens up the problem of divine strictness. Can a loving father "righteously" punish a creature that is guilty of defamation by allowing the very creature to become a murderer?

Decidely more important, however, is the basic problem itself. If it is true that we do not escape God's power of disposal ("non podemos salir del poderío de Dios" [p. 231]), how is it possible that we sin at all? The only answer is the theory of the inexplorable election that Augustine already formulated.[54] Thus, the text's ideas already imply everything that followed, when half a century later an Augustinian monk took up again the answer that had been formulated at the beginning of the career of monotheism.

However, the archpriest avoids this most basic aspect of the problem in which he finds himself. During the rest of the chapter, he concentrates on a less fundamental although considerable problem. Here, too, he unintentionally discloses the problem's insoluble character by trying to evade it with the help of metonymical shifting. The problem consists in the good person burdened by the *malum.*[55] The rather simple but consistent answer goes as follows: The good person who suffers distress is in fact not a good person but a skillful hypocrite who is punished by God for his hidden misdeeds.[56] Martínez then adds a long passage on one kind of hypocrite with reference to his book's main concern—an illustrating example, or so he claims. In fact, it rather seems like a means of the shifting mentioned above: There are men that give the impression of the greatest virtue by systematically staying away from women but who in fact commit carnal sins much worse than those of the normal hedonistic people. The archpriest wisely avoids the soundness of his argument being tried, that is, the proof that God indeed does punish all carnal sinners *contra naturam* in this world. The very passage, however, gives him the opportunity to depict a panorama of especially depraved sinfulness in drastic and disapproving, although at the same time suggestive, words.[57]

Martínez closes the chapter as he nearly always does, with a few unambiguously orthodox statements: God has three different motives, he says, for making people suffer, or rather for allowing their suffering. The first variant is punishment of sinners ("los malos," "los [. . .] perversos" [p. 243]). The second one is a warning for good people to always be aware of the weakness of their flesh and of the existence of God ("permite los buenos ser castigados porque le non desconoscan" / "He allows for the good people to be punished so that they do not misjudge Him [His nature, i.e., His omnipotence]" [p. 244]). The third variant is called *tribulatio* (trial) in official terminology:[58] The severe suffering up to sickness and death is supposed to give the person affected the opportunity to prove his faithfulness to God. The suffering thereby becomes a means of salvation.[59] It is characteristic of the conceptual dubiousnesses in which Martínez got stuck while trying to belatedly correct his not very orthodox little book that he presents the three variants according to a grading of relevance which is just the opposite of their actual importance in orthodox teaching. The first variant is, stricto sensu, un-Christian. It is a relic of the Jewish belief in law. The Christian God does not punish in this world. However, it has been an element of popular preaching at all times. The second variant that contains the element of warning is an orthodox one. Nevertheless, it is not relevant for the problem of severe earthly suffering, which is of actual interest. The only theory of evil that can be called orthodox in the full sense is the last one. Its purview, however, is restricted by the archpriest to apostles, saints, martyrs, and the like who, according to him, still exist in his times, "aunque pocos, por nuestros pecados" / "even if only a few, because of our sins" (p. 245).

The second chapter of the *media parte*[60] consists of a version of a story taken from *De casibus virorum illustrium.* It is about the battle of the personified allegories of Fortuna and Probeza[61] which, as the story has it, took place in the dim and distant past and which ended with Poverty's victory and Fortuna being sentenced to permanent captivity. It would definitely be interesting to discuss the differences between this version and the original story by Boccaccio. However, the argument that is followed up here would only gain in marginal aspects. The closing chapter of this part and at the same time of the whole text comes back to the point that was already discussed in the first chapter of this fourth book. Thereby, this shows how unsatisfactory the solution attempted here remains. The precarious theodicy is repeated again, that in case someone is afflicted by misfortune it is always just punishment for sins that he committed earlier. And here, too, one might say that the attempts Martínez makes to "amend" the answer already given finally lead to an aggravation of the problem which was implied in this answer. The archpriest asks his readers to consider that often one does not know what sin one is punished for because God in his mercy gives the sinner not only a day, not only a year, but often many years to repent before punishing.[62] Thereby, Martínez plunges the reader into an absolute uncertainty, into a state of not knowing about the world and his own life that could nearly be called the generalization of the Aristotelian model of tragedy.

Like many medieval texts, particularly those which are not organized in the form of narrating a continuous story, the *Arcipreste de Talavera* seems not very coherent. Rather, it appears to be a hotchpotch of this and that which is only loosely held together by the topic of the "loco amor." However, this impression is distorted; lastly, it is only true of the surface of what is being said, a surface which shows clear residues of orality, as do many texts of that period.[63] But the intellectual matrix of the treatise is tremendously coherent and compelling, and above all, it seems representative of the epoch: The reference to determinism is the unavoidable result of the conflict between the (Aristotelian) epistemology which is based on the senses and the dogma (of the original sin) which is hostile to the senses. There cannot be a coherent connection of perception, cognition, volition, and action if the means of perception are at the same time agents of those impulses of the soul which systematically contradict what has been gained in knowledge on the level of cognition, especially if these impulses of the soul in the end are more powerful than anything that can be achieved by experience, even wisdom. Nevertheless, it can be observed that there are variants on the level of behavior. Sensual desire does not impose the same patterns of behavior on all people. It is therefore consistent that action is moved to the realm of dependency on external influences (external in reference to the individual and its perceptions and cognitive acts): It is these external forces, be it the stars, or rather the temperaments determined by them, be it divine will, that decide on how each individual manages with the promptings of his senses.

Of course, determinism cannot be a satisfying answer to the whole question, which is what the archpriest's text shows, too. For reasons that cannot be discussed in this essay, determinism as the most consistent consequence of monotheism is a pattern always present in the history of the Occident, although it has so far never become dominant.[64] What remains at the end of the *Arcipreste de Talavera* is again only the appeal to reason, that is, to cognition and volition that resume to sensory perceptions ("Por ende, amigos, [. . .] *nos apercibamos,* [. . .] e de los vicios nos corrijamos" / "Therefore, my friends, . . . *let us become aware of* . . . and let us free ourselves from our vices" [p. 278]), although it has been convincingly demonstrated before how precarious they are.

And finally, there is a two-page epilogue that contradicts the semantic axis of what was said before in such an obvious way that these two pages have often been denied their authenticity.[65] In this epilogue, the author tells us that after finishing his little book, he had retired to his bed in the evening. In a dream that he had that night, more than a thousand very beautiful ladies appeared to him. They beat him and whipped him and demanded of him to answer the following question: "Loco atrevido, ¿dó te vino osar de escrebir ni hablar de aquellas que merescen del mundo la victoria?" / "You mad presumptuous person, how dare you write and speak about those that deserve the first place in the world?" (p. 280). After some time, he woke up bathed in sweat and regretted what he had written: "-¡Guay del que duerme solo! [. . .] con arrepentimiento demando perdón dellas [de las señoras]" / "Woe betide him who sleeps alone! . . . with regret I ask for their [the women's] pardon" (p. 281). From the point of view of my interpretation of the text, this palinode, which indeed would seem strange in a modern text, is nothing but the reflex of the fundamentally paradoxical relation to the senses which seems to be the very characteristic of the epoch in which the text was written.[66]

A (hysterical) swinging between extremes, circularity of the train of thought, lastly the decisive questions being left unanswered without even an indication of the possibility to follow up this thought, which means stagnation—these are the main characteristics of the *Arcipreste de Talavera* which I have tried to bring out. These categorizations obviously imply evaluations, and these evaluations have been made from a point of view which conceives of coherence, vectorial trains of thought, and dynamics as positive values. In short: From a modern point of view—how else could it be? Therefore, the readers of this essay will possibly neither deny the legitimacy of evaluation in general, nor perhaps this very specific evaluation. It is possible, though, that my reading of the *Arcipreste de Talavera* as representative for the epoch of the "Middle Ages" might be rejected and even more, as I suppose, the notion implied in my description, that is, that the distance between the Middle Ages and Modernity is an enormous one. If I wanted to discuss these two aspects, however, I would have to present a complete literary history of the European Middle Ages and in addition a general history of the Occident from 500 AD up to now.

Therefore, it shall suffice to say that I do give a certain credit to the hypothesis that the characteristics mentioned above are representative of medieval literature to a certain extent. I would like to add just one remark, admittedly a bold one, concerning the following question: What does moral philosophy look like under the conditions of Modernity? In my opinion, there are two models. One of them seems to be most clearly realized in Kant: The principles of right action are not founded on experience based on the senses, but on transcendental premises. The second model is distinctly realized for the first time in Montaigne: We have nothing but the experience based on the senses, but this experience is not capable of systematically grasping the law of mobility of the social world. In the end, right action is thereby only possible by not acting at all. What remains otherwise is *reflecting* upon actions *afterwards;* its moral use is mainly to occupy a human being's time, which otherwise would be dedicated to inevitably problematic new action.

Notes

1. This is certainly not the right place to discuss the question why the Middle Ages were inclined toward an Aristotelian epistemology rather than toward a Platonic one, although Plato's philosophical tenets are much closer to Christian dogma than Aristotle's (as was already advocated by Augustine). One of the many reasons for this is, of course, the myth of incarnation. The incarnation implies a revalorization of the material world, which, for Plato, was nothing but a multitude of *eidola,* whereas for Aristotle it is the concrete material world that matters. This line of argument, by the way, would also be able to explain the waning importance of Aristotelianism from the fifteenth, sixteenth, and seventeenth centuries onward: As soon as dogma and epistemology are no longer put into an hierarchical relation but begin to be considered as two different discourses—which is one basic feature of the period we call Renaissance—it is no longer necessary to valorize epistemologically what is essential from the standpoint of dogma.

2. According to this variant the reason why the human mind has a higher faculty of abstraction than the minds of animals is solely based on the fact that the human brain is able to process the sensory data in a better and faster way; the difference between human and animal cognition is therefore only one of degree.

3. See esp. *De anima* III, 5, 430a.

4. Concerning the reception of Aristotelian epistemology in the Middle Ages, see Harry A. Wolfson, "The Internal Senses in Latin, Arabic, and Hebrew Philosophic Texts," in *Harvard Theological Review* 28 (1935): pp. 69–133; E. Ruth Harvey, *The Inward Wits: Psychological Theory in the Middle Ages and the Renaissance* (London, 1975); Leen Spruit, *Species Intelligibilis: From Perception to Knowledge*, vol. 1, *Classical Roots and Medieval Discussions* (Leiden, New York, and Cologne, 1994); J. S. Wilkie, "Body and Soul in the Aristotelian Tradition," in *The History and Philosophy of Knowledge of the Brain and Its Functions: An Anglo-American Symposium, London, July 15th–17th, 1957* (Oxford, 1958), pp. 19–28.

5. The materialistic variants flatly deny the existence of "higher," purely intelligible items of cognition (*intelligibilia*). As briefly shown above, the other variants mobilize transsensual instances in order to explain the cognition of the intelligible. With respect to these latter ones, Christianity seems to offer nothing but their continuation, but when taking a closer look it proves a qualitative leap. The extent of this leap becomes clear when taking into consideration the fact that from a Christian perspective, *ratio* is only responsible for the cognition of this world, and it is the transrational, or in other terms, the irrational category of belief which accounts for the cognition of all higher truths. This becomes most obvious in the archetypal biblical scene of a form of cognition that has shed the basis of what is perceptible by the senses. It is the moment when the risen Christ meets the disbelieving Thomas: "Dixerunt ergo ei [Thomae] alii discipuli: Vidimus Dominum. Ille autem dixit eis: Nisi videro in manibus ejus fixuram clavorum, et mittam digitum meum in locum clavorum, et mittam manum meam in latus ejus, non credam. Et post dies octo [. . .] venit Jesus [. . .] et [. . .] dicit Thomae: Infer digitum tuum huc, et vide manus meas, et affer manum tuam, et mitte in latus meum, et noli esse incredulus, sed fidelis. Respondit Thomas et dixit ei: Dominus meus, et Deus meus. Dixit ei Jesus: Quia vidisti me, Thoma, credidisti; *beati, qui non viderunt et crediderunt*" (John 20:24–29). The corresponding conceptual pattern is continued in the Eucharist. The senses are not capable of perceiving the higher "being" of the consecrated substances; more precisely: Of these substances, the senses perceive only what is absolutely irrelevant from the point of view of the higher truth.

6. *Eth. Nik.* 1099b.

7. I will mention only two especially important reasons for this reevaluation: One is the already mentioned concept of original sin; since the "soul" of every individual is considered to be created by God "in his likeness," it would be difficult to conceive of it as the "seat" of sinfulness. Of necessity, the body is the corrupt part. The postlapsarian human soul is affected by the corruption of the body; while this latter feature is an inevitable one, the corruption of the soul, though, can be palliated (by baptism, by partaking of the Eucharist, etc.). The second reason which is connected to the first stems from Pauline rhetoric (Paul seems to be the "inventor" of the concept of original sin). Confronted with the necessity to establish Christianity's identity, that is, to differentiate the newly created sect

from the mainstream of Jewish orthodoxy, Paul systematically recurs to the (asymmetrical) dichotomy of Jews as "mere flesh" and Christians as "spirit," in the sense that for a Christian believer the bodily impulses that still exist can be, or rather should be, superseded by the "spirit," which, at the same time, is the individual, God-like soul and the Spirit as one of the three "personae" of God (see chapter 8 of this volume).

8. Although he does not fully agree with Plato's concept of the tripartite human soul (*Politeia* 435a ff., esp. 437b ff.), Aristotle adopts Plato's concept of "desire" (*epithymia*); in *De anima* II, 2, 413b 23f., he says that whenever there is "sensory perception" (*aisthesis*), there is *epithymia,* and he classifies the connection as a "necessary" one (*eks anagkes*); the concept of *orexis* (perceived of as a "faculty" [*dynamis*] of the soul) comprises *epithymia* (see *De anima* II, 3, 414b 2).

9. See Romans 7:7ff., and *De civitate Dei* XIV, 16–19.

10. As far as this aspect is concerned, the main difference between the ancient pagan and the Christian viewpoint is mainly based on what I have described in the parenthesis above: From an ancient pagan, secular perspective, the senses can become a means of self-destruction only if they manage to enforce their claims to an immoderate degree. *Ratio,* however, can (nearly) always fend off this absolute unrestrainedness. At least as far as *luxuria* is concerned, a slight prompting of the senses, which in the same quantity might be considered moderate, even healthy, from an ancient pagan perspective, is already considered as deadly sinful from a Christian perspective.

11. The concept of the "hysterical" is not only meant in the sense of the current use of the word, that is, as an obsessive behavior characterized by an extreme wavering between two ways of acting which are logically contradictory. I would suggest that the medieval attitude toward the senses could be described, at least to a certain extent, with reference to the concept of hysteria as developed by Sigmund Freud and Josef Breuer in *Studien über Hysterie* (Leipzig, 1895/1922). As Freud and Breuer explain in the "Vorläufige Mitteilung" ("Über den psychischen Mechanismus hysterischer Phänomene"), hysteria is the result, respectively the product of the attempt to resolve the unsolvable conflict between impulses of desire and their repression by means of a compromise; this attempt is necessarily doomed to fail—hence the obsessiveness that is so characteristic of hysterical phenomena.

12. When I use the term "modern" with reference to history, it is always in the sense of pre-postmodern, that is, referring to the period between the middle of the seventeenth to the middle of the twentieth century. In postmodern times, to give a rough account, we experience a renaissance of the ancient evaluation of the senses.

13. One may definitely doubt that the senses and the sensual were less relevant in reality during epochs influenced by Cartesianism than in the periods before—this may or may not be the case. But there is no doubt that the senses become less relevant for anthropology, for self-reflection.

14. The text has the following epigraph: "Libro conpuesto por Alfonso Martínes de Toledo, Arcipreste de Talavera, en hedat suya de quarenta años. Acabado a quinze de março, año del nascimiento de nuestro salvador Jesuchristo de mill e quatrocientos e treynta e ocho años. Syn bautismo, sea por nonbre llamado 'Arcipreste de Talavera,' dondequier que fuere levado" / "Book, written by Alfonso Martínes of Toledo, in the fortieth year of his life. Finished on March 15, in the year 1438 after the birth of our redeemer Jesus Christ. Without baptism, it shall be called 'Archpriest of Talavera,' wherever it might be taken to." The text is quoted from the edition of Joaquín Gonzalez Muela (Madrid: Clásicos Castalia, 1970), here: p. 39). All translations are mine.

15. The incunabulum was produced in Seville, 1498.

16. The structure that I refer to is also present in other, lyrical or narrative, texts (courtly romance, mainly *Perceval;* Petrarch, *Canzoniere;* Boccaccio, *Decameron;* Fernando de Rojas, *Celestina,* etc.). Less important than this general structure seems to me the fact that in some of these texts it is the condemnation of sensuality which is at the center of attention (as is the case with *Arcipreste de Talavera*), whereas in others it rather seems to be the praise of sensual pleasures. What is remarkable, independent of this dominance, is the copresence of aspects that contradict themselves.

17. I myself have held this opinion ("Welterfahrung und Selbsterfahrung im *Arcipreste de Talavera,*" in *Romanistisches Jahrbuch* 50 (1999): pp. 364–400); for a similar view, see Marina S. Brownlee, "Hermeneutics of Reading in the *Corbacho,*" in Laurie A. Finke and Martin B. Shichtman, eds., *Medieval Texts and Contemporary Readers* (Ithaca and London, 1987), pp. 216–223), although hers is based on a different argumentation. In her essay, Brownlee makes explicit what is also true for my reading at the time: They are readings that consciously take up a hermeneutic position, readings that "update." Insofar, the rather archaeological reading that I am attempting now has different premises than my earlier one.

18. In the end, the same argument is valid for those cultures whose way to Modernity does not lead them via rationalism but empiricism. This is because the empirical method and the Aristotelian-medieval epistemology differ insofar as empiricism is based on the doubt that the "pictures" which the singular acts of sensory perception supply are reliable: Only when one perception has been confirmed by many perceptions of a similar kind, can the perceived be considered reliable, and even then only for the time being. An unconditioned esteem of the senses, as was the case under the Aristotelian auspices, is out of the question here. Modernity considers the senses either fundamentally unreliable or susceptible to errors to such an extent that they are not able to supply anything of importance without permanent systematic control by rational principles.

19. Unless otherwise noted, emphasis in quotations has been added.

20. This formula—the appeal to the perception of that which is and has hardened into experience—can be found passim throughout the whole of the text; here, I will quote only a small choice: "cada día por esperiencia veemos que [. . .]" /

"every day we see from experience that . . ." (p. 50); "E muchas veses veemos [. . .]" / "and often, we see . . ." (p. 56); "como veemos [. . .] de cada día" / "as we see every day" (S. 56); "¿Quántos, di, amigo, viste o oýste dezir que [. . .]?" / "How many, tell me, my friend, did you see or did you hear say that . . ." (p. 58); "E esto por experencia lo podemos de cada día veer" / "And this we can see every day from experience" (p. 61); "por quanto nunca vi, nin viste, nin veer esperas, [. . .]" / "therefore I never saw, nor did you see, nor do you hope to see, . . ." (pp. 63f.); "por experiençia lo verás" / "from experience you will see" (p. 64); "lo veemos de cada día por esperiencia de fecho" / "we see this every day from actual experience" (p. 69); "por quanto experiencia muestra que [. . .]" / "therefore experience shows that . . ." (S. 81); "Asý lo verás de cada día en los logares do byvieres" / "So you will see it every day, in whatever place you might live" (p. 85); "E jamás verás a ninguno avrir la mano a fazer franqueza synón a su coamante" / "and you shall never see anyone who opens his hand in order to be generous if not to his lover" (p. 104); "de cada día veemos que [. . .]" / "every day we see that . . ." (p. 146). A complete list of the respective statements would take up pages; the entries in the *Concordancias del "Arcipreste de Talavera,"* ed. Ralph de Goro and Lisa S. de Gorog (Madrid, 1978), on the verbs of sensory perception are a useful means for gaining a quick overview of this quality of the text.

21. In this article I will not discuss the question of misogyny of the *Arcipreste de Talavera;* I may only add that the text has been the aim of such reproaches in Modernity, which was to be expected (see especially, the "Introducción" by E. Michael Gerli, which precedes his edition of the text [Madrid, 1987]). On the other hand, there are also voices that award the book by Martínez de Toledo a nearly profeminist tendency judging by the standard of the time (see, e.g., David O. Wise, "Reflections of Andreas Capellanus's *De reprobatio amoris* in Juan Ruiz, Alfonso Martínez, and Fernando de Rojas," in *Hispania* [Journal of the AATSP] 63 (1980): pp. 506–509). The latter is likely to be exaggerated. However, the derogatory statements about women quoted above are matched by statements about men that exactly correspond to the first ("bestia desenfrenada" [p. 55], etc.), and after all, the text contains one out of four parts dedicated exclusively to the sins of the flesh of the men (the *tercera parte*). As to be expected from his educational background and his profession, Martínez de Toledo supports the Christian principle of equality: All humans, indifferent of their sex, age, origin, and status, are subjected to the same conditions since they are creations of one and the same God. Things look different—and this is a manifestation of antifeminism that is inevitably inherent in the text as a text of that time—when looking at the sins of the flesh of men and those of women with respect to honor, reputation, i.e., the evaluation from the point of view of society. Here, in agreement with the patriarchal principle, the sins committed by men are tolerated ("tolerado") to a certain extent while a woman loses her reputation for the rest of her life when committing only one single offence (see I, 8; quotation: p. 60).

22. In the sense of the dominant anthropological model of man.

23. A single chapter (I, 37) is dedicated to the topic of "Cómo el que ama pierde todas las virtudes" / "How the one who loves loses all of his virtues," and in this chapter there are only two pages (pp. 111f., and in addition a passage of three lines on p. 116) on which Martínez deals with the "amor loco" and the seven virtues.

24. *Studien zur Geschichte der spanischen und portugiesischen Nationalliteratur* (Berlin, 1859), pp. 232–235.

25. (Madrid, 1905), pp. 110–120; other important representatives of the same view, though sometimes their emphasis differs from that of Wolf and Menéndez Pelayo: Erich v. Richthofen, "Alfonso Martínez de Toledo und sein *Arcipreste de Talavera,* ein kastilianisches Prosawerk des 15. Jahrhunderts," *Zeitschrift für Romanische Philologie* 61 (1941): pp. 417–537, here: pp. 457–460 and pp. 530–533; Dámaso Alonso, "El Arcipreste de Talavera a medio camino entre moralista y novelista," in idem, *De los siglos oscuros al de Oro* (Madrid, 1958), pp. 125–136; E. Michael Gerli, *Alfonso Martínez de Toledo* (Boston, 1976), esp. pp. 74f.

26. See Matthew 4:1–11, and Luke 4:1–8.

27. This loss of order is to be seen in the light of the "right" order of the senses' function for cognition and desire, which was still guaranteed in ancient anthropology, while Christianity accepts this only for the God incarnate (and at best for Mary as the theotokos).

28. *Weimarer Ausgabe* 51, 126, 7ff.

29. In the case of the author, this would be the fame he wants to achieve with his book.

30. In the following, Martínez de Toledo refers back to this justification. In a sense, he does so in order to protect himself; compare, e.g., II, 10: "Por ende, a todo buen fin se dize. A buena parte, por Dios, lo tome el que lo leyere [. . .]; que el mundo es oy tan malo que byen dezir es muerte, mal dezir es gloria delectable. Esto sea quanto a mi escusación [. . .]." / "And therefore everything will be said to a good end. And pray God that he who reads it takes it for the good . . . ; because the world today is so bad that saying something good means death and saying something bad is worthy of praise. So much for my excuse" (p. 165).

31. Most of all, this is because the "classic" sins *luxuria* and *avaritia* are integrated into the story about the queen in Barcelona under the heading of *concupiscentia.*

32. As one example among many, I quote a woman's complaint about her husband reducing her spendings on clothes due to acute financial difficulties:

> E sy el marido con menester enpeña alguna aljuba o manto della, o cinta, o otra alfaja, aquí son los llantos; aquí son los gemidos, los reçongos, los çaferíos, lágrimas, e maldiciones, diziendo: -¡Ay, sin ventura de mí! Non ove yo ventura como mi vezina; que en guar de medrar desmedro. En guar de fazerme paños nuevos enpeñástesme estos captivos que en la boda me distes, e tales quales ellos son. ¿Esto esperava yo medrar conusco? ¿Asý medran las

otras? ¿Asý van adelante? -En buena fe, nunca desta casa salga y para que ayan que dezir! Ya non tengo con qué salir.-¡Ay, triste de mí! Pues, tomaldo todo [. . .]; vendedlo todo; e después syquiera esté yo enparedada e nunca salga; que vos por esto lo avedes. Pues, yo vos fartaré; yo vos contentaré; que yo vos prometo que por aquella puerta non me veáys sallir más. Yo sé qué digo. Séame Dios testigo.

And when her husband pawns one of her coats or a cape, or a ribbon or a piece of jewelry, then you hear the complaints; then you hear the sighs, the grumbling, the clamor, tears and curses, and she says: "Oh, how unlucky I am! I did not have my neighbor's luck; instead of becoming richer, I become poorer; instead of making me new clothes you pawned those fine ones you gave me for our wedding, and just like they are. Was I supposed to expect that this would happen to me? Does it happen to other women? Is this the way they walk around? By God, I never want to leave this house again, only for the others to gossip! I have nothing left to put on! Oh, poor me! There, take everything . . . ; and then, at least I want to be in my own four walls and never go out again; this is what you get! I shall satisfy you; I shall make you happy; and I promise that you shall never again see me walk through this door. I know what I am saying. God be my witness." (p. 128)

For reasons of appropriate restriction I will not go into detail concerning the portraits of the other female sins (or rather the female weaknesses, as one would have to call them according to my analysis) as there are talkativeness and a tendency toward spreading slander, especially about other women (II, 2); again material desire ("cobdicia"), although this now has become an end in itself and has lost the obligation of giving something in return (II, 3); envy of other women, especially if they are more beautiful (II, 4); fickleness and unreliability (II, 5); two-facedness and a tendency toward falseness (II, 6); disobedience and unruliness (II, 7); pride and overestimation (II, 8 and 9); a tendency toward lying (II, 10); alcoholism (II, 11); the incapability to keep secrets (II, 12); being fickle in their affection (II, 13).

33. See especially the story of the wife, the husband, and the lover in II, 10, p. 163.

34. For the poetics of the realist novel, see Joachim Küpper, *Ästhetik der Wirklichkeitsdarstellung und Evolution des Romans von der französischen Spätaufklärung bis zu Robbe-Grillet. Ausgewählte Probleme zum Verhältnis von Poetologie und literarischer Praxis* (Stuttgart, 1987).

35. As this essay is not about nineteenth-century realism, I will not discuss these other registers; it might suffice to say that for all the authors mentioned above, the paradigm of "science" (from historiography to medicine and biology) guarantees the "truth" of the narrated.

36. "[P]orque fasta aquí el amor de las mugeres fue reprovado, conviene quel amor de los onbres non sea loado. E sy las mugeres amar quisyeren los onbres,

vean quién aman" / "since the love of women has been reproved until now, it is only appropriate that the love of men shall not be praised. And if women wished to love men, then let them see who it is they love" (pp. 178–179).

37. As far as the reasons for this different treatment of the two sexes are concerned, Martínez stays rather schematic. He refers to the "general opinion" and to the Aristotelian understanding of the difference between the sexes: "E por quanto comúnmente los onbres non son reprehendidos como las mugeres so reglas generales—esto por el seso mayor e más juyzio que alcançan—, conviene, pues, particularmente fablar de cada uno segund su qualidad; e esto non se puede saber syn natural materia de los estrólogos naturales" / "And this is why men are not commonly reprimanded in this as women are, that is, according to general rules—because of the greater sense and faculty of judgment they achieve—therefore, it is necessary to speak about each man according to his nature; and this you cannot know without the natural science of the astrologers" (p. 179).

38. In III, 6, the archpriest explicitly refers to the *Secreta secretorum* (p. 186).

39. Pp. 199–203; however, the archpriest tries to maintain at least parts of a moralizing façade by constantly repeating that he is concerned with the problem of marriage ("matrimonio"). But the point of view from which he judges the four possible couplings is that of sensual pleasure alone, and he does not only know but also presents the orthodox theory of matrimonial sexuality in several passages of the book: The union of husband and wife serves the purpose of procreation; if it is practiced with the intention of gaining pleasure, it is sinful even though its conditions are "legitimate."

40. Pp. 202f.

41. Possibly in order to avoid a violation of the orthodox commandment that is too obvious, the archpriest resorts to the proceeding of only mentioning the "carnal cópula" of the model couple without going into further detail. But he portrays the other three couplings with more detail and obviously enjoys presenting all of their repulsive aspects.

42. Or, rather, it is no longer striking if one accepts my thesis. (Materialistic) determinism is the only answer to the question opened up by the *primera parte:* What is it, in essence, that causes human beings to do what they should do on no account if they followed what the *aisthesis*-based experience teaches them?

43. This is not the place to discuss the relation of the determinism that follows from a certain view of Christian dogma with deterministic aspects that are already contained in ancient pagan philosophy and moral philosophy. If we look at the first elaborate manifestation of this pagan-ancient determinism, i.e., Plato's idea of man as the "puppet of the gods" (*Nomoi* 644d; see also 645a–b, and further 803c and 804b), then we find that in the end, this statement has a different focus than the Christian idea of predestination; at least in the case of the passage just quoted, what is at stake is not an established statement but rather an assumption of the kind of a hypothesis of thought (from which conclusions are drawn afterwards; however, these are not of interest to us at the moment). Every ideological system

that works with the supposition of the existence of gods contains elements of determinism. What sense would it make to postulate the existence of gods if their power was not greater than that of the humans and if they were not able to guide the latter by it, or at least influence them? But this thought may only become a truly "hard" determinism if the omnipotent authority is to be understood as one and only one authority, which, indeed, is the case in the first commandment of the Decalogue. It is not the case with Plato, and basically with no ancient thinker, because with them it is not clear in the end what parts of the speech of "God" and at the same time of "the gods" are to be considered truth and what parts are to be seen as metaphorical.

44. Marcella Ciceri has claimed in her edition of the text (2 vols., Modena, 1975), which does without an interpretation, or a literary commentary, but which is the most exact of the recent editions, that the term *media parte* goes back to a series of mistakes by the copyists. Originally, as she says, the autograph had a simple Latin "quarta" (iiija) in its place (vol. 2, p. 8). Colbert I. Nepaulsingh presents an alternative which in my opinion seems rather bizarre. See "Talavera's Imagery and the Structure of the *Corbacho,*" *Revista canadiense de estudios hispánicos* 4 (1980): pp. 329–349, here: pp. 332–335.

45. "Aquí comiença la media parte desta obra e deste libro, que fabla del común fablar de fados, fortuna, sygnos, e planetas" / "Here, the middle part of this work and of this book begins, which deals with the widespread opinions on fortune, fate, the signs and the planets" (as the heading puts it, see p. 207).

46. "[E] desta materia non se deven las personas mucho curar nin disputar, especialmente los que deólogos mucho fundados non son, segund en el libro *De vita Christi* dixo maestre Francisco Ximenes, frayle menor" / "and the people shall neither concern themselves much with this matter nor shall they debate about it, especially those who are not established theologians, says Master Francisco Ximenes, Brother of the Minorites, in his book *De vita Christi*" (pp. 212f.). Albert G. Hauf identified the passage which Martínez quotes here and reprinted the respective passage of Eiximenis's *Vita Christi.* See "Fr. Francesc Eiximenis, O. F. M., *De la predestinaçión de Jesucristo,* y el consejo del Arcipreste de Talavera 'a los que deólogos mucho fundados non son,'" in *Archivum Franciscanum historicum* 76 (1983): pp. 239–295, here: pp. 251–253.

47. "[N]uestro Señor Dios es el que faze todas las cosas e non otro fuera dél. Pues, luego, fados, planetas, sygnos nin ventura non han este poder; que antes, como suso dixe, son regidos e governados por El [. . .] Pues, déxate de fablar de planetas e sygnos, fados e fadas, e venturas e fortunas; que todo es nada synón sólo Dios todopoderoso" / "it is Our Lord who controls everything and nobody but Him. Therefore, neither fortune nor planets nor signs nor fate have this power; rather, they are controlled and ruled by Him, as I said above . . . so this is why you shall stop to speak of planets and signs, of fortune and fairies and of fate and luck; for all of this is nothing, and only God is omnipotent" (pp. 225f.).

48. Martínez, or rather his fictitious interlocutor sets up an example of a sin-

ner who remains in his sinful state and a sinner who repents as background for posing the following question: Why does God, if He is the one who arranges and permits everything in the end, make the one repent and the other become obstinate? "Sy demandas por qué esto, responde Sant Agustín: 'Porque al Soberano asý plaze'" / "If you ask, why is this so? then Saint Augustine answers: 'Because it pleases the Almighty'" (pp. 213f.; quotation: p. 214). Further see pp. 221f., where the implications of rejecting the belief in fate are made explicit: "pues nuestro señor Dios da ser e permanecer e obrar e finir, e da sus costelaciones a las planetas e sygnos, e dél proceden todos los [movi]mientos que fazen [. . .], pues, ¿quién dubda sy Aquel que rige a tu planeta e sygno, (que) rige mayormente a ty?" / "because Our Lord gives living and staying and creating and ending, and sets the planets' and the stars' paths, and all movements that they make come from him . . . ; so who doubts that He who controls your planet and your sign of the zodiac the more controls you?"

49. As we know from the history of the version of Christianity that drew the consequences from what Martínez discusses here.

50. See esp. p. 221 and passim.

51. See p. 226.

52. "E asý nuestro Señor, segund la su grand begnidad, nos castiga por mortandades, malos tienpos, adversydades, sequedades de pocas aguas, guerras, enfermedades, pasyones, dolores de cada día e afanes. [. . .] Estas cosas e otras veemos de cada día por nuestros pecados e merescimientos" / "And therefore Our Lord punishes us, according to his kindness, with epidemics, thunderstorms, adversities, droughts caused by water shortage, wars, illnesses, passions, daily pains and efforts. . . . These and other things we witness day by day, are things that are caused by our sins and because we deserve them" (pp. 230f.).

53. "[P]or pecados, mal diziendo, mal de otros fablando o murmurando, profaçando, detratando [. . .]" / "for sins, swearing, saying bad things about others, slandering, treating badly . . ." (p. 227). If the punishment was not a graver sin, then it would lead to nothing but remaining in the first sin.

54. Martínez quotes the Augustinian *theologumenon* and without further ado equates it with the belief in the stars and in fate. As it were, the archpriest considers it over and done with from then on. The belief in stars implies *necessitas,* which, however, is not tenable for reasons of the divine omnipotence. Thereby, all other assumptions that amount to *necessitas* become untenable: "E sería venir a la fuerte materia de los precitos e predestinados, diziendo que los unos de nescesario han de ser salvos, los otros dañados" / "And this would mean getting back to the strong matter of the damned and predestined and to state that necessarily some have to be saved while the others have to be condemned" (p. 212). The question whether Martínez was not aware of the inversion of his argument he performs here or whether it was clear to him that the rejection of the *necessitas* controlled by the stars, a rejection by means of the omnipotence-argument, finally leads to the theory of a *necessitas* controlled by God (and whether Martínez foregrounds

this connection by means of his logically illicit argumentation) forms one of the abysses of the text on which we cannot throw light *ex post.*

55. "¿[Q]ué justicia o qué razón es, que el malo prospere e biva e que el bueno padesca e muera?" / "What kind of justice would it be and what sense would it make if the bad person prospered and lived, and the good person suffered and died?" (p. 219).

56. "Que desto nuestro Señor sabe quál es el malo e quál es el bueno, quál byve byen, quál byve mal; que [a] Él non se le esconde nada, e a las gentes sý" / "Because Our Lord knows who is bad and who is good, who lives well and who lives badly; because you cannot hide anything from him, but you can hide things from your fellow men" (p. 233).

57. See pp. 233f.

58. See, for example, the especially detailed explanation in Thomas Aquinas's *Reportatio super Evangelium Matthaei* VI, 5.

59. "Ay otros buenos que nuestro Señor permite que sean punidos por merescer más gualardón" / "And there are other good persons whom God allows to be afflicted by misfortune so that they can earn themselves an even greater reward" (p. 244).

60. Due to a lack of space I will leave out two thematic strands of this chapter that are quantitatively subordinate. One of them is a piece taken from popular theodicy inspired by Stoicism: The question of divine justice is answered by the "proof" that earthly happiness is in fact nothing but unhappiness. The happy person only hardens up toward his fellow men. He is more attached to life than the poor person, so that to him, death is considerably more painful. Most of all, though, he is envied. There is no one around him, neither his spouse nor blood relations who do not wish him to die so that they can have the earthly possessions at their own disposal (see pp. 247f. and pp. 255–257). The second strand is the quotation from orthodox teaching about the influence of the stars on earthly doings (which cannot be denied completely in the light of the Ptolemaic worldview): The stars have power over everything that ranks below them in the hierarchy of being. Concerning man, this is his body. The soul ranks above the stars because it is created by God and in God's image. Therefore, the stars cannot influence free will, while the latter in turn can in principle control the body (see pp. 249f.).

61. Martínez himself refers to Boccaccio (see p. 251), and Erich v. Richthofen has identified the exact source ("Alfonso Martínez de Toledo," pp. 478–482, with a reprint of Boccaccio's version [*De casibus virorum illustrium* III, 1]). Harriet Goldberg has compared the two versions by Boccaccio and Martínez and has come to the conclusion that the two authors' intentions and the two versions' messages are quite different. Goldberg is of the opinion that Martínez is concerned with the propagation of the notion of free will (this is absolutely true, although it opens up questions that Goldberg does not see), while Boccaccio, according to her, refers to the concept that everyone is responsible for his respective misfortune. See "Fifteenth-Century Castilian Versions of Boccaccio's Fortune-Poverty Contest,"

in *Hispania* 61 (1978): pp. 472–479. In his article on the parallel, E. Michael Gerli has mainly concentrated on an aspect which, mutatis mutandis, is also true for the relation of the *Arcipreste de Talavera* and Andreas Capellanus: The Spanish version is considerably longer than its source; here, as elsewhere, Martínez uses the method of a wealth of details which is so typical of his style. See "Boccaccio and Capellanus: Tradition and Innovation in *Arcipreste de Talavera,*" in *Revista de estudios hispánicos*" 12 (1978): pp. 255–274, here: pp. 260–265.

62. See p. 276.

63. This style's main features are redundancy of thought, a tendency toward digression and a stereotyped manner of expression. It is known that the author produced texts of a similar kind in oral form when he was court chaplain of Juan II. The style of the *Arcipreste de Talavera* has therefore often been categorized as "preaching style"—which would be reasonable if it did not include the opinion that the text's argumentation was on the level of naïve lay preaching didactics (see esp. Gerli, *Alfonso Martínez de Toledo,* pp. 77–107 ["The Whip and the Pulpit"]).

64. This is the difference between Christian and Islamic monotheism, and this difference might be a serious obstacle to coexistence. It looks like either the West has to accept determinism and thereby revoke Modernity completely, or Islam has to renounce its "hard" monotheism in favor of a semi-syncretism and -polytheism whose flexibility (as I assume) accounts for the enormous success of the Western model. Although I now do not want to start that discussion here, as a rudimentary hint let me add that the Occident's resistance to determinism can on the one hand be explained by its reception of the Greek philosophical tradition already in early Christianity, and continuously from then on; on the other hand, a lot is due to the fact that in the beginning, Christianity was a (Jewish) sect. Whether the etymology (*sequi*) is true or not, sects demand a *decision* to follow the respective teaching. The ideological basis of sects is always elitist, and they keep their antideterministic elements that are bound to the freedom of choice of each individual even when they become a "generally" accepted, predominant system to explain the world. This elitist and activist feature might, by the way, also be a viable explanation for Judaism's highly developed adaptability to an ever-changing world; Judaism shares with Islam the concept of a "pure" monotheism (as compared to Christianity); but in contrast to its Islamic counterpart, the Jewish version of monotheism is not universalist. It is a "communitarian" monotheism, which is a logical contradiction and from a historical perspective hints to the status of Judaism as a monotheism in the state of emergence.

So, the two logically precarious variants of the three monotheisms known to us seem to be more effective; this might be astonishing at first sight, but perhaps monotheism as the logically most coherent version of the belief in gods needs elements to counterbalance what may be an excess of logicalness. In view of Protestantism, the variant of Christianity which gives more significance to determinism than Catholicism, I will only add very briefly that its understanding of determinism is always a "hidden" one: The Protestant believer is determined in either way, but he never knows for certain in which way. Because of this not-knowing, he acts as if he had alternatives of action; he tries to act as though he would if he were an *electus.*

65. For a documentation of the discussion, see Gerli's edition of the text, "Introducción," p. 26, including the annotations, and the detailed report by Mercedes Turón, "La enmienda de *El Arcipreste de Talavera* escrita por Martínez de Toledo," in *Revista del Instituto de lengua y cultura españolas* 4 (1988): pp. 99–128.

66. It is true that where the text is concerned with a positive valorization of the faculties of the senses, it foregrounds their cognitive capacities. However, particularly in the portraits of men and women, the *segunda* and the *tercera parte* contain many passages that praise rather freely the senses as means of desire and its fulfilment. And finally, one might ask whether this can be achieved at all: to ascribe an unreservedly positive (cognitive) function to one and the same component of the comprehensive system called "human being," here, to the senses, and at the same time unreservedly anathematize these very senses as the gate of entry to doom.

8 Christian Sovereignty and Jewish Flesh

David Nirenberg

In the fall of 1449 a university graduate of obscure lineage and no previous literary experience took up his quill in Toledo. He was writing under pressure. Outside the gates were ranged the forces that would tomorrow capture the city. But today he wrote in defense of his actions and those of like-minded compatriots. He wrote, that is, in defense of Toledo's rebellion against its king, and of the peculiar form that rebellion had taken: the killing of neighbors descended from the many Jews who had converted to Christianity over the past sixty years, and the passage of a municipal ordinance barring any such people from ever holding public office.

The "Bachiller Marcos" knew himself to be in a difficult position, one so difficult that even his choice of address was a tortured one:

> [I address this letter] to the very Holy Father . . . , and to the very high and powerful king or prince or administrator to whom, according to God, law, reason and right there belongs the administration and governance of the realms . . . , and to all other . . . administrators in the spiritual and temporal [affairs] of the universal orb, in the Church militant, which is the congregation and university of faithful Christians, [that is, those] truly believing in the birth, passion and resurrection [etc.] . . . , [but I do not address it to] the unbelieving and the doubtful in the faith, who are outside of us and in confederation [*ayuntamiento*] with the synagogue, which is to say a congregation of beasts, for since such bind themselves like livestock to the letter, they have always given and still give false meaning to divine and human scripture. [In short, I address this letter to those] attesting to the truth and saying: "the letter kills, the spirit vivifies (2 Cor 3:6)."[1]

In the Bachelor's discriminating salutation we recognize a political distinction between a community that lives the purely carnal and material life of animals, and one that exists for the sake of a higher good.[2] The Bachelor writes only to "administrators" in the latter community, the "congregation and university of faithful Christians." Specifically excluded are those who live as "Jewish" beasts. Creatures of carnality, they have lost the human right to participate in the republic, and whatever power they wield is by definition tyrannical, not sovereign. We know exactly who he had in mind: the royal favorite cum prime minister Alvaro de Luna, the King Juan II who supported him, and even the pope, if he ended up rejecting the Bachelor's appeal and ruling in favor of the king.

Onto the oppositions of "Jew" and Christian, beast and human, material life and spiritual life, tyrant and legitimate magistrate, the Bachelor maps yet another: killing letter and vivifying spirit. Through this formulation, borrowed from St. Paul, the Bachelor proposes a literacy test for citizenship.[3] Those who read like Jews, literally after the flesh, deprive themselves of legitimate authority and exclude themselves from the human community, becoming beasts of the synagogue. If no prince can be found who reads like a Christian, the treatise concludes, then the city should place itself directly under the governance of the Holy Spirit.

The royalists soon retook Toledo, and the Bachelor was hanged in the public square. His treatise became a founding document of the Castilian ideology of "purity of blood," hence of importance to anyone interested in the history of racial ideologies in Spain and its colonies. But it is as an example of a particular logic of revolution that his claim on our time is both more urgent and more general. Sovereignty and freedom, as the Bachelor expounded them, required the "spirit" to achieve the political subjection of flesh and the hermeneutic subjection of letter. The reverse produced, not sovereignty, but tyrannical materialism. Within the Bachelor's political theology this materialism was best understood as "Jewish," and the struggle for sovereignty could best be represented as a struggle against the "Jews." The political perfectibility of the world therefore required, as a very different revolutionary put it more famously some four centuries later, "*the emancipation of society from Judaism.*"[4]

The quote from Marx is meant only to suggest the degree to which variants (sometimes secularized) of the Bachelor's political theology saturated Enlightenment and Modernity. With the triumph of "American materialism," the globalization of economic systems, and the emergence of the state of Israel as a focal point for the aspirations to sovereignty of Muslims across the world, that saturation is in some ways even more complete today. It may well be that at present more people than ever before understand their struggles, whether against racism, the institutions of global capitalism, or political oppression, in terms of resistance to domination by materialist "Jews" and their "agents." All the more pressing is the need for a history of the terms, ideas, and discourses through which this understanding is conceived and expressed.[5]

It should already be evident that this history has deep philosophical and theological roots. In order to uncover these roots I will describe how the fruitful flesh of the Jew nourished the growth of a theory of reading into a theory of politics central to the expression of early Christian (and early Islamic) aspirations to sovereignty.[6] We will then explore briefly some implications of this exceptional status of the Jew for the development of Christian politics in the medieval monarchies of Western Europe.[7] My claim, of course, is that this history is crucial to any understanding of the places assigned to Jews and Judaism within later Christian (and Muslim) ideologies. The modern trajectory of these ideas I leave to extrapolation, but the Bachelor himself dictates our starting point. "The letter kills, but the spirit gives life": we must begin with Paul.

Reading through Jewish Flesh

Saul's fall upon the road to Damascus, and his subsequent recovery as Paul, transformed the meaning of Jews and Judaism forever. As soon as he was healed he began to preach, first to the Jews and then to the gentiles, about (among many other things) the relationship of the Jews to Jesus. The interpretation of the textual records of this preaching (i.e., the Pauline Epistles) bristles with complexity.[8] Paul, like other early Christians both Jewish and gentile, confronted two important "Jewish questions." The first had to do with the past. How was the ancient covenant given to Abraham, and its textual expression in the form of the Hebrew Bible, related to the new promise of Jesus? Could it be appropriated? Rejected? The second was a subquestion of the first. How should followers of Jesus act in the present? Should they, or should they not, observe Jewish practices and rituals?[9]

Paul's letters to the Galatians and the Romans provide the earliest surviving treatment of these questions. In them he articulated a fierce universalism aimed at all the particular identities that his society held most sacred.[10] "God shows no partiality" (Gal. 2:6). "There is neither Jew nor Greek, there is neither slave nor free, there is neither male nor female; for you are all one in

Christ Jesus" (Gal. 3:28). Such universalism was not entirely novel. It was underwritten both by Pharisaic beliefs in the messianic ingathering of gentiles, and by a widespread philosophical dualism (often called "Neoplatonic") that stressed the existence of an idealized brotherhood in the spirit, and emphasized the superiority of that spiritual state over the many differences of body and of circumstance that marked the flesh of living beings. But Paul (or at least his later readers) came to define his universalism against one particular status that had previously been almost entirely ignored by the Greek philosophical tradition. Not gender or condition of liberty, but Judaism, served as the constant target of Paul's eloquence. This is clear even in the structure of Galatians 3:28 cited above, which concludes in pointed fashion: "And if you are Christ's then you are Abraham's offspring, heirs according to promise." Of all the antinomies of identity from which it was constructed, the category of Jew, of descendent of Abraham, most needed to be expanded in order to make room for other "heirs." Paul's universalism was articulated in terms of a struggle for control over the Jewish past and future. It is in this struggle that later generations carved out the exceptional space occupied by Jews and Judaism in Christendom.

To the extent that Jews refused to surrender their ancestors, their lineage, and their identity, they became emblematic of the particular, of stubborn adherence to the conditions of the flesh, enemies of the Gospel. Paul did not believe this enmity to be permanent.[11] It was necessary that the Jews stumble, for their "rejection meant the reconciliation of the world." But they will receive mercy, be grafted back again, and their reacceptance will mean "nothing less than life from the dead" (Rom. 11:1–15). His is a message of a necessary but temporary blindness, a hardening of heart like Pharaoh's, produced by God for the salvation of the world (Rom. 9:17). Hence Paul's extraordinary conception of "Jewish enmity": "As regards the Gospel, they are enemies, but for your sake; but as regards those who are God's choice, they are still well loved for the sake of their ancestors" (Rom. 11:28). Jews who do not recognize Jesus as Messiah are the exemplary enemies of Christ's followers, but also the beloved foundations of their salvation: a charitable enmity whose political depths will be plumbed in the following pages.[12]

Paul's position was motivated in part by the tension between two convictions: that of the ongoing relevance of God's promise to Abraham, and of the extension of that promise beyond Abraham's descendents in the flesh. Had Paul desired to abandon Judaism or condemn its scriptures as false (as many would soon do), Judaism might have become no more important to ancient

Christians than any other of the myriad ethnic identities they were capable of ignoring as spiritually insignificant. But he did not, and Judaism became a key term in Christian hermeneutics. Paul's letters were primers for a practice of reading meant to transform the meaning of Abraham's biography:

> For it is written that Abraham had two sons, one by a slave and one by a free woman. But the son of the slave was born according to the flesh, the son of the free woman through promise. Now this is an allegory: these women are two covenants. One is from Mount Sinai, bearing children for slavery: she is Hagar . . . she corresponds to the present Jerusalem, for she is in slavery with her children. But the Jerusalem above is free, and she is our mother. . . . Now we, brethren, like Isaac are children of promise. . . . But what does scripture say? "Cast out the slave and her son; for the son of the slave shall not inherit with the son of the free woman." (Gal. 4:22–30)

Abraham's families, one slave, one free, here unleash a chain of allegorical significations. Hagar and Ishmael represent flesh and slavery, Sarah and Isaac promise and freedom. Thus far the reading would not have shocked. But next comes an earthquake. Hagar and Ishmael, flesh and slavery, are associated with the law given on Mt. Sinai and historical Jerusalem. Sarah and Isaac are a new covenant and a heavenly city. One allegorical stroke reverses the traditional readings of this story. The Mosaic Law and the people and polity that observe it are, insofar as they reject Jesus, not the heirs of God's promise to Abraham, but are condemned as "of the flesh," sentenced to slavery and exile. This terrestrial Jerusalem is replaced by the spiritual Jerusalem set free by faith in Jesus. The same technique Paul applies here to the covenant with Abraham he applies elsewhere to the specific practices through which that covenant was announced. Abraham's circumcision, for example, emerged from under the pressure of Paul's stylus as merely a "sign or seal of the righteousness which he had by faith while he was still uncircumcised" (Rom. 4:11).

The style of reading through which Paul achieved this translation from promise in the flesh to promise in the spirit was not a novel one. Word and meaning were arrayed against each other in a hierarchy explicitly parallel to that of flesh and spirit. The task of a reader was to penetrate beyond the "letter," the sign, the outer body (*soma*) or literal meaning of a text, and into its inner or spiritual meaning. Such reading practices were standard amongst both Jews and gentiles familiar with Hellenistic philosophy.[13] What was surprising about Paul were not his methods but his conclusions: once the inner meaning was understood, the literal meaning could be dispensed with. As he put it in Romans 7:5–6, "For when we were still in the flesh, our sinful passions, stirred up by the law, were at work in our members to bear fruit for death. But now we are fully freed from the law, dead to that in which we lay captive. We can thus serve in the new being of the Spirit and not the old one of the letter." It is not just the law that is left behind by the spiritual believer and reader, but also the companions that Paul everywhere associates with it: the letter, and even flesh itself.

Paul valued the spiritual world much more highly than the phenomenal one through which it was perceived. He was convinced that the end of the material and the beginning of the messianic world was near. But he did not represent the material world and its organic necessities as evil. In his letters to the Corinthians, for example, the body (*soma*) appears, not as the "tomb" (*sema*) favored by so many authors, but as a sheltering tent (2 Cor. 5:1–4). And if on the one hand, Christians "long to be exiled from the body" and "look not at the things which are seen, but at the things which are not seen" (2 Cor. 5:8, 4:18), yet conversely the spiritual requires the physical. "If there is a physical body, there is also a spiritual body. . . . But it is not the spiritual which is first, but the physical, and then the spiritual" (1 Cor. 15:42–50).[14] Still, on the topic of Judaism Paul's dualism was more systematic, his condemnation of flesh more severe. The first of two difficulties that pushed him toward extremes has already been mentioned: the need to distinguish between the fleshly and the spiritual heirs of Abraham. To this end Paul characterized the many Jews who did not believe in Jesus as pure flesh. This Israel could not even be said to be truly alive. A branch cut from the vine (Rom. 11:17–24), she was an inanimate form, a body without spirit. Into this vessel Paul repeatedly poured the dangers of reading and believing "after the flesh."

The carnality of Israel comes into sharpest polemical focus only when Paul confronts a second difficulty, the question of gentile Christian adherence to the mandates of Jewish law. Among Jewish believers in Christ such adherence was for Paul at best commendable—perhaps even required—at worst a matter of indifference.[15] Among gentile converts, however, it was a horrifying symptom of literalism, evidence that they had not understood Christ's message, nor the practice of interpretation that conveyed it. When, for example, the non-Jewish Christians of Galatia circumcised themselves they placed significance in the sign rather than in what it signified, and thereby revealed themselves as "severed from Christ" and Spirit by the "desires of the flesh" (Gal. 5:4, 16–18). Gentiles, Paul insisted, ought to become heirs of Abraham in the spirit without becoming Jews in the flesh. "To set the mind on the flesh is death, but to set the mind on the Spirit is life and peace. For the mind that is set on the flesh is hostile to God . . . and those who are in the flesh cannot please God" (Rom. 8:6–8).

It is not the evils of Judaism that Paul is here concerned with, but those of gentile *Judaizing*. Paul himself invented the word in Galatians 2:14, in order to describe gentile Christian observance of Jewish laws and rituals.[16] As he presents it in Galatians and Romans, the danger is not that Jews seduce Christians to their ways, but that gentile Christians are attracted to the old honors of Israel: "the glory was theirs and the covenants; to them were given the Law and the worship of God and the promises. To them belong the fathers and out of them, so far as physical descent is concerned, came Christ who is above all" (Rom. 9:4–5). These privileges are real, but the gentile who yields to their attractions expresses doubt in the power of Christ's grace, and thereby becomes infected by the flesh. As Paul put it in a different context, "do you not know that only a little yeast leavens the whole batch of dough?" (1 Cor. 5:6). Paul's rhetoric against Torah grows most heated when he attempts to quarantine its temptations for gentiles. It is only in those moments that Judaism emerges as the antipode of spirit, as dead letter, killing flesh.[17]

Sharpening Enmity: Gospel Hermeneutics and Jewish Hypocrisy

There is a vast and contentious literature on how the authors of the Gospels, all writing after Paul, after the destruction of Jerusalem and its Jewish Temple in 70 CE, and for an audience now largely gentile, transposed and amplified these themes.[18] For our purposes we need remember only three points. First, all the Gospel authors stress the prophetically ordained enmity of those Jews who rejected Jesus (or some representative subset of them, such as the Pharisees) not only toward the Messiah and his followers, but also toward God. Their hatred proves the truth of Jesus's message, and defines his community as one of spirit. "You stubborn people . . . you are always resisting the Holy Spirit. . . . Can you name a single prophet your ancestors never persecuted? They killed those who foretold the coming of the Upright One, and now you have become his betrayers, his murderers" (Acts 7:51–53. Cf. Acts 28:28; John 8:44–47).

Second, that enmity is conceived of hermeneutically, in terms of a disjuncture between seeming and being, outer and inner moral state, form and meaning. Matthew and Luke explore this disjuncture repeatedly through the theme of the Pharisees (mentioned twenty-nine times in Matthew, twenty-seven in Luke) and their hypocrisy. In the Sermon on the Mount, for example, Jesus preaches "the seven woes of the Pharisees," seven indictments that describe in deafening crescendo the different ways in which the Pharisees confuse appearance with reality (Matt. 23:25–32). Let the sixth be representative: "Alas for you, scribes, and Pharisees, you hypocrites! You are like whitewashed tombs that look handsome on the outside, but inside are full of the bones of the dead and every kind of corruption. In just the same way, from the outside you look upright, but inside you are full of hypocrisy and lawlessness." The Pharisees pride themselves as heirs of the prophets and guardians of their tombs, when in fact they are tombs themselves, about to prove their own corruption and hypocrisy by sending yet another prophet to his grave. Here, as elsewhere in the Gospels, the tension between body and spirit resolves in the direction of the empty carnality, the living death, of the Jews.[19]

Third, the conception of Jewish enmity in terms of hypocrisy allowed Matthew and Luke to develop what we might call a theory of infection, an anxiety about the ease with which "Pharisaic" attributes could overwhelm the Christian. They summarized this theory in an apt biological metaphor: "Be on your guard against the yeast of the Pharisees—their hypocrisy. Everything now covered will be uncovered, and everything now hidden will be made clear" (Luke 12:1–2). Matthew uses similar words, but provides a terrifying example:

> The disciples, having crossed to the other side, had forgotten to take any food. Jesus said to them, "Keep your eyes open, and be on your guard against the yeast of the Pharisees and the Sadducees." And they said among themselves, "It is because we have not brought any bread." Jesus knew it, and he said, "You have so little faith, why are you talking among yourselves about having no bread? Do you still not understand? . . . How could you fail to understand that I was not talking about bread? What I said was: Beware the yeast of the Pharisees and Sadducees." Then they understood that he was telling them to be on their guard, not against yeast for making bread, but against the teachings of the Pharisees and Sadducees. (Matt. 16:5–12)

Here, at the very moment that Jesus warns his closest associates about the dangers of "Pharisaism," they act like "Pharisees" themselves. Rather than understanding his statement metaphorically and spiritually they understand it literally and materially, in the context of their own bodily hunger. The danger is inherent in the nature of language itself. How can we know if Jesus spoke literally or metaphorically of "yeast," of "bread," or of "Pharisees"? Because the authors of Matthew and Luke understood the relationship between the "thing" a word referred to and its "higher meanings" (metaphor, allegory, etc.) in terms of the relationship between perishable flesh and eternal spirit, these linguistic questions encapsulated for them the difficulty of understanding the relationship between the material world and the divine Word. At the crossroads of these questions, representing the possibility of confusion in its purest form, they placed the Jews.

Dualism versus Incarnation: The Theological Labor of Jewish Flesh

For the Gospel authors this confusion may have been sociological as well as exegetical. The fourth Gospel's stark vocabulary of Jewish enmity, for example, is often attributed to the trauma of the Johannine community's expulsion from their local synagogue.[20] The utility of Jewish enmity for the Christian communities of the second and later Patristic centuries, however, derived much more exclusively from philosophical questions about the relationship between matter and spirit that had little to do with real Jews, though they were expressed in terms of Judaism. One of these many questions concerned the status of the Messiah himself. Was Jesus Christ a man or a god? The question was in some ways as difficult for the increasingly gentile and Hellenistic believers of the second century as it had been for the Jews of Jesus's day. Readers in the Greek Platonic and Aristotelian philosophical traditions were not accustomed to thinking of the highest deity in material terms, or as suffering change. How then to approach Jesus Christ? Many pathways were proposed. At one extreme were the various groups who held that Jesus was a human being of flesh and blood, not born of a virgin, who was chosen (or adopted) by God to carry out His will on earth. At the other were those who believed Christ to be entirely a god, incapable of suffering or death, only appearing human for the sake of His audience. In between were many communities holding a variety of positions, including some that seemed to many contemporaries paradoxical and incoherent but that we now think of in retrospect as orthodox, namely, that Jesus was both fully man and fully God.[21]

Perhaps the most influential opponent of such paradox was a second-century Christian named Marcion (fl. 139–156). The tension that Marcion saw between flesh and spirit was so severe that it called for complete separation. Not only could the highest god not assume a corruptible body, he could not even produce one, for to do so would be to suffer change. An evil "creator" god was the author of the flesh and everything material. The savior god was a "stranger" to the world, concerned only with soul and spirit. And just as there were two creations there were also two scriptures.[22] The god of matter's scripture was the Hebrew Bible. The Stranger's scripture was a Gospel (Luke, according to Irenaeus) and ten Pauline Epistles, all purged of any "Jewish" traits (such as quotations from the Hebrew Bible) that might lessen the starkness of the oppositions Marcion understood them to contain.[23]

Marcion read Paul as a dualist. What we today may want to characterize as Paul's ambivalence toward flesh, Marcion and many others saw as utter condemnation.[24] Marcion systematically expressed his rejection of material creation in terms of a rejection of letter, law (meaning Jewish scripture), and above all, Judaism. In this again he believed he was following Paul, whose clear opinions had been obscured by the textual tampering of Judaizing Christians intent on concealing the message of the savior god. So far as we know, Marcion's predilection for distilling the evils of flesh into Judaism had nothing to do with his experiences of, or competition with, real Jews. Rather it was driven by his readings of those Pauline passages, especially in Galatians and Romans, which described the existence of a "law of the flesh" and expressed the dangers of that law in terms of Judaizing. The importance of this reading cannot be overemphasized, for it turned Jews and Judaism into a popular arena for contests over the relationship between matter and spirit, man and God, and over the texts and sacraments that mediate between them.

One of the most important of these contests was over the content and the meaning of scripture. Marcion entirely rejected the books of the Jews, attributed their authorship to the evil creator of the material world, and purged his own collection of any references that obscured the sharp distinctions he saw between the scriptures of spirit and the scriptures of flesh. His was, in fact, the first systematic attempt to delineate the form and boundaries of a Christian scriptural canon, and it precipitated an explosion of debate and activity, ranging from forgery to philology, out of which the canonical "New Testament" was born.[25]

The largest question Marcion raised about the shape of the Christian canon was over the status of the Hebrew Bible. As Tertullian put it in 207 CE, "The separation of Law and Gospel is the primary and principal exploit of Marcion. . . . For such are Marcion's *Antitheses,* or Contrary Oppositions, which are designed to show the conflict and disagreement of the Gospel and the Law, so that from the diversity of principles between those two documents they may argue further for a diversity of gods."[26] It was in its response to this separation, and in defense of the unity of scripture both Old and New, that Christianity elaborated its most fateful attitudes toward the Jew. Justin Martyr, a contemporary and outspoken opponent of Marcion's, is exemplary in this regard. His rebuttal of the dualists, an inspiration to like-minded polemicists for centuries to come, was staged in the form of the "Dialogue with Trypho the Jew" (circa 150 CE). According to Justin, the dualists reject the Hebrew Bible and its God because they do not know how to read it. Understood literally, the Law is indeed carnal. God gave it in this literal form because of the Jews' hardness of heart, but meant it to be read allegorically, and its true meaning was always spiritual. The circumcision of the heart, the Sabbath in Christ, these were the true messages revealed through the ancient prophets. The Jews themselves had never grasped this. Because they read literally and believed carnally, they failed to see that the preincarnate Christ had authored their scriptures (or "rather not yours, but ours") in order to proclaim His truth, and failed as well to recognize their God when He walked among them in the flesh. The dualists, in their literal reading of the Law, simply repeat this error. Tertullian's later formulation of this position was characteristically pithy: "Let the heretic now give up borrowing poison from the Jew."[27]

The Jewish focus of these antidualist polemics was a strategy to defend an "orthodox" Christian reading of Hebrew scripture from the dualists' charge of Judaizing and demonic carnality, and to return that same charge to the dualists themselves. For Justin, Tertullian, Origen, and others, the Law understood literally was indeed a curse, but spiritually a blessing. Because the Jews had never understood this, they had never been the true Israel. The Law's spirituality was concealed only by the blindness of its readers. If the Marcionites could not see it, this was because they were like the Jews, creatures of pure carnality.

In short, these theologians saved the prophets from the dualists' attack by using allegory to deprive the Jews of their scriptures, and the scriptures of their Jews. From their point of view such thoroughgoing "de-Judaization" had two great, if somewhat contradictory, virtues. On the one hand it countered dualist readings of the Law's carnality, casting such readings as themselves "Jewish." On the other, it widened the gap between literal meaning and spiritual truth, and therefore served as a powerful antidote to the concern with Judaizing that preoccupied Christian exegetes of the Law since the days of Paul. But the reader who would hold these virtues together in one hand had to fend off irony with the other. For insofar as they radically devalued the literal, historical, and carnal meanings of scripture, the allegorists themselves risked becoming dualists.[28]

Exiling the Jew into Letter and Flesh

That this risk was keenly felt is evident in the controversy over the biblical interpretations of Origen (ca. 185–252/3). According to Origen biblical texts often did not make sense, or even proved false, on a literal level. This was especially true of large parts of the Old Testament, but also of bits of the New. Their divine Author clearly meant us to understand that these texts had no literal sense or truth, but only a spiritual one.[29] These truths Origen set out to provide. His allegories, first in Greek and then in Rufinus's Latin translation, crashed like waves over the fourth-century Church.[30] It is upon their crests, for example, that St. Jerome, author of the standard Latin translation of the Bible, rode to prominence. Others, however, emphasized the danger rather than the sport inherent in such readings. Chief among these was a young North African bishop, a fervent debater of heretics and himself a recovering dualist, the future saint Augustine.

Augustine entirely agreed with his predecessors about the dangers of language, and expressed them with characteristic clarity in his *De doctrina christiana* (III.9): "The ambiguities of metaphorical words . . . demand extraordinary care and diligence. What the Apostle says pertains to this problem. 'For the letter killeth, but the spirit quickeneth.' That is, when that which is said figuratively is taken as though it were literal, it is understood carnally. Nor can anything more appropriately be called the death of the soul than that condition in which the thing that distinguishes man from beasts, which is the understanding, is subjected to the flesh in pursuit of the letter." Like Justin Martyr before him and the Bachelor Marcos after, Augustine concurred that to read *carnaliter* was to become a beast like the Jews. But he disagreed strongly with those who would solve the problem by eliminating literal meaning, and by extension the Jews who symbolized it. The nature of this disagreement becomes especially evident in the series of letters (dating from 395 to 404) he exchanged with Jerome, letters that reveal the dangerous potential of the fleshy Jew lurking in the Christian text.

Augustine insists that passages of scripture can never be accounted literally untrue, lest "nowhere in the sacred books shall the authority of pure truth stand sure" (Ep. 28.4, cf. Ep. 40, 3.3). Denial of literal truth opens the door to heretics like the Manichees, "perverse men" who dismiss Pauline passages awkward to their cause as falsehoods uttered for some strategic purpose rather than literal truths. "I would devote all the strength which the Lord grants me, to show that every one of those texts which are wont to be quoted in defense of the expediency of falsehood ought to be otherwise understood, in order that everywhere the sure truth of these passages themselves may be consistently maintained" (Ep. 28, 3.5).[31] Augustine concentrates his efforts upon a text often cited by the allegorists precisely because it synthesized the problem of Judaizing and the problem of reading into one conflict both potent and apostolic. The text was Paul's exhortation to Peter in Galatians 2:11–14: "If you, though a Jew, live like a Gentile and not like a Jew, how can you compel the Gentiles to Judaize?" Following Origen, Jerome denied that Peter could ever have required gentile Christians to live according to Jewish law (Ep. 75, III.7, citing Acts 10:10–16). It was absurd to believe that either Paul or Peter would have recognized the ongoing validity of the Law and its practice, either for Jewish Christians or for gentile ones. Paul had merely said these things in order to "soothe troublesome opponents," just as he sometimes pretended to observe Jewish law, not out of principle but in order to escape persecution (Ep. 28, 3.4; 40, 3.3).[32]

Augustine's position was a radically different one. "Paul was indeed a Jew; and when he had become a Christian he had not abandoned those Jewish sacraments which that people had received in the right way, and for a certain appointed time" (Ep. 40, 4.4). Paul, like Peter, observed Jewish laws, "but with this view, that he might show that they were in no wise hurtful to those who, even after they had believed in Christ, desired to retain the ceremonies which by the law they had learned from their fathers." Peter's error consisted only in this: out of fear he had agreed to compel gentile converts to observe Jewish ceremonies, and in so doing gave the false impression that these were "still necessary for salvation."

Perhaps the best evidence for the sting of Augustine's argument was the grace with which it was met. For years Jerome did not answer Augustine's letters, judging them "tainted with heresy" (Ep. 72, I.2). When in 404 he finally did reply, it was ungenerously. Augustine was insisting, Jerome claimed, that Jewish law remained binding on all Jews, even after they converted to Christ. In this he was "reintroducing within the Church the pestilential heresy" of the Ebionites and other Judaizing sects. If such opinions were countenanced, Jerome warned, the ongoing conversion of Jews to Christianity would destroy the Church. "If . . . it shall be declared lawful for them to continue in the Churches of Christ what they have been accustomed to practice in the Synagogues of Satan, I will tell you my opinion in the matter: they will not become Christian, but will make us Jews" (Ep. 75, IV.13).

Jerome's ferocity was symptomatic but unwarranted. Augustine did not claim that observance of the Law was binding on converts from Judaism. What he did say, most clearly in the treatise "Against Faustus the Manichee" (*Contra Faustum*) of 398 as well as in his correspondence with Jerome, was that such observance was not prohibited to the apostolic generation; that it was understandable as the product of habit and custom; and that the apostles had favored it as a theologically advisable approach toward the Torah, "lest by compulsory abandonment it should seem to be condemned rather than closed" (*CF* XIX.17). The ritual practice of the apostolic generation served as widow's weeds, a reminder of the Law's place in sacred history and a reproach to those who would deny that it had ever been beloved. But such behavior was acceptable only for these first generations. After the burial of the Synagogue, Torah observance became a type of necrophilia, the fruitless loving of an empty letter.

Augustine claimed Hebrew scripture for Christianity by turning Jews into the living dead. Jews after the killing of Christ were like Cain after the killing of Abel, both hypercarnal and alienated from the world (*CF* XII.9–13). Not even their Law would give them fruit any longer: "they continue to till the ground of an earthly circumcision, . . . while the hidden strength or virtue of making known Christ, which this tilling contains, is not yielded to the Jews. . . . The veil which is on their minds in reading the Old Testament is not taken away." Carnal as they are, the Jews are in the end alienated even from their own mortal flesh, as Cain had been: "So Cain . . . said: . . . 'I shall be a mourner and an outcast on the earth, and it shall be that everyone who finds me shall slay me.' . . . 'Not so,' [God] says; 'but whosoever shall kill Cain, vengeance shall be taken on him sevenfold.' That is . . . not by bodily death shall the ungodly race of carnal Jews perish. . . . So to the end of the seven days of time the continued preservation of the Jews will be a proof to believing Christians of the subjection merited by those who . . . put the Lord to death."[33]

The Marcionites, Manicheans, and other dualists had stripped Christ of His flesh and Christianity of Hebrew scripture. Their "orthodox" opponents retained both flesh and scripture, but did so by stripping the latter of its Jews, that is, of its literal and historical meaning. Against both of these Augustine posed a historical realism, one that restored a literal and spiritual value to the Torah and its people.[34] His hermeneutic domesticated (though it could not entirely tame) the tendency of letter and meaning, flesh and spirit, "Old Testament" Jew and "New Testament" Christian, to fly toward opposite poles. But it did so by alienating the Jews who walk the earth after Jesus from their own texts and history, converting them into corporeal shells of flesh without spirit. A series of linguistic metaphors drives home the point. "Like milestones along the route the Jews inform the traveler, while they themselves remain senseless and immobile." The Jews are "living letters of the Law," "desks" of the Christians, adhering fruitlessly to "Jewish form" (*forma Iudaeorum*) but knowing as little of its content as a blind man knows of his face in the mirror.[35] More than any other Church Father Augustine was master of the paradoxical union of material and divine. Yet he achieved his alchemy in the same alembic as Paul, Marcion, or Jerome, distilling the danger of flesh and letter into an exceptional condensate of the Jew.

From Language to Politics: Sovereignty of Spirit, Tyranny of Flesh

Thus far the focus has been semiotic, the goal to explore some hermeneutic consequences of the dialectical tension in early Christian thought between the visible, carnal, and literal, on the one hand, and the invisible, spiritual, and nonliteral, on the other.[36] Throughout, the claim has been that ideas about "Jews" and "Judaism" play a crucial role in this dialectic. The same centrality of "Judaism" is evident in early Christian political thought. This centrality should not be surprising, given that Hellenistic political thought was fashioned out of the same distinctions of body and soul as Hellenistic hermeneutics. Aristotle articulated a key distinction, between the corporeal politics of bare life and the higher politics of the good: "Men form states to secure a bare subsistence; but the ultimate object of the state is the good life."[37] The "natural" relationship of soul to body as ruler to subject provided a powerful political analogy. "[A]lthough in bad or corrupted natures the body will often appear to rule over the soul, because they are in an evil and unnatural condition. . . . It is clear that the rule of the soul over the body . . . is natural and expedient" (*Politics* 1254b). For Aristotle and the tradition that followed him, the chief function of the sovereign was to guide politics away from the demands of the body toward those of the immortal soul. As Aristotle put it in the *Nicomachean Ethics:* "we must not follow those who advise us, being men, to think of human things, and being mortal, of mortal things, but must, so far as we can, make ourselves immortal" (1177b). He realized, of course, that many rulers did indeed reverse these priorities, placing worldly gain ahead of a common and immaterial good, and he represented this reversal not as sovereignty but as its most basic distortion, tyranny. Tyranny, in other words, consisted of a perverted preference for self-interest over the commonwealth, for the mortal over the immortal, for flesh over spirit.[38]

These distinctions had long been commonplace in Hellenistic and Roman political thought by the time they were translated into Christian terms, and the relationship in early Christianity between the politics of flesh and the politics of spirit proved every bit as dialectically tense as that between carnal and spiritual hermeneutics. The energy released by this tension, like its hermeneutic analogue, had a tendency to seek ground in the Jew. We can see how great the potential force of this tension was by focusing on an important early Christian debate, that on the relationship of secular to divine power. There were many apostolic positions available in this debate. Paul, in Romans 13:1ff., had refused to distinguish between the two, treating secular magistrates as God's appointees and agents: "Let every soul be subject to the governing authorities."[39] The author of Matthew 22:21 drew a clearer distinction: "render unto Caesar the things that are Caesar's, but unto God the things which are God's." The Gospel of John went further, and imagined sharp conflict between the power of the Word and the "prince of this world" that would only be resolved with the defeat and disappearance of the latter (12:31, 14:30, 15:18). Early Christian exegetes developed these positions and many others.[40] All, however, shared a tendency to think of the princes and principalities of this world in carnal terms. And all mapped their distinctions onto the same dualities of flesh and spirit, Old Dispensation and New, which had pointed hermeneutics so fatefully toward the Jew.[41]

Origen, for example, adapted the same distinctions that informed his exegesis to the question of politics, dividing mankind into three classes: the hylic (from *hylē,* "matter"), or materialists, who were pagans and Jews; the psychics (from *psychē,* "soul"), who corresponded to the average Christian; and the pneumatics (from *pneuma,* "spirit"), who included only the most spiritual and ascetic of Christians.[42] Caesar's claims were only on the body, and only those who were of the body had to render unto him: Jews, pagans, and average Christians, but not pneumatics, not those who dwelt truly in the Spirit. Hence Peter and John had nothing to render unto Caesar ("Gold and silver have I none," Acts 3:6), for they had no business in the world.[43]

It has been justly said of Origen that "in his politics the state is related to the Church, very much as in his exegesis the letter is related to the spirit." The same general claim could be made of many other theologians, both Latin and Greek, who came after him. One seldom noted consequence of this analogy is the tendency to discuss political error (that is, an improper balance between material and spiritual) in the same terms used to assess hermeneutical error: Judaism and Judaizing. Origen himself occasionally did so.[44] But the most famous example of such slippage, and the most revealing, comes from more than a century later, when the conversion of the Empire, or at least of its emperors, to Christianity had sharply raised the stakes involved in questions about the relationship between Princely and Episcopal power.

Judaizing Secular Power

In 388 a crowd of monks burned down a Jewish synagogue and a Valentinian (heretical Christian) church in the town of Callinicum. The military Count of the East ordered their punishment, and instructed the local bishop, who had apparently incited the attacks, to pay for the reconstruction of the synagogue. The incident would have remained a local and minor one, were it not for the intervention of St. Ambrose, bishop of Milan, teacher of Augustine, and leading churchman of his age. In letter and sermon addressed to Emperor Theodosius, Ambrose opposed these orders. The first five paragraphs of Ambrose's letter sketch the outlines of a model of sovereignty with which Christian political history would become familiar. The monarch has the power to compel obedience "in state causes," the priest has the obligation to state the will of the King of Kings, "one whom it is even more perilous to displease" (Cf. Matt. 10:19–20). "For this is the difference between good and bad princes, that the good love liberty, and the bad slavery. And there is nothing in a priest so full of peril as regards God . . . as not freely to declare what he thinks."[45]

Only once he has established this framework of dual offices, imperial and priestly, with their incipient dual sovereignties and freedoms, does Ambrose take up the case at hand. It is not some overzealous bishop in an obscure province who ordered the synagogue burning. The synagogue "began to be burnt by the judgment of God." Behind this judgment stood the entire Church. The bishop and his monks were but the instruments of God's justice, their violence a proclamation of His sovereignty, for insofar as the synagogue represented a space outside the law of Christ, its existence diminished that sovereignty. Ambrose transforms a conflict over the relative power of governor and bishop, emperor and church, into a struggle for sovereignty between Judaism and Christianity. Should Theodosius rebuild the synagogue "the . . . Jews will set this solemnity amongst their feast days, . . . in memory of their having triumphed over the people of Christ." Any defense of the Jews, no matter how small, represents a Jewish victory that must not be granted.

The emperor and his count believed the synagogue affair to be a matter of public order, and acted to defend that order and their own sovereignty from the monks' claims to place both themselves and their victims outside the law. Ambrose's response is breathtaking. He claims that this very insistence on upholding the letter of the law is Judaizing, and pointedly reminds the emperor of his predecessor's unhappy fate. "Maximus . . . hearing that a synagogue had been burnt in Rome, had sent an edict to Rome, as if he were the upholder of public order. Wherefore the Christian people said, No good is in store for him. That king has become a Jew." The threat rests in implication: a monarch who reads literally, upholding the letter of the law over the demands of spirit, deserves deposition as a Jew.

Ambrose placed the Jew entirely outside the law. According to him, they themselves "deny that they . . . are bound by the Roman laws," and by rejecting God's Son they have set themselves outside His law as well. "Will God the Father avenge those who do not receive the Father, since they have not received the Son?" By asserting the Church's power to exclude the Jews from the protection of public law, Ambrose sought to articulate a hierarchy within Christian politics. Imperial will is sovereign only insofar as it accords with the will of God, "Who is rightly set before even emperors," and with the Church that communicates that will. The Jews, with their peculiar status as enemies of God and vessels of letter, law, and flesh, seemed to him a decisive point of engagement in the struggle for sovereignty between divine and secular power. Ambrose did succeed in obtaining the revocation of the count's order, but his victory was anything but decisive. For the project he had set himself—the assertion of the supremacy of heavenly over earthly law through the complete exclusion of the Jews—proved just as problematic as its hermeneutic analogue: the attempt to purge Christian letters of "Jewish" literalism.

Again it was Augustine who pointed the way, not toward a solution, but toward a more durable paradox, assigning to the Jews an exceptional political space congruent with their semiotic one. In an exegesis of Psalm 59 aimed at the "Origenist" Pelagius, Augustine explained that God had poured his message into two vessels, one of mercy, the other of wrath, the former perceptible through the latter.[46] "For so God, willing to show wrath, and to manifest His power, has brought in with much patience the vessels of wrath, which have been perfected unto perdition" (citing Rom. 9:22). These vessels of wrath were God's enemies the Jews, destroyed spiritually but nevertheless preserved in the flesh ("dead men") and protected in the polity so that His sovereignty might be known. Exiled yet ubiquitous, conquered but still a distinct nation, enemies of God that adhere to His laws, the Jews' exceptional status served as the best evidence for the nature of Christ's sovereignty over the world, and as a lesson for heretics everywhere. Hence, according to Augustine, the Psalmist sang, "Slay them not, lest sometime they forget your law" (*En. in Ps.* 59.17–19). And hence (as he put it in the *Contra Faustum*) "no emperor or monarch who finds under his government the people with this mark [of Cain] kills them, that is to say, makes them cease to be Jews, separate in their observance and unlike the rest of the world."

For heuristic reasons then, Augustine assigned to the Jews the exceptional role of "included exile,"[47] a status that many historians believe made possible the continued survival of the Jews in Christendom. But this status had constitutional consequences as well. Insofar as the power of both divine and imperial law was manifested through the Jews' peculiar status, they became a potential focal point for debates over the nature of that power.[48] Indeed Augustine's transformation of the Jews into living monuments of God's law, combined with their placement under the sign and power of earthly legislators, created political difficulties analogous to and even sharper than the exegetic ones created by holding together the Old Testament and the New. Analogous, in that in order to articulate God's sovereignty the laws of "Emperor or monarch" had to contain Judaism within themselves, much as Christian scripture needed to contain the Hebrew Bible. Sharper, in that unlike biblical exegesis (which has at least the potential to lead toward the divine), Augustine understood terrestrial politics to take place always beneath the curse of Cain, its first practitioner. Like Cain, the founder of every polity is of necessity "a fratricide" (Augustine gives the example of Romulus). Like Cain, who sinned by subjecting his reasoning soul to the desires of his flesh, every earthly city "has its good in this world, and rejoices in [the material world] with such joy as such things can afford," so that it will at the end of time be "committed to the extreme penalty." Secular power operated under Cain's conjoined significations, as both "founder of the earthly city" and "a figure of the Jews."[49] Sovereigns therefore trod a path haunted by monsters of Judaism even more ferocious than those that beset readers of biblical texts. Augustine did not seek to slay these monsters. Instead he immured them, like the furies under Aeschylus's Athens, at the foundations of the Christian hermeneutic and political order.

Toward a Medieval Resistance Theory

We have already seen, in the world of exegesis, that Christians were sometimes willing to release these furies in order to deploy them against their Christian rivals through accusations of Judaizing. The same is true in the world of politics, where we can speak at the very least of a latent potential, under particular conditions of conflict, for the violent release of the "Jew" against the sovereign. This release, foreshadowed by Ambrose, was occasionally suggested in Late Antiquity and the early Middle Ages. But we can find particularly coherent examples of this political discourse after the year 1000, when newly robust monarchies began to emerge throughout Western Europe. Among the first prerogatives established by these young monarchies was the power of decision over the Jews. Even the Papacy, upon which royal claims to sovereignty so often foundered in this period, did not often contest the monarch's special powers over a people explicitly excluded from the Ecclesia. The king's position as protector of the Jews became a commonplace of medieval law.[50] The sovereign decided the Jews' fate, and any attempt by other Christians to circumscribe that power of decision through violence became a violation of the king's rights. As King John of England famously put it in his edict forbidding attacks on Jews, "If I give my peace even to a dog, it must be kept inviolate."[51]

Insofar as the Jews represented regalian rights in their most concentrated form, the Jews' diffusion could help kings expand those rights. In the twelfth and early thirteenth centuries, for example, a number of the great magnates of France who gave only token recognition to Capetian suzerainty harbored Jews on their lands. In 1230 King Louis IX issued the Ordinance of Melun, claiming the right to prohibit one lord's Jews from emigrating to the domains of another, even when neither domain belonged to the Crown. The French Crown claimed the right to adjudicate between lords in all such disputes. Moreover, the Ordinance asserted that any lord who resisted these claims could be punished as a rebel: "If any barons do not wish to observe them, we shall compel them. . . . We and our other barons have sworn to compel the rebels to observe the aforesaid statutes." William Jordan has called this "the first piece of treason legislation in French history," as well as the first example of French legislation since the Carolingians. Such arguments not only extended royal authority over Jews who belonged to other lords, they also provided an entry point for new forms of monarchical power (such as the charge of treason and lèse majesté) that would later find much broader application.[52] By the thirteenth century, control over Jews had become a defining characteristic differentiating monarchy from lower forms of political authority.

These articulations of royal sovereignty through the idiom of the Jewish exception were met by an increasingly powerful critique of monarchy as protector of Jews. As Peter the Venerable put it in the mid-twelfth century to King

Louis VII of France: "Has that which a certain holy king of the Jews once said escaped the notice of the king of the Christians? 'O Lord,' he said, 'shall I not hate those who hate you and be consumed with enmity for your enemies?' (Psalm 139:21)."[53] Royal protection and toleration, critics increasingly argued, gave the Jews an opportunity to act out their eternal hatred of Christians through usury, blasphemy, and murder.[54] The consequences of this imagined Jewish enmity widened over time. Jewish usurers were portrayed sucking the blood of Christian peasants. Jewish blasphemers were said to desecrate hosts and murder Christian children. Jews were believed to cause plague and disease, either actively through poison, or passively because Christian toleration of their malignity angered God and roused Him to punishment.

Within this discourse the decisions of princes were presented as a choice between a corrupt materialism that endangered the land or a piety that protected it, between "Jewish" carnality and Christian spirit. Medieval Europe developed a number of ways of representing the potential hypercarnality of monarchs. Stories about host desecration and ritual murder, for example, first began to circulate in twelfth-century England before spreading to the continent, where they remained an important tool of political mobilization until the seventeenth century. And though their rise has often been explained in terms of the increasing importance of Eucharistic devotion and Marian piety, it is more important for our purposes to stress their birth as a form of political critique. Through a narrative about Jews physically tormenting the Eucharistic flesh of Christ and the living flesh of Christian children, ritual murder and host-desecration accusations gave flesh to the charge that the material greed of princes tormented Christian society.[55] Throughout the 1380s, to choose but one example, the town council of Prague fought with King Wenzel of Bohemia over his protection of money lending. "Oh kings, kings! Be shamed for such a crime . . . in which you yourselves are proven to be accursed usurers." During Holy Week 1389 the conflict escalated. The Jews of Prague were accused of chanting "stone him, for he pretends to be God's son," and throwing rocks at a Eucharist carried in procession. Since the king wrongly tolerated such "nefarious acts against Christ's faithful," the people took it upon themselves to exact vengeance, eviscerating and dismembering the Jews, burning their bodies and their habitations.[56] By representing their actions in these terms, the people of Prague asserted that theirs was not a rebellion against divinely appointed monarchy, but rather what St. Ambrose might have called legitimate resistance to Jewish tyranny.

If tales of murder and host desecration provided one way of representing the dangers of royal "love" for Jews, tales of real love, carnal and passionate, provided another.[57] Perhaps the most revealing of these stories was told about Alfonso VIII, king of Castile (1158–1214) and grandfather of France's St. Louis:

> After the king Alfonso was married . . . he departed to Toledo with his wife. And while there he saw a very beautiful Jewess, and he became so attached to her that he left the queen his wife and secluded himself with the Jewess . . . for seven months, so that he paid no attention to himself or his kingdom or anything else, and they say that this great love that he bore the Jewess was caused by love magic and spells that she knew how to make. But the counts and knights and rich men, seeing how the kingdom was in such danger . . . agreed together how they would resolve such a bad and unconscionable situation. And the agreement was that they would kill her. And with this intention they entered to where the king was, pretending that they wished to speak to him. . . . While some spoke to him the others entered to where the Jewess was and . . . they cut her throat and did the same to the others who were with her. . . . And then some of his vassals took him and transported him to a place called Illescas. . . . And as he lay one night preoccupied by the affair of this damned Jewess there appeared to him an angel who said to him: how now, Alfonso, are you dwelling on the evil you have done, from which God received great disservice? You do ill, for know that He will charge you dearly for it, you and your kingdom . . . because it consented.[58]

Though this account was often rewritten for the benefit of early modern and modern audiences moved by *mesaliances,*[59] the medieval version was not a romance but a morality tale, an erotic allegory for medieval Christian ideas about the peculiar and perilous nature of relationships between monarchs and Jews. The tale splits those potential relationships into two relatively extreme positions. On the one hand the philo-Semitism of the king, in this case carnal as well as political, puts Jews at the center of the kingdom's affairs. The king's barons espouse the opposing view, favoring the extermination of what they perceive to be a dangerous Jewish influence. God's angel agrees with the barons, and even heightens the revolutionary implications of that agreement by promising God's punishment not just against the king, but also against the kingdom, "because it consented" to his sin. Kingdoms that allow their kings to love Jews will suffer. The barons' only error was in not having taken action earlier.

The history of medieval rebellions is peopled with "Jew-loving" rulers. In Castile alone the list is revealing: the civil war against Alfonso X ("the Wise," r. 1252–1284) was fueled, in part, by complaints that he was a Jew-loving tyrant. The aristocratic factions that deposed and murdered King Peter "the Cruel" in the mid-fourteenth century justified their actions by portraying him as a favorer of Jews, and even claimed that he was a cuckoo, the son of a Jewess adopted by the queen mother to conceal her inability to provide an heir. Prince Henry (IV) rebelled against his father Juan II claiming that he favored the Jews (it is in this revolt that we met the Bachiller Marcos). He himself would later be ritually deposed, accused of favoring Jews and of living like a Muslim. Even the "Catholic monarchs" Ferdinand and Isabel, conquerors of Granada, founders of the Inquisition, expellers of the Jews, were said by some of their subjects to be descended from Jews and to favor them in their policies.[60]

"Royal Judaizing" was particularly useful as a revolutionary discourse in late-medieval Castile, where mass conversions and intermarriage had created an unusually potent confusion of bloodlines and hermeneutics. But there was nothing peculiarly "Hispanic" about the discourse itself.[61] It was rather the pan-Christian product of a genealogy of morals that rooted extremes of spirituality and carnality, of love and enmity, of metaphor and letter, of freedom and tyranny, in the one lineage that had simultaneously produced the flesh of God and of his enemies, the lineage of the Jews. The Bachiller Marcos, besieged by royalists and with time for only one more salvo, did not call for some new weapon in his moment of greatest need. He reached instead for a fundamental insight of Patristic pyrotechnics: the language of sovereignty burns hottest in the presence of Jewish flesh.

Notes

1. Text in E. Benito Ruano, "El Memorial del bachiller Marcos García de Mora contra los conversos," *Sefarad* 17 (1957): 314–351, here pp. 320–321. With the occasional exception of some biblical, classical, or Patristic passages for which widely available translations exist, all translations are the author's own unless otherwise noted.

2. According to Aristotle the natural life of subsistence we share with animals, but the human has a higher goal: "born with regard to life, but existing essentially with regard to the good life," *Politics* 1252b, 30. Cf. 1278b, 23–31; 1252a, 26–35. On the *Politics* in Spain during this period, see A. R. D. Pagden, "The Diffusion of Aristotle's Moral Philosophy in Spain, ca. 1400–ca. 1600," *Traditio* 31 (1975): 287–313.

3. This is not the same as Aristotle's distinction between *logos* and *phonē*, language and voice. Animals have voice, but only humans have language, the precondition for moral judgment and political life (1253a, 10–18). Paul's distinction

discriminates among men as Aristotle's does not: all humans have language, but only some read correctly, according to the spirit.

4. K. Marx, "Zur Judenfrage," in *Karl Marx, Friedrich Engels, Werke,* Bd. 1 (Berlin, 1981 [1956]), S. 347–377, here p. 377, final sentence (italics in the original). Cf. J.-P. Sartre, *Anti-Semite and Jew* (New York, 1965), pp. 148–150. These positions are (to my mind) secularized products of the political theology this essay seeks to describe.

5. The bibliography of each of these claims is so vast that it defies footnoting. Since that on the contemporary linkage of anti-imperialism, antiglobalization, and anti-Americanism with anti-Judaism remains most fragmentary, I provide a few examples of its analyses: Pierre-André Taguieff, *La nouvelle judéophobie* (Paris, 2002); Mark Strauss, "Anti-Globalism's Jewish Problem," *Foreign Policy* (Nov.–Dec. 2003: www.foreignpolicy.com). For an example of its invocation, see the President of Malaysia (Mahathir bin Mohamad), "Address at the Opening of the Tenth Session of the Islamic Summit Conference," Putrajaya, Oct. 10, 2003.

6. Though this essay will not touch directly on the subject, the absorption of much Christian material into early Islam influenced use of the Jews as negative foils for Muhammad's prophetic and political sovereignty. For one particularly important example among many see the Qur'an, Surah II, al-Baqarah. For a modern Islamist interpretation of this Surah that explicitly adopts the terms we are interested in, see Sayyid Qut.b's monumental *tafsīr* first published in 1952: *Fī Z.ilāl al Qur'ān,* English translation: *In the Shade of the Qur'ān,* vol. 1 (London, 1999).

7. The word "exception" is a term of art in discussions of sovereignty today, one that moves in the twin gravitational fields of Carl Schmitt, with his claim that "he is sovereign who decides the exception" (e.g., *Political Theology* [Boston, 1985], p. 5), and Walter Benjamin, with his emphasis on the undecidability of the exception (e.g., *The Origin of German Tragic Drama* [London, 1998], p. 71). These positions will both prove useful in understanding the exceptional political function of the Jew, but neither will govern this essay.

8. My attention to the scholarship will necessarily be limited. I will not touch at all upon the many fruitful rereadings of Paul that seek to underwrite philosophy or theology in our own time (such as Badiou or Agamben). I will enter only briefly into the heated debate about how Paul himself understood his words. My interest is primarily in the main streams of debate that Paul's texts made possible for the many historical communities that read them, both in his own and later times.

9. These questions were not Paul's alone. Cf. Acts 10:10–16 and Galatians 2:11–13 on Peter.

10. On some consequences of this universalism, see Kathy Gaca, "Paul's Uncommmon Declaration in Romans 1:18–32 and Its Problematic Legacy for Pagan and Christian Relations," *Harvard Theological Review* 92, no. 2 (1999): 165–198.

11. In contemporary political philosophy the term "enmity" seems always to gesture toward Carl Schmitt, who understood it as the fundamental political con-

cept. Schmitt, however, rarely treated Judaism explicitly as a "political enmity," for all that he saw politics as a secularized form of theology. The oversight is curious in someone who lived through Weimar and National Socialism. It has been pointed out, first by J. Taubes in his *Ad Carl Schmitt: Gegenstrebige Fügung* (Berlin, 1987), and more recently by J. Derrida, *Politics of Friendship* (London, 1997), pp. 84–85.

12. This reading of Romans is not much like the "politico-theological" reading maintained by Jacob Taubes in his debate with Schmitt. (For Taubes Romans was "a political declaration of war" and Paul an archtheorist of enmity: *Die Politische Theologie des Paulus,* ed. A. Assmann and J. Assmann [Berlin, 1993], pp. 27, 72.) It is rather the result of contemporary attempts to read Paul in his historical and rhetorical context. For a synthesis of these rereadings of Romans, see J. Gager, *Reinventing Paul* (Oxford, 2000), pp. 101–143. Of course the Patristic period and the Middle Ages had their own very different traditions of reading these much debated texts. See, inter alia, P. Gorday, *Principles of Patristic Exegesis: Romans 9–11 in Origen, John Chrysostom, and Augustine* (Lewiston, 1983); F. J. C. Iturbe, "Et sic omnis Israel salvus fierit, Rom 11,26-su interpretación por los escritores cristianos de los siglos III–XIII," *Estudios Biblicos* 21 (1962): 127–150; and above all J. Heil, *Kompilation oder Konstruktion? Die Juden in den Pauluskommentaren des 9. Jahrhunderts* (Hannover, 1998), pp. 140–158.

13. A generation before Paul, for example, the Jew Philo of Alexandria stressed the need to read for "the hidden meaning that appeals to the few who study soul characteristics, rather than bodily forms," and discussed the signification of circumcision in terms very similar to Paul's, though written a generation before (Abr. 147). But for Philo circumcision's spiritual meaning increased, rather than lessened, the necessity of the outer practice. *On the Migration of Abraham* 92–93: "we should look on all these [outward observances] as resembling the body, and [these inner meanings as resembling] the soul. It follows that, exactly as we have to take thought for the body, because it is the abode of the soul, so we must pay heed to the written laws. If we keep and observe these, we shall gain a clearer conception of those things of which these are the symbols." On Philo's (and later Origen's) Neoplatonic use of the analogy of body and soul for text and meaning, see D. Dawson, "Plato's Soul and the Body of the Text in Philo and Origen," in *Interpretation and Allegory,* ed. Whitman (Leiden, 2000), pp. 89–107. See also A. J. M. Wedderburn, *Baptism and Resurrection: Studies in Pauline Theology against Its Graeco-Roman Background* (Tübingen, 1987).

14. In all the passages cited here Paul uses the term *soma* for body, but it is not the only term in his vocabulary. In Gal. 5:16 and elsewhere, e.g., he uses *sarx* (σαρξ). The difference is important, but lies beyond our reach here. On Philo's body as tomb, see D. Winston, ed. and trans., "Philo and the Contemplative Life," in *Jewish Spirituality from the Bible through the Middle Ages,* ed. A. Green (New York, 1988): 198–231, here p. 212. D. Boyarin, *A Radical Jew: Paul and the Politics of Identity* (Berkeley, 1994), pp. 57–85, emphasizes Paul's "moderate" dual-

ism; and G. Caspary, *Politics and Exegesis: Origen and the Two Swords* (Berkeley, 1979), pp. 108–116, illuminates the generative potential of the Pauline polarities.

15. This, in any event, is the reading favored by those many scholars who have accepted the implications of E. P. Sanders's *Paul and Palestinian Judaism* (Minneapolis, 1977), L. Gaston's *Paul and the Torah* (Vancouver, 1987), and J. Gager's *The Origins of Anti-Semitism: Attitudes toward Judaism in Pagan and Christian Antiquity* (Oxford, 1985).

16. Gk. Ἰουδαΐζειν Latin *iudaizare.* The Douay Rheims translation expands a bit: "how dost thou compel the Gentiles to live as do the Jews?"

17. In letters of undisputed Pauline authorship, the few passages that articulate an unambivalent view of Jewish enmity have come under scrutiny as later interpolations. See, e.g., 1 Thess. 2:13–16: ". . . the Jews, who killed both the Lord Jesus and the prophets, and drove us out, and displease God and oppose all men by hindering us from speaking to the Gentiles that they may be saved." On this passage, see Birger A. Pearson, "I Thessalonians 2:13–16: A Deutero-Pauline Interpolation," *Harvard Theological Review* 64 (1971): 79–94; Gager, *Origins,* pp. 255–256.

18. The dating of the New Testament's books is much debated, but there is a scholarly consensus (e.g., W. G. Kümmel, *Introduction to the New Testament* [Nashville, 1975]) at which all revisions aim. The genuine writings of Paul come first, circa 45–60 CE. (For a revised dating of the letters, see G. Luedemann, *Paul, Apostle to the Gentiles: Studies in Chronology* [Philadelphia, 1984].) The Gospel of Mark is often characterized as the earliest Gospel, written shortly before or after the destruction of the Temple in 70 CE, followed by Matthew later in the first century (W. R. Farmer's reversal of the two in *The Synoptic Problem: A Critical Analysis* [Dillsboro, 1976] has not altered the consensus). Luke is sometimes treated as contemporaneous with Matthew but is probably later, since Acts, written by the same author, is generally dated to circa 100 CE. John has almost universally been treated as coming last, though recent revisionists argue instead for its priority (see, e.g., J. A. T. Robinson, *Redating the New Testament* [London, 1976]).

19. Without plunging into a vast literature, the reader can get some sense of current debates about Gospel representations of Jews in W. Farmer, *Anti-Judaism and the Gospels* (Harrisburg, PA, 1999). For the Sermon on the Mount, see W. D. Davies, *The Setting of the Sermon on the Mount* (Cambridge, 1964).

20. On the Johannine community, see J. L Martyn, *History and Theology in the Fourth Gospel* (New York, 1968); J. Townsend, "The Gospel of John and the Jews," in Davies, *Anti-Semitism and the Foundations of Christianity* (New York, 1979), pp. 72–97; W. Meeks, "'Am I a Jew?' Johannine Christianity and Judaism," in *Christianity, Judaism and other Greco-Roman Cults,* ed. J. Neusner (Leiden, 1975), pp. 163–186. For A. Reinhartz, however, Christology drives sociology. See her "The Gospel of John: How 'The Jews Became Part of the Plot,'" in *Jesus, Judaism and Christian Anti-Judaism: Reading the New Testament after the Holocaust,* ed.

A. Reinhartz and P. Fredriksen (Knoxville, 2002), pp. 99–116. For the Matthean community, see D. C. Sim, *The Gospel of Matthew and Christian Judaism: The History and Social Setting of the Matthean Community* (Edinburgh, 1998).

21. See, e.g., the creed in Ignatius's letter to the Ephesians, 7: "There is one Physician possessed both of flesh and spirit, both made and not made, god existing in flesh, true life in death, both of Mary and of God, first possible and then impossible."

22. Irenaeus, *Adversus haereseos* 27.2. There were many other important early Christian thinkers (e.g., Valentinian) whose knowledge of Greek philosophy led them to argue for the separation of the highest god from the god of Genesis and the Jews. My focus on Marcion is meant to be heuristic, not exclusive.

23. A. von Harnack, *Marcion: Das Evangelium vom fremden Gott,* 2nd ed. (Leipzig, 1924); J. Knox, *Marcion and the New Testament: An Essay in the Early History of the Canon* (Chicago, 1942); E. C. Blackman, *Marcion and His Influence* (London, 1948); S. G. Wilson, "Marcion and the Jews," in *Anti-Judaism and Early Christianity,* vol. 2, ed. S. Wilson (Waterloo, ON, 1986), pp. 45–58.

24. Indeed in the second century the apostle to the gentiles seems to have been more popular among dualists than among those we consider proto-orthodox. See E. Pagels, *The Gnostic Paul: Gnostic Exegesis of Pauline Letters* (Philadelphia, 1975), pp. 1–13.

25. H. Von Campenhausen, *The Formation of the Christian Bible,* trans. J. A. Baker (Philadelphia, 1972), p. 148; cf. B. Metzger, *The Canon of the New Testament: Its Origin, Development, and Significance* (Oxford, 1987), pp. 90–99; B. Ehrman, *The Orthodox Corruption of Scripture: The Effect of Early Christological Controversies on the Text of the New Testament* (Oxford, 1993).

26. *Adversus Marcionem* 1.19, ed. and trans. E. Evans (Oxford, 1972), vol. 1, p. 49.

27. *Adversus Marcionem* 3.7, vol. 1, p. 191.

28. Tertullian was among those theologians who argued strongly against too sharp a differentiation between the figurative interpretation and the literal reality. His words in *Adversus Marcionem* 4.40, e.g., are suggestive: "figura autem non fuisset, nisi veritatis esset corpus. Ceterum vacua res, quod est phantasma, figuram capere non posset." Or as he writes of the prophets in *De resurrectione carnis* 19, they expressed themselves in flesh as well as in allegorical shadows: "nec omnia umbrae, sed et corpora." How this caution affected his polemics against Judaism (e.g., in his *Adv. Iudaeos*) remains unexplored.

29. As he put it in his commentary on the sacrifice of Isaac, "sicut in Domino corporeum nihil est, ita etiam tu in his omnibus corporeum nihil sentias; sed in spiritu generes." *PG* 12, 209b.

30. See E. A. Clark, *The Origenist Controversy* (Princeton, 1992); K. Jo Torjesen, *Hermeneutical Procedure and Theological Method in Origen's Exegesis* (Berlin, 1986); H. de Lubac, *Histoire et Esprit: L'intelligence de l'Écriture d'après Origène* (Paris, 1950). More tangential to our topic, see also N. R. M. de Lange, *Ori-*

gen and the Jews: Studies in Jewish-Christian Relations in Third-Century Palestine (Cambridge, 1976).

31. For an example of the strength Augustine devoted to the task, and a restatement of his motives for doing so, see his work from the 410s, the *De Genesi ad litteram* (*On the Literal Interpretation of Genesis*) CSEL 28, 8.1, pp. 231–232. He had undertaken but not completed a similar project in 393, *De Genesi ad litteram liber imperfectus* (CSEL 28.I).

32. On Origen's theory of scriptural deception, see J. W. Trigg, "Divine Deception and the Truthfulness of Scripture," in *Origen: His World and His Legacy,* ed. C. Kannengieser and W. Peterson (Notre Dame, IN, 1988), pp. 147–164; and D. Satran, "Pedagogy and Deceit in the Alexandrian Theological Tradition," in *Origeniana Quinta,* ed. R. Daly (Louvain, 1992), pp. 119–124.

33. This exegesis was much cited in the Middle Ages, on which, see G. Dahan, "L'Exégèse de l'histoire de Caïn et Abel du XIIe au XIVe siècle en Occident," *Recherches de Théologie ancienne et médiévale* 49 (1982): 21–89, and 50 (1983): 5–68, here (1982): 25–27. Augustine treats Cain quite differently in *De civitate Dei* 15.7, where Cain is the founder of the earthly city. On this contrast, see the beautiful passage of P. Brown, *Augustine of Hippo: A Biography* (London, 1967), p. 321. On the evolution of Augustine's views on religious coercion and his turn to other prooftexts (such as Psalm 59:11, "slay them not"), see P. Brown, "St. Augustine's Attitude to Religious Coercion," *Journal of Roman Studies* 54 (1964): 107–116, and J. Cohen, *Living Letters of the Law: Ideas of the Jew in Medieval Christianity* (Berkeley, 1999), pp. 54–55.

34. Cf. Paula Frederiksen, "Divine Justice and Human Freedom: Augustine on Jews and Judaism, 392–398," in *From Witness to Witchcraft: Jews and Judaism in Medieval Christian Thought,* ed. J. Cohen (Wiesbaden, 1996), pp. 29–54, here p. 48.

35. Milestones: Sermo 199.I.2, PL 38:1027. For other examples, see Cohen, *Living Letters of the Law.* Compare Qur'an 62:5, with its image of the Jews as donkeys carrying books.

36. In this sense I am following a path parallel to that of Erich Auerbach in his essay "Figura," in *Neue Dantestudien* 5 (Istanbul, 1944), pp. 11–71.

37. See n. 2, above.

38. E.g., *Politics* 1279b.

39. Elsewhere Paul seems less monistic: cf. 1 Thess. 5:1–11, 1 Cor. 3:5–4:5, 15:24; 2 Thess. 1:1–12.

40. Tertullian, e.g., opposed Church and Empire as castle of light to castle of darkness: *De idolatria* 19.1 (CC 2:1120). Similarly for Hippolytus of Rome "the kingdom of this world" "rules through the power of Satan" (*Eis ton Danila* 4.9, cited by Caspary, *Politics and Exegesis,* pp. 137–138). The argument that earthly kingdoms are Godly institutions for the utility of the pagan un-Godly emerges in the second century author Irenaeus, *Adversus haereseos* 5.24.2. Those gathered at the council of Antioch in 341 thought of earthly kings as *exterae potestates,* nei-

ther demonic nor salvific, but simply external and natural powers appointed for those who do not belong to the people of God (Canon 5). On the issues treated in the following paragraphs, Caspary, *Politics and Exegesis,* chap. 4, and L. Field, Jr., *Liberty, Dominion, and the Two Swords* (Notre Dame, IN, 1998), are especially useful.

41. Of course within a Christian logic the Jews chose Caesar's kingship over God's when they executed Jesus, as Pseudo-Cyprian put it. Ps.-Cyprian, *Adversus Iudaeos* 42, 54 (CC 4.271, 273), and *De montibus* 7 (CSEL 3.3.111). See also Justin, *Dialogus* 41.1, and Melito of Sardis's Homily on the Passion. On debates over the dating (212?) and authorship of the *Adv. Iud.,* see the works listed in Field, *Liberty, Dominion, and the Two Swords,* n. 60, p. 280.

42. *Com. Rom.* 9.25, 1226B. See Caspary, *Politics and Exegesis,* p. 142; H. Crouzel, *Théologie de l'image de Dieu chez Origène* (Paris, 1954), pp. 193–196.

43. This position is less antinomian than it sounds. Origen also stressed (tropologically) that since all bodily things "bear the bodily image of the Prince of Bodies," all men must pay "tribute to Caesar." Only Jesus's flesh did not bear upon it the stamp of the Prince of this world: Caesar had no rights over him. Hence Jesus had to draw from the mouth of a fish the coin with which he paid the tax collector (Matt. 17:24ff.). *Com. Rom.* 9.25, 1226B on Peter and John. *Com. Mat.* 17.27, 659f.: "imaginem enim Caesaris habet omnis res corporalis." On the fish, *Com. Mat.* 13.11, 208f.

44. The quote is from Caspary, *Politics and Exegesis,* p. 9. Caspary uses the term "fleshly envelope" to refer to Origen's view of the relationship of state to Church (p. 181). For examples of Origen's "Judaizing" political error, see *Com. Mat.* 17.27, 659f., where he calls those Christians who err by refusing to acknowledge the debts of the flesh "Pharisaei"; or his characterization in his commentary on Romans of Pneumatics, who resist the earthly powers with material force as Judaizing Zealots.

45. A position eventually adopted as imperial law: cf. *Codex Iustinianus* 1.4, *De audentia episcopali* 26.5 (*Corpus iuris civilis,* ed. Paul Krüger, Theodor Mommsen, and Wilhelm Kroll, [Berlin, 1900–1950], 3 vols., here 2.43). Ambrose's letter is preserved in two versions: the finished form (Ep. 74) and an original or earlier draft. I quote from the latter, Ep. 1a *extra collectionem,* in Ambrose, *Epistulae et acta,* ed. O. Faller and M. Zelzer, CSEL 82.1–4, 4 vols., (Vienna, 1968–1996), vol. 3, pp. 162–177. See generally, N. B. McLynn, *Ambrose of Milan: Church and Court in a Christian Capital* (Berkeley, 1994), pp. 298–315.

46. For a sustained reading of Pelagius as an Origenist, see Clark, *The Origenist Controversy.*

47. Cf. Giorgio Agamben's discussion of "included exclusion" in *Stato di eccezione* (Turin, 2003), a discussion which I heard at UCLA in preliminary form. Curiously, some Roman authors had described the Jews' status in the Empire in similarly paradoxical terms, i.e., Seneca (circa 70 CE) in his lost *De supersti-*

tione: "The vanquished have given their laws to the victors" (*victi victoribus leges dederunt*). The text survives only in its citation by Augustine, *De civ. Dei* 6.11 (= GLAJJ, I, no. 186). Compare Augustine's contemporary Rutilius Namatianus: "And would that Judea had never been subdued / by Pompey's wars and Titus' Military power! / The infection of this plague, though excised [*excisae pestis*] still creeps abroad to more: / and 'tis their own conquerors that a conquered nation keeps down." *De reditu suo* I, 391–398 (= GLAJJ 2, no. 542).

48. The paradoxes of exile as a status constituted by the law as outside the law had long been fertile ground for ancient legal theorists. See, e.g., G. Crifò, *L'esclusione dall città: Altri studi sull'exilium romano* (Perugia, 1985).

49. *De civ. Dei,* 15.4–5, 7. Cain's politics give priority to flesh, "that part which the philosophers call vicious, and which ought not to lead the mind, but which the mind ought to rule and restrain by reason." Augustine's prooftexts here come significantly from Galatians (5:17) and Romans (7:17, 6:13).

50. One widespread expression of this was the legal notion that all Jews in whatever kingdom they were found were "slaves/serfs [*servi*] of the king's chamber." But regardless of specific legal form, the king's prerogatives over Jews became emblematic of royal power at its most absolute. On these issues, see most recently D. Abulafia, "The Jews in the Municipal Fuero of Teruel (1176–7)," in *Jews, Muslims and Christians in and around the Crown of Aragon: Essays in Honour of Professor Elena Lourie,* ed. H. J. Hames (Leiden, 2004), pp. 97–123; idem, "The Servitude of Jews and Muslims in the Medieval Mediterranean: Origins and Diffusion," *Mélanges de l'École Française de Rome, Moyen Âge* 112 (2000): 687–714. For the particularly stark case of England, see also J. Watt, *The Jews, the Law, and the Church: The Concept of Jewish Serfdom in Thirteenth-Century England,* Studies in Church History, Subsidia 9 (Oxford, 1991).

51. Quoted in Cecil Roth, *A History of the Jews in England* (Oxford, 1964), p. 33.

52. W. C. Jordan, "Jews, Regalian Rights, and the Constitution in Medieval France," *AJS Review* 23 (1998): 1–16, here p. 7. The ordinance is published in the *Layettes du Trésor des Chartes,* ed. A. Teulet et al., 5 vols. (Paris, 1863–1909), vol. 2, no. 2083, pp. 192–193.

53. Peter the Venerable, *Epistulae* 130, in *The Letters of Peter the Venerable,* ed. G. Constable, 2 vols. (Cambridge, MA, 1967), vol. 1, pp. 327–330. Without contradicting Augustine, Peter pushed him to an extreme. "Slay them not," he conceded, "for God does not wish them to be entirely killed and altogether wiped out, but to be preserved for greater torment and reproach, like the fratricide Cain, in a life worse than death." On Peter, see Cohen, *Living Letters of the Law,* pp. 245–270.

54. As Ramon Martí put it in the thirteenth century, "what do you think the devil can accomplish through the Jews, who are so numerous, almost all educated and most adept at trickery, so well endowed with the good life and the usuries al-

lowed them by Christians, so loved by our princes on account of the services they provide and the flatteries they spew forth, so scattered and dispersed throughout the world, so secretive in their deceptions that they display a remarkable appearance of being truthful?"

55. In the earliest surviving narrative of ritual murder (Thomas of Monmouth's account of William of Norwich's death in 1144), royal complicity is already an important element. The king's sheriff blocks the investigation, and the king is skeptical of the charges. See *The Life and Miracles of St. William of Norwich by Thomas of Monmouth,* ed. A. Jessopp and M. Rhodes James (Cambridge, 1896); G. Langmuir, "Thomas of Monmouth: Detector of Ritual Murder," *Speculum* 59 (1984): 822–846. Telling a similar story long after the Jews had been expelled from England, Chaucer's Prioress still remembered royal perfidy as an indispensable detail: "In Asia once there was a Christian town / In which long since a ghetto used to be / Where there were Jews, supported by the Crown / For the foul lucre of their usury, / Hateful to Christ and all His company."

56. I am here conflating the claims of a number of sources (notably the "Passio judaeorum secundum Johannes rusticus quadratus" and the "De caede judaeorum pragensi") that are analyzed in M. Rubin, *Gentile Tales: The Narrative Assault on Late Medieval Jews* (New Haven, 1999), pp. 135–140.

57. Guibert of Nogent, for example, excoriated the Count of Soisson for his affair with a Jewess: *De vita sua* III.16 (English translation in J. Benton, *Self and Society in Medieval France: The Memoirs of Abbot Guibert of Nogent* [New York, 1970], pp. 209–211). Count Thibault of Blois brought his dalliance with the Jewess Pucellina to a brutal conclusion by burning a number of her coreligionists on charges of ritual murder in 1171: see most recently, S. Einbinder, *Beautiful Death: Jewish Poetry and Martyrdom in Medieval France* (Princeton, 2002), pp. 45–49. According to Polish legend, King Casimir the Great (1310–1370) expanded Jewish privileges in 1334 because of his love for the Jewess "Estherke" (Esther): H. Bar-Itzhak, *Jewish Poland: Legends of Origin* (Detroit, 2001), pp. 113–132; Ch. Shmeruk, *The Esterke Story in Yiddish and Polish Literature: A Case Study in the Mutual Relations of Two Cultural Traditions* (Jerusalem, 1985) (my thanks to Magda Teter for this last reference).

58. I am citing from the Crónica de 1344, Biblioteca Nacional, Madrid, ms. 10,815, fol. 145 r–v. For an extensive treatment of this story, see my "Deviant Politics and Jewish Love: Alfonso VIII and the Jewess of Toledo," *Jewish History* 21 (2007): 15–41. This story of love between Jewess and Christian king has an obscure history, on which, see most recently G. Hilty, "Die Jüdin von Toledo: Entstehung und Frühgeschichte des Motivs in der spanischen Literatur," in *Verlust und Ursprung, Festschrift für Werner Weber,* ed. A. Maass and B. Heinser (Zürich, 1989), pp. 241–267. The tale first appears around 1292, in a "mirror for princes" written by King Sancho IV (*Castigos e documentos para bien vivir,* ed. A. Rey [Bloomington, IN, 1952], p. 133).

59. Most notably in Lope de Vega's (1617) and Franz Grillparzer's (1851) plays, and in Lion Feuchtwanger's novel (1955). On these and others see, inter alia, J. Castañeda, *A Critical Edition of Lope de Vega's "Las paces de los reyes y judía de Toledo"* (Chapel Hill, 1962).

60. On the accusations made by Castilian bishops against Alfonso X, see P. Linehan, "The Spanish Church Revisited: The Episcopal *Gravamina* of 1279," in *Authority and Power: Studies on Medieval Law and Government Presented to Walter Ullmann on His Seventieth Birthday,* ed. B. Tierney and P. Linehan (Cambridge, 1980), pp. 127–147. On complaints about Peter's favor toward Jews, see C. Estow, *Peter the Cruel of Castile: 1350–69* (Leiden, 1995), pp. 154–179; and on his Jewish mother, M. Kriegel, "Histoire sociale et ragots: sur l' 'ascendance juive' de Ferdinand le Catholique," in *Movimientos migratorios y expulsiones en la diáspora occidental* (Pamplona, 2000), pp. 95–100. For Henry IV's difficulties, see most recently F. Foronda, "Le prince, le palais et la ville: Ségovie ou le visage du tyran dans la Castille du XVe siècle," *Revue Historique* 305 (July 2003): 521–541; A. Echevarria Arsuaga, "La conversion des chevaliers musulmans dans la Castille du XVe siècle," in *Conversions islamiques. Identités religieuses en Islam méditerranéen,* ed. M. García Arenal (Paris, 2001), pp. 119–140. On Isabel as "protector of the Jews and daughter of a Jewess," see the account of the Polish traveler Nicolas Popplau, in J. Liske, *Viajes de extranjeros por España y Portugal en los siglos XV, XVI, y XVII: colección* (Madrid, 1878).

61. In England, e.g., it stoked (among others) the famous rebellions against King John that produced Magna Carta. See clauses 10 and 11 of that document (both omitted from the version reissued by John in 1216).

9 Paradoxes of the Senses

Gabrielle M. Spiegel

Christian thought in the Middle Ages always struggled with the question of the senses as the source of knowledge, pleasure, and desire. Heir to the Aristotelian principle that all knowledge begins in the senses as well as the Neoplatonic distrust of the body and its carnal modes of knowing, and itself committed to the principle that preternatural and supernatural sources of knowledge were available and meaningful, it was difficult for Christian thinkers to reconcile this classical legacy with its own physics and metaphysics. Insofar as medieval thought remained wedded to ancient theories of the senses, there existed intrinsic conflicts that beset the medieval understandings of perception, cognition, and volition by virtue of their reliance on an epistemology fundamentally at odds with the Christian metaphysics of the Incarnation. If Christian thought aimed, ultimately, at a purely spiritual apprehension of God, it nonetheless acknowledged that, in this life at least, such aspirations of the soul necessarily relied upon the cognitive modalities supplied by the body, whose own imperatives ultimately posed insurmountable obstacles to the achievement of genuine and pure spiritual knowledge. The three essays discussed below explore the multiple paradoxes generated within medieval considerations of the place of the senses in an epistemological understanding of man as reliant upon the senses for knowledge, but whose proper goal was to overcome the implications that this fundamental belief had for the deeper search for a truth that lay beyond sense perception.

Thus, in chapter 7, Joachim Küpper demonstrates how, insofar as late medieval thinkers relied upon Aristotle's epistemology that delineated and joined the perception of the senses and reasonable action, thus linking—in humans anyway—the sensory data processed by the cognitive senses through the "passive intellect" to "higher" forms of cognition, produced through the "illumination" offered by the consciousness of the immaterial *intellectus agens,* or active intellect, they were bound to founder in the face of the central mystery of Christian dogma: the fact that the sacrificial death of Christ only makes sense if there is no other way of resolving the possibilities of right action. In other words, Christ's redemptive sacrifice required the idea of original sin, and original sin, in turn, meant the weakening of *ratio*—of rational judgment governing perception and behavior—to such an extent that the desire prompted by the human senses and sensuality could not be controlled. That intrinsic—and necessary—fallibility of reason left Christians in the grips of the permanent rebellion of desire against reason, distinguishing thereby Christian from ancient pagan moral philosophy.

Moreover, since—quite obviously—the senses could not be abandoned or bypassed, for they were the means whereby embodied beings acquired cognition of the world and therefore were necessary for self-preservation (*conservatio sui*), the very thing that preserved life led inexorably to a failure to recognize truth, and thus to metaphysical self-destruction. The senses thus functioned in the Christian Middle Ages, he argues, at one and the same time as the basis of embodied life and the cause of spiritual death. This paradox, which had its corollary in the dual valorization of the activity of the senses (compared, say, to Cartesian modernity) and equally strong repudiation of the senses as the locus of desire, meant that medieval Christians were trapped in what Küpper calls a "*hysterical*" relation to the senses, by which he means a cognitive and moral impasse, an inertia or inability to move fully in either direction, either to transcend the senses or to abandon the self to them in the form of unregulated desire.

The fundamental and unresolvable incoherence at the core of medieval theories of cognition are, he then goes on to show, staged and modeled in the text of the *Arcipreste de Talavera,* by Alfonso Martínez of Toledo, completed in 1438, in which emphatic praise of the senses and sensual pleasure is accompanied by an equally harsh denunciation of them. What this demonstration indicates, is that we have perhaps misunderstood the source of such contradictory procedures as they appear in a host of medieval texts, from Andreas Capellanus to the *Roman de la Rose.* Instead of seeing the renunciations that so frequently appear at the end of such texts as a kind of moral cover for otherwise frankly sensuous treatments of the body, the senses and sexuality,

Küpper argues that they are inescapable contradictions endemic to medieval epistemology, which relies upon the mediation of experience by the senses to produce knowledge of the world, but which at the same time produces the concupiscence that is the source of evil, including cognitive evil. This is the ultimate impasse of medieval anthropology and epistemology, contradictory in themselves (and not, therefore the product of a *dualistic* philosophy or theology), making man a being that finds itself in permanent struggle with itself. In contrast to ancient, that is, Aristotelian, epistemology, where the cognitive faculty governs desire, in Christian dogma, it is desire that governs the cognitive faculty. Small wonder that medieval thought so often relies upon a reflex of determinism to escape the unavoidable moral consequences of this cognitive dilemma.

Küpper's analysis offers, I think, a perfect analytical framework for approaching the cognitive and moral struggles of figures like Paul, Augustine, even Origen, that are taken up in chapters 1 and 8, by Eugene Vance and David Nirenberg, respectively, but before passing on to those essays I would like to pose the following question: To what extent was a writer like Alfonso Martínez of Toledo aware of the *sources* of the contradictory impulses which his text staged; or did he see the problem in more narrowly theological terms, and hence tended to enact it as a dualism, rather than a paradox? Can one generalize from Alfonso Martínez to other authors whose works betray the same hysterical tendencies?

In significant ways, Vance's wonderful essay on Augustine's struggles with the senses—and his own sensuality—and his lifelong (or at least postconversion) desire for a spiritual apprehension of God enacts a problematic very close to that outlined by Küpper, only in this case it is the Platonic scorn of the body, rather than an Aristotelian epistemological embrace of the senses as the origin of knowledge, that figures as its source. Moreover, as Vance indicates, Augustine's reckoning with these questions was less systematic than it was dynamic, evolving as his personal and political needs changed, making it impossible to identify any single, definitive stance that informed the various positions he staked out, a phenomenon that equally informs Nirenberg's sensitive treatment of Augustine and the carnality of the Jews. The paradoxes that seem characteristic of all such ventures begins in Augustine himself, whom Vance identifies as a Pauline (hence Neoplatonic) Christian who was at the same time a sworn enemy of the Platonists, against whom he defended the radical Christian doctrine of the resurrection of the body, as purified flesh, in frontal assault on the Platonist desire for an afterlife in which the soul is freed entirely from its body and stationed in eternal contemplation of the truth of uncreated forms, that is, of God as the "It-Itself" (*Idipsum*).

I will not rehearse here Vance's precise and complex unpacking of Augustine's theory of cognition, in particular of "extramissive vision" and the mediating role of memory, all of which he has so powerfully explained. What strikes me as most interesting—or at least the aspect that most overlaps with the other chapters—is his analysis of Augustine's varying attempts, from the *De musica,* to the *Confessions,* to the *De Genesi ad litteram* and, finally, *The City of God,* to at once preserve the senses as a source of cognition and spiritual joy and to deny and/or transcend their capacity, in giving rise to the passions, to draw the soul away from God and into a state of decadence, that "metaphysical self-destruction" noted by Küpper. Indeed, Vance sees the *Confessions* as Augustine's attempt to negotiate with the experience of all the corporeal senses and to demonstrate his own power to address the claims of the bodily senses and to consign their truth to the realm of the body, thereby transcending them in spiritual knowledge. What Küpper identified as the "literary realism" intrinsic to representations of the senses in Christian thought, Vance sees as Augustine's prescriptions for subjugating them. One solution to this problem, in the *Confessions,* was to focus on the *imagines* gathered by the senses, imprinted on memory and stored as *phantasmata*—that is, as Vance explains, as figments of carnal thinking. In that sense, for Augustine, the senses, whose role in this life as the source of knowledge of the world cannot be gainsaid, must remain both viable yet subordinate to the free will and judgment of reason. But the difficulty for Augustine, of course, was the powerlessness of the will and the distortion of reason effected by original sin. As narrated in the *Confessions,* it was only after Augustine's encounter with Christian Platonists and the allegorical mode of reading Scripture that he was able to understand the need to turn inward to the realm of the "inner senses" of the soul—the "ears" of the heart and the "eye" of the mind. Yet even here, the soul's apprehension of its own spiritual nature is mediated by sense perception, for in man's embodied life in the world, the *invisibilia* of God are understood only via the things which are made, the *visibilia,* hence dependent on sense perception.

A more successful approach, perhaps, was Augustine's attempt to meet the contradiction head on, by defining the senses and the world they make visible negatively, as that which is not God. The *visibilia,* the world of sensible things, according to this mode of reasoning, presents itself as other, that is as a *sign*—"a thing" that "makes something other than itself come into our thought." Signs—signifiers—thus function in the alienated world of man's *regio dissimilitudines* as that which point—negatively—to the "other" which is It-Itself, that is, God. They do so as images of the sensible world that become subject to the purely mental things in memory that are not *sensibilia* but *intelligibilia.* Thus far in the development of Augustine's thought, we are told, Platonism is alive and well.

But the ever restless Augustine, by the time he was finishing the *Confessions,* became wary of a spirituality that erased the literal truth of the Creation—its physics—and sought to show how Creation might be understood spiritually, that is, metaphysically. For Augustine, the crux of the problem was posed by the doctrine of the Resurrection, which functions in his evolving thought much as the sense-based epistemology of Aristotle does later for the *Arcipreste de Talavera:* as the bodily carnality that must, somehow, be incorporated into a Christian metaphysics of the spiritual, requiring, therefore, that the bodily senses be reintegrated into spiritual apprehension, in contradiction of the Platonists' certainty that physical resurrection of the body is impossible. Augustine, ever sensitive to the promptings of the body, proposes, against the assertions of his old enemies, that resurrection is not just of the inner person, but of the fleshly body itself, as in the assertion that "yet in my flesh shall I see God." To dissolve this inhering paradox of Christian doctrine, Augustine displaces it, claiming (in no less a paradoxical way), that the flesh, qua flesh, is nonetheless purified in its resurrected state, so that while the bodily senses are truly sensual, even in heaven, flesh then shall be spiritual and subject to the spirit. And in this purified state the body complements, rather than impairs, the participation of resurrected Christians in their vision of God. Flesh and spirit, spiritualized flesh and embodied, "carnalized" spirit—these same themes reappear in Nirenberg's penetrating analysis of the Christian hermeneutics and politics that revolve around the figure of the Jews as both prophets of the spirit and, post-Incarnation, dead letters of the flesh. Yet again, a central Christian dogma makes paradox abound.

Ranging widely through the first centuries of Patristic thought and writing, Nirenberg suggests that the "fruitful flesh" of the Jews nourished the growth of a theory of reading, of a specific Christian hermeneutic practice founded by Paul, which ultimately inflected, or, on his reading, perhaps even constituted, later Christian theories of sovereignty. Instead of simply jettisoning the Jews as historically and spiritually irrelevant after the Incarnation (as Christian dualists like Marcion were more than willing to do), Paul sought to maintain the ongoing relevance of God's covenant with Abraham and the figure of Isaac as prophet of the spirit. In keeping the Jews "legible" as prophetic *figurae,* yet insisting on the supersession of the New Testament over the Old, dualistic tendencies in Paul's thought came to the fore, turning Jews into emblems of carnality and pure flesh, from whom the spirit that had once informed the Chosen People had been evacuated.

Although Paul argued that gentiles should become heirs of Abraham in the spirit, without becoming Jews in the flesh (an argument that bespeaks the enduring significance of Abraham and Isaac, a point to which I shall return), the underlying logic of his hermeneutics established a stark distinction between flesh and spirit, Old Testament and New, Law and Grace, and all the other antinomies with which medievalists are familiar. One unnoticed consequence of Patristic hermeneutics, Nirenberg argues, was to make the Jews an emblem of carnality, a metaphor taken up and carried to extremes in subsequent Christian polemics. To be sure, Augustine, despite or perhaps because of his early Manichean leanings, sought instead, as Vance showed in other contexts, to keep the literal, and hence the flesh, visible by adopting, in Nirenberg's words, a "historical realism . . . that restored a literal and spiritual value to the Torah and its people." Yet the price for this legibility, Nirenberg argues, was the alienation of Jews who lived after the Incarnation, who were converted into corporeal shells of flesh without spirit.

The metaphorics of Christian hermeneutics, whether dualistic or figural, thus transformed "Jews" into repositories of flesh and it was *as flesh* that Jews entered the realm of politics and contributed to evolving ideas of Christian sovereignty. Here, once again, Augustine provides the conceptual "myth" (to borrow Lévi-Strauss's term) with which to think philosophical questions about the relationship between matter and spirit. Augustine, Nirenberg demonstrates, assigned to the Jews an exceptional political space as the vessels of God's wrath who, like Cain after the slaying of Abel, nonetheless were not to be put to death, but maintained to toil the earth, figures of the "bare life," protected by sovereigns precisely as testimony to Christ's regnant sovereignty over the earth. The political complement to this semiotic role of the "Jews" was royal prerogative over, hence protection of, Jews. In their exceptionality—the essence of sovereignty if one follows Schmitt—protection of Jews became emblematic of royal power at its most absolute, and the idiom through which royal sovereignty itself was articulated. Thus Nirenberg can argue that Jewish carnality became a means of representing the hypercarnality of monarchs (St. Louis would not be pleased with the formulation, I am sure) and, when things went wrong, were liable to being equated with Jews, as he compellingly shows. On both the hermeneutic and political level, therefore, Judaism, as bare life and letter of flesh, became the focal point for the articulation of Christian order.

Doubtless, this abbreviated version of Nirenberg's rich and nuanced essay does not do it justice. But given the limited time, let me go on to pose a few questions. If we accept his analysis, it still remains a puzzle to me why Jews should have been so persistently literalized and carnalized in Christian hermeneutics. Once Paul had determined to keep Abraham and Isaac, covenantal Judaism and the like "legible" as prophecies of the spiritual world (and one might point out that in a thinker like Eusebius, they are more than prophecies; indeed Abraham figures among the patriarchal *christi*—but that is another subject), why do they not retain a positive value? If, as Nirenberg argues, for Justin Martyr, Tertullian, Origen, and others, the Law (OT) understood literally was indeed a curse but spiritually a blessing, why, indeed, is the Law not seen, as Augustine saw it, as closed but not condemned? I can think of a score of historiographical texts (many of them indebted to Eusebius) in which Israel as the Chosen People figures metaphorically, when applied, for example, to the Saxons by Bede, as a wholly positive image. In other words, by keeping the Old Testament, Jews as God's Chosen People, and Isaac and the Law legible as prophecies and *models* of Christian life, to what extent is the positive resonance intrinsic in this procedure evacuated, or not? Nirenberg suggests completely, but I wonder.

Similarly, while I think the argument about Jewish exceptionality as an emblem of the exceptionality of sovereignty is brilliant, and helps to explain certain vulnerabilities of medieval monarchs, can this really be the essence of Christian theories of kingship? What, may I ask, has happened to sacral kingship, to the king not only as the protector of Jews but as the vice-gerent of God on earth? Do we lose something by modeling sovereignty only on the basis of what I am tempted to call its Jewish exceptionality?

The three essays discussed here are powerful demonstrations of the complicated relationship that Christian thinkers as diverse as Paul, Augustine, and Alfonso Martínez of Toledo posited between the senses on which man, as an embodied creature, relied for knowledge of the world and of his spiritual nature and destiny. The impossibility of bypassing sense perception in favor of a purely spiritual apprehension of God meant that all created beings were caught, to one degree or another, in the epistemological impasse inherent in the very nature of human life in the world. Paul's figuration of the Jew as "pure flesh" is, in a sense, only the most radical formulation of one pole of this necessarily dual understanding of man in relation to God, an understanding that Augustine continually contested and problematized, while struggling to resolve it, throughout the course of his life. No purely philosophical stance, whether Aristotelian, as in the case of Alfonso Martínez of Toledo, or Platonic, as in the case of Augustine and Paul, offered adequate paths through the field of paradoxes generated by the physics of the body in service to the metaphysical aspirations of the spirit. What each author has shown us in his chapter, is the heroic lengths to which medieval thinkers went in attempting to resolve the contradictions that such a conception of man entailed. Bound by body to a reliance upon the senses, both material and immaterial, yet at the same time awakened by them to the possibilities of spirit, medieval thought was caught in the paradoxes generated by human nature itself.

10 *Representation and Participation*

Some Remarks on Medieval French Drama

ANDREAS KABLITZ

In the midst of life—right in the middle of a lively town, in fact—Pieter Brueghel chooses the setting for his depiction of Christ bearing the cross (fig. 10.1). Even a fleeting glance will reveal that historical truth is not a major concern here. Doubtless, the figures mourning in the foreground can be taken to allude to well-known iconographic traditions; Mary is easily identified. But the town life surrounding the scene is based on Brueghel's own times, especially the clothing.

The message conveyed by this painting is open to various interpretations. Thus it is at first quite difficult to detect the central action: the bearing of the cross. It almost gets lost in the hustle and bustle of this town—as if the painting were shouting at its beholders: "Look at the careless way in which you treat the salvation wrought by Christ." For it can scarcely be sustained that all those shown in the painting are interested in Christ and his cross. Indeed, this is another reason for the striking difference in pictorial representation between the group of mourners and the other persons shown. The biblical characters are the only ones who exhibit appropriate behavior. They are set off from the others, who either seem to regard Christ suffering and collapsing under the weight of the cross as a spectacular exhibition, or are not interested in Him at all. But the borrowings from Brueghel's contemporary world which are visible here seem to have yet another meaning: Christ's passion is still being enacted amongst you; you are still hurting Jesus who brought about your salvation.

Establishing so strong a link between past and present may seem an anachronism, if looked at from an historically informed point of view. It seems

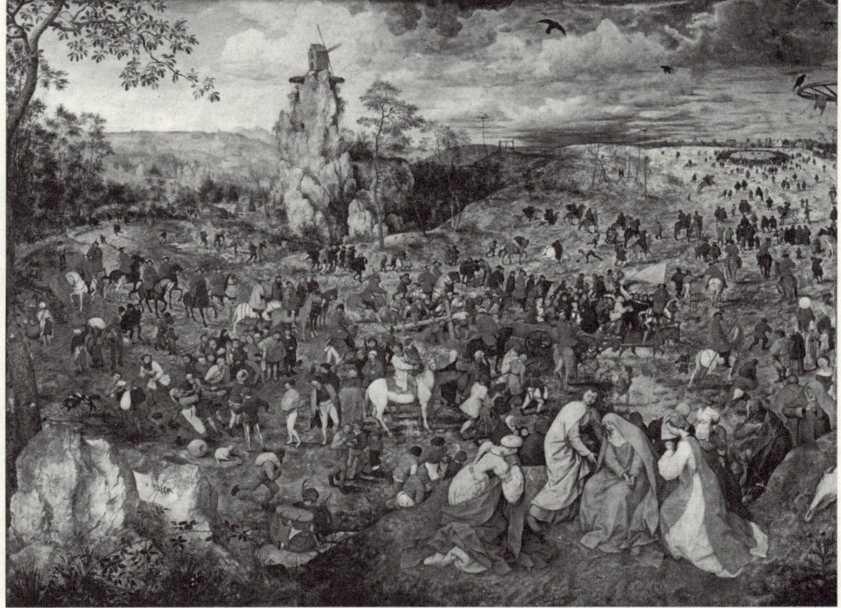

Figure 10.1. Pieter Brueghel the Elder, *The Procession to Calvary* (1564). Kunsthistorisches Museum, Vienna.

inadmissible to bring together different periods in such a way. But even historicism, which thrived on such distinctions, had to admit that chronology sometimes thwarts the project of a clear differentiation of historical constellations. This explains the famous formula of the simultaneity of that which is not simultaneous (die Gleichzeitigkeit des Ungleichzeitigen).

Yet, in this case the seeming historical inappropriateness between the event painted in Brueghel's picture and the setting of it appears to be a different one. At first sight, the nothing-but-curious relationship between present and past proves, at a closer look, a consequence or a symptom of one of the basic features of Christian thought, that is to say, the relation between truth and time. Christian truth, as revealed in the holy book, as related in the Bible, is substantially based on narration. The Bible tells the story of salvation, opening with the Creation and the Fall of Man, and ending with Man's Redemption and the history of early Christianity as reported in the Acts of the Apostles. However, the substantial link between narration and past, simultaneously, implies also one between past and truth. It is exactly here that one of the crucial questions of Christian thought originates: For a Christian, the salvation of man implies that the facts narrated in the New Testament are not simply things of the past, but live on in the present. The importance of this problematic relationship is constantly growing as long as the apocalypse, in other words Christ's return to earth and the subsequent end of the world as it was predicted in the Gospel, does not happen. Thus, one of the major concerns of Christian thought is to be found in the very question of how to transport the biblical past to contemporary life.

The respective relationship between truth and time proves quite different in philosophical systems which rely on a set of abstract assumptions—as, for instance, in Platonic or Aristotelian metaphysics. Abstraction itself guarantees timelessness, and this advantage of philosophical thought probably leads to one of the most fundamental reasons why Christian thought has been so much interested in an initially astonishing synthesis of the truth of Revelation and pagan philosophy. For this synthesis, the appropriation of a rational system of thought transforms a story, being as such unavoidably bound to time, into a theological system that overcomes time—creating simultaneously a quite unique and specific combination of empirical and analytical truth. The goal to establish timelessness of truth, therefore, appears indeed to be one of the major motivations for the Christians' interest in the heathens' thought. Yet this strategy, perhaps best observed in scholastic theology, which aims to free truth from time, reveals, at the same time, the ultimate base of all theology. The truth of theology requires as its proof the wording of the Gospel. Theology, therefore, relies ultimately on exegesis, thus initiating the specific Christian interference between systematic thinking and exegetic practice.

In this regard, it is interesting to observe that exegesis of the Bible itself aims to match the narration's dependence on time and the timelessness of truth. In one of the most prominent and influential texts on the theory of exegesis, in St. Augustine's *De doctrina christiana,* the author attaches great importance to defining the conditions under which the wording of the Bible requires an allegorical interpretation:

> Demonstrandus est igitur prius modus inveniendae locutionis, propriane an figurata sit. Et iste omnino modus est, ut quidquid in sermone divino neque ad morum honestatem, neque ad fidei veritatem proprie referri potest, figuratum esse cognoscas. Morum honestas ad diligendum Deum et proximum, fidei veritas ad cognoscendum Deum et proximum pertinet.[1]

"Neque ad morum honestatem neque ad fidei veritatem": whenever the text of the Bible does not refer explicitly to a moral rule or to a principle of the faith it is to be understood allegorically. Defining a segment of the wording of the Bible that does not need any further interpretation allows one to secure the self-interpretation of the holy text. For, whatever the meaning of allegorical parts of the Bible may be, this sense has necessarily to be found elsewhere in the same biblical text, for it is the only source of all truth. In the passages of the holy text, where Christian doctrine becomes evident, all allegorical meaning from other parts of the Bible must be included. Narration again proves to be insufficient for the revelation of truth. On the contrary, it has to be integrated in this truth, becoming explicit elsewhere.

It might appear as if the Christian service, the celebration of mass, gives greater significance to narration. Indeed, the reading of several parts of the Bible plays an important part in this ceremony. And even the very center of mass, the consecration of bread and wine, becoming Christ's flesh and blood, resembles a re-presentation of the Last Supper. Yet it cannot be denied that the structure of the mass itself is not at all a mimetic one. Its highly symbolic status seems even to avoid all narrative representation. This becomes all the more clear if we take into consideration that a greater presence of mimetic representation is restricted to only a few liturgical exceptions, especially in the services of the Holy Week. (And interestingly in the same week, in which the consecration of bread and wine will no longer take place, namely, on Holy Friday. Nonetheless, it is not more than a speculation that there is a substantial link between the absence of the sacrament and the increase of mimetic representation in the liturgy.) That is to say, furthermore, that the Christian liturgy does not actually make evident the presence of the events narrated in the Holy Text; it does not—with the one exception of transubstantiation—guarantee the presence of the past. This is, as I will try to argue in this essay, exactly one of the major tasks of the mystery plays. The, at first sight, astonishing combination of past and present in Brueghel's picture corresponds precisely to the basic structures of the mystery play. By its very semiotic construction, it succeeds in bridging the gap between a biblical past and an actual everyday life, that seems to take place quite far from the biblical stories. The mystery play demonstrates that later generations continue to participate in the events of the life of Christ.

Let me give you as a first example for this concept of the ongoing presence of the history of salvation, a little scene coming from what might be regarded as a transformation of the mystery play, a transformation that survived the break in history caused by the Reformation. I mean the enactment of Christ's passion in the form of an oratorio, or, to be precise, Bach's *St. Matthew Passion.* Jesus, having sat down for the Last Supper with his disciples, announces that one of them will betray him during the following night. The text reads—I quote the Authorized Version—"they were exceeding sorrowful, and began everyone of them to say unto him: 'Lord, is it I?'" And when Judas asks him, "Master, is it I?" Jesus answers: "Thou hast said." Bach set all this to music as printed. But just before Judas speaks, there is a break in the setting of the Gospel in Bach's score; a chorale is interpolated at this point. When the apostles ask, "Lord, is it I?" the congregation comes in with its own, sung answer: "It is I, I should atone, My hand and feet bound in hell." The treason committed against Jesus by each and every sin is still taking place, and thus Judas is still present in every faithless Christian. But all of those sinners can also, by the same token, be regarded as sitting at the table of the Last Supper. Guilt and salvation are moments of participation, and this participation in the history of salvation cancels the differences of time. What is told in the Gospel—as becomes evident in the respective scene of Bach's *St. Matthew Passion*—is not a story of the past, nor is it a story about others or—even less—about strangers; it is and remains alive in the present, in which everyone participates, whether they want it or not. For even the unbelievers are part of this story. In the story of Christ's passion this part is enacted by the Jews who urge Pilate to pass judgment in a way that runs counter to his actual wishes.

This constellation, the ongoing presence of past history, can be seen in the opposite of the history of salvation as well, as it has been elaborated by Christian theology: in the concept of original sin. Original sin means that the fall of man is more than just a single event in the past, it is something that remains true in the present. The genealogy of man as descending from Adam is also his generic definition as a sinner: Man is (and remains) known as "the old Adam."

I should like to use this view of time in a context of the history of salvation and grace as my point of departure for a brief look at what can still be regarded as the most remarkable contribution made by German "Romanistik" to research on the mystery play. I mean Rainer Warning's habilitation thesis *Funktion und Struktur. Die Ambivalenzen des geistlichen Spiels.* This book is nowadays more discussed by students of German literature than by those specializing in Romance literatures. The central thesis brought forward by Warning can be resumed in the author's own words as follows: "The mystery play tends to re-mythologize the history of salvation on a monumental scale. It redirects the story enacted into the very dimension against which its *kerygma* was constituted in the first place: The biblical acts of salvation are present there in a mythical, archetypal form."[2]

In the background of this thesis, a special interpretation of time may also be detected. The *kerygma* directs all attention (in Warning's words) "to the expectation of future fulfilment of a promise made by and in an historic event in the past (or an event believed to be historic)." Myth, on the other hand, which is determined by its inception rather than its goal, directs all attention to the origin. The tendency back toward myth, which Warning observes in the type of *mimesis* specific to the mystery play with its reenactment of the past, mobilizes a certain pagan potential: Back to mythology means back to paganism. The context of this article does not allow a more detailed analysis of the various implications of Warning's thesis. Let me just mention that it implies a certain concept of aesthetics as well. The mystery play, like all plays free from the constraints of everyday life, shows this freedom by resisting all things official, and thus it seems to have a natural tendency toward negation or even subversion. I am not convinced that such a concept of the aesthetic, obviously due to a modern theoretical framework, can provide an adequate framework for a characterization of the profoundly premodern, medieval mystery play. But this issue cannot be discussed in detail here. I would rather like to concentrate on the semantics of time on which Warning's thesis rests.

It cannot at all be denied that the expectation of the last judgment, and thus an eschatological moment, is of crucial importance for all varieties of the Christian faith. Yet, I do not hold an opposition between pagan myth with its orientation toward origins, and the *kerygma* with its orientation toward future fulfilment, to be an adequate instrument to allow us to understand the complexity of the Christian interpretation of time. For such a reading overlooks the fact that the events narrated in the New Testament are themselves fulfilments of anterior promises. This is borne out by the frequency of the formula "that it might be fulfilled which was spoken by the prophet"—especially in the narratives of Christ's passion. In fact, as it has been pointed out so perfectly by Erich Auerbach,[3] all of the Old Testament was read in a figural sense with regard to the New Testament. But to read the events narrated in the New Testament as *implementa* of the *figurae* found in the Old Testament, means seeing them as the fulfilment of a promise, and this imparts a sense of presence to the events of the *Novum Testamentum* which differs from the structure of myth. In this regard, it is, by the way, not without interest that myth becomes calculable from the very moment of incarnation. In the Old Testament, the creation of the world is situated in a mythical past without coordinates. But this situation changes with the Advent of the Son of God. In the Christmas entry of the Roman calendar of feasts, the birth of Christ is given an exact date, it is related chronologically both to the foundation of

Rome and to the creation of the world. Thus, it is the enduring presence of salvation itself, and not the later orientation toward the eschatology of fulfilment, that makes the old concept of myth disappear.

Again, it is the protestant Bach who provides us with a clear case in point: In the fifth cantata of his Christmas oratorio, the cantata for the Sunday after New Year, where we hear about the magi coming to Jerusalem from the East, there is a trio, in which the soprano and tenor parts give a rather chromatic, somewhat whining rendering of the following verses: "Oh, when will the time appear, oh, when will He comfort His children?" And then suddenly the alto interrupts in an almost angry tone and sings with great determination: "Be silent, He is here already." The effectiveness of salvation is more than just a promise for the future, it is something that is alive in the present, and it means enduring participation in the saving grace, the workings of which are told in the New Testament.

This conception of time according to Christian thought is also central to the mystery play. Indeed, it is a point against an interpretation of this genre or phenomenon as a pagan remythologizing of Christianity. The complex structure of the Christian conception of time does not describe the mystery play as a genre that simply recalls biblical happenings to the present: Rather, it makes tangible what is implied anyway, it shows the ongoing presence of these happenings which in itself is independent of such recall. This has at least one important consequence: The mystery play not only transports the past into the present, it also localizes the present in a biblical past that is only apparently so. By its very construction, both past and present are freed from time.

If we follow this thesis, we have to envisage some important consequences for what might be called the semiotic arrangement of the theatrical form developed by the mystery play. Its peculiarities can be grasped by contrasting them with the variety of theater that is probably best known to most of us; let me start with the arrangement of space.

The theater of our times can be described as a heterotope—to use a word of Michel Foucault which seems to be much in fashion these days. The space of theater is divided from the world of everyday life by a border which we can only cross with the help of an admission ticket, usually more or less hard to get. Yet, within the theater, there is another border which partly cancels the first one: For the everyday world excluded by the former now comes back to us on the stage—but with a crucial difference: It returns in a symbolic mode. By this change, it gains great potential, for a symbolic world has almost infinite elasticity—for example, as regards the treatment of time and space.

Now, it seems to me that the mystery play is characterized by a more or less complete absence of this type of distinction. There is no significant border between the space of the everyday world and the space of the mystery play. The "stage" is identical with the space of everyday life. From a teleological point of view it might look as if this situation represents a lower state of development within the history of theater. But, this is not the case, for the lack of difference has a quite precise function in the construction of the medieval theater, as we shall see.

To mention another kind of distinction, this involves the very difference between actors and spectators. As is well known, this kind of drama was not performed by professionals, but by laymen. This fact has at least one major consequence for our context: The actors can thus be taken to represent the community surrounding the performance of which they are a part. Especially in American research and especially with reference to the Corpus Christi plays, medievalists have put forward the thesis that the mystery play is a social enactment in which the town community represents itself as a Christian community. I think this thesis identifies a very important aspect of the mystery play. But it is the concept of representation that is of particular weight here. The actors representing the social community to which they belong are deputies acting on behalf of other potential actors—they are deputies a little like the members of a modern-day parliament.

Jan-Dirk Müller has rightly emphasized the need to keep up a distinction between play on one side and worship or cult on the other—even though a certain continuity between the two phenomena cannot be denied.[4] Nonetheless, I should like to mention an element common to both, and it can be found in the aforementioned role of the deputy. The institution of the mass is characterized by the presence of deputies for the congregation at the altar, such as acolytes. In a similar way, the lay actors of a mystery play stand in front of a community of which they nevertheless form a part. Representation and participation coincide in this case.

Let me repeat that much can be said in favor of the thesis quoted above, which takes the mystery play to be a social enactment, a kind of theatrical self-portrait, of a Christian community. On the other hand, this view seems to name but one half of the construction on which this genre is based. For the double relation of representation and participation in which the actors stand with regard to their social community holds just as well for the characters enacted by them. The actors represent certain biblical characters, but (as we have seen), owing to the continuing presence of biblical history, they participate in the being of these biblical personalities even outside their role play. The relation between person and role is thus not just an occasional one, but a substantial one—another decisive difference between medieval and modern theater. In every human being that sins and thus betrays Jesus, there is a part of Judas. But insofar as we are saved, Christ's love has given us a part of His person as well, for St. Paul says that we are reborn in Christ.

Thus, the semiotic construction at the base of the mystery play can be understood as doubling the relation between representation and participation. The actors represent the social community to which they belong, and they represent characters, or rather: persons within the history of salvation, of which they are also a part. Taken together, these two aspects show the mystery play to be an institution with the help of which a community ascertains the continuing presence of salvation history and its own participation in it, bridging the gap between (narrative) truth and presence. Yet, it is important to take into consideration, that this effect of presence is not *produced* by the mystery play, but that the play makes evident what also holds elsewhere: the ongoing—although latent—presence of the biblical (narrative) past. If that is indeed the case, one may ask why such ascertainment is necessary, seeing that participation in salvation is already guaranteed by the sacrament which forms the center of mass. The mystery play, however—and this is the salient difference as well as the surplus afforded by it—brings salvation history to the space where the life of a community is lived. And the reverse is also true: The mystery play marks the fact that the world of social life belongs to salvation history. It is not only at the privileged place of worship, in the heterotope of the church building (the border of which can only be crossed by undergoing a reduced form of a purgation ritual by holy water), but everywhere within the space occupied by community life, that the mystery play affords a tangible demonstration of the presence of salvation, to be enacted by members of this community in front of each other and for each other.

And this is why I think that Warning's thesis concerning an alleged remythologizing and repaganization unduly modernizes the mystery play. But at the same time, I think that the traditional view, which Warning rightly challenges, the view of the mystery play as a merely didactic genre, plays down and indeed misses some of the most interesting aspects of this form of drama: By ascertaining the community's participation in salvation, the mystery play activates a central element within the fabric of Christian thought. It attempts to present a solution for one of the basic problems of Christian culture: It offers a chance to bridge the gap between truth and time.

This concludes the systematic part of my remarks. However, I should like to work out my thesis in somewhat greater detail by analyzing a few peculiarities of at least one example of the medieval mystery play. For this purpose I have chosen the *Passion Sainte-Geneviève.* The complete title of the 1974 edition is *Le Mystère de la Passion Nostre Seigneur du manuscrit 1131 de la Bibliothèque Sainte Geneviève.* The language of the play seems to indicate the fifteenth century as its date of composition; scholars opt mostly for the year 1440. As to its place of origin—and thus the traces of dialect to be discerned in it—the text shows important traits of the *koinè* formed by the Parisian dialect of the fourteenth and fifteenth centuries; some anomalies indicate the North-East of France.

I have put forward the thesis that the mystery play allows the community enacting it to ascertain the continuing presence of salvation and its participation in it. One of the strategies used for this purpose can be compared to a certain technique of biblical exegesis. In both cases, a narration is typically made susceptible to the attribution of a *sensus moralis.* In this way, the story narrated can be turned into a plan of action. And this is exactly what our passion play does. Toward the end of the prologue, which is little else but a summary of the passion story up to the morning of Easter Sunday, its speaker addresses the audience. For the narration of the various epiphanies of the risen Christ, who showed himself first to Mary Magdalen, and then to all his disciples together, this narration leads to the punch line that it pays to serve the Lord. And so the audience is invited to do just this. And the prologue ends with a prayer to the Lord to afford us the possibility of being of service to Him.

It is interesting to note that immediately after the prologue, the action of the play sets in with a scene that demonstrates the disciples' readiness to be of service. Jesus is about to set forth for Bethany. He asks three of His disciples to accompany Him: Judas, John, and James. This is quite unimportant for the development of the main action. But it becomes important, because the positive reaction of each of the three is worked out as a demonstration of obedience. All of them—the traitor Judas must obviously be understood to be lying—all of them stress their willingness to obey Jesus's words and back this up by very precise reasons: out of love to Jesus—or because they want to obey His law in every respect. Jesus's simple request for company is moralized by turning it into a question of obedience. From the very beginning, in the correspondence between the end of the prologue, which is addressed to the audience, and the beginning of the passion story, which is centered around Jesus's request to obtain the service of His disciples, we see a marked continuity between the theatrical situation and the dramatic action, that is, the passion story.

This is all the more true since the willingness exhibited by the disciples in the Bible itself is undoubtedly ambiguous. Not only is there Judas's false claim that he will follow Jesus out of love. Even James, who professes his faith with an honest heart, will be dissuaded by fear from following Jesus when the latter is taken prisoner. Thus the text offers a potential for identification that includes the possibility of failure or of sin. And this means that from the outset, the historical action and the world of the audience stand in direct relation to each other.

Let me discuss one more strategy of this passion play which again aims at highlighting the presence of the salvation brought about by Christ's incarnation and death. It is a feature of this text (and of many others of the same type) that it treats the words of Scripture rather freely. Not only do these texts enrich the story narrated by interpolating passages from other sources, such as apocryphal texts or the liturgy. It is also quite remarkable that their authors feel free to change the order of action as told in the Gospel. That Jesus goes to Bethany one more time before His passion—that is something that can be read in the New Testament; John, Matthew, and Mark report it. In the Gospel according to John, Mary Magdalen then approaches and pours oil on His head—this is taken in ill humor by the disciples, who maintain somewhat sourly that the money spent for the oil would have been of more use if given to the poor. In Luke's version there is a report on an invitation to the house of a Pharisee, much earlier, in chapter 7. During the meal, an anonymous woman, a known sinner, accosts Jesus, bathes His feet with her tears and dries them with her hair—upon which Jesus forgives all her sins. The *Passion Sainte-Geneviève* throws the two episodes together. The text links the scene in which the repentant sinner washes Jesus's feet and the one in which oil is poured on His head. Why this change?

A first (if perhaps somewhat superficial) answer could be that, in our mystery play, the narrative of Christ's passion becomes a kind of compendium of the New Testament. Presumably this would lead into the right direction, but it has to be taken into account which choices have been made for this compilation. In this case, it seems that a direct link is forged between Christ's death and the forgiveness of all sins. But the most striking effect achieved by this rearrangement is revealed by another change made in the Gospel text.

Immediately after the scene that combines the anointing of Jesus with the forgiveness of all sins, there follows the episode of the resuscitation of Lazarus.

The only exact account of this scene is found in the Gospel according to John, but there it precedes the anointing scene in Bethany. So why the rearrangement in the *Passion Sainte-Geneviève*? Perhaps we can get nearer to an answer by looking closely at the circumstances. When Martha complains about the serious illness of her brother Lazarus, Magdalen, just converted, suggests that Jesus should be called. It is thus by her intercession that Lazarus, who has died in the meantime, is then awoken from the dead—which event, of course, prefigures Christ's own resurrection. Recognition of sin and forgiveness therefore lead to the raising of Lazarus, which is in turn a prelude for the Easter morning. The change in the order of events demonstrates the immediate effectiveness of Magdalen's good deeds, or: of the service she offers to the Lord.

This is another element of the strategy of moralizing the passion story, calculated to let all those involved in its enactment experience their participation. From the resurrection of Christ there is a direct way back via the raising of Lazarus to the penitent sinner, and her repentance is identified as the *via regia* to eternal bliss as early on in the performance as during the recitation of the prologue.

The effectiveness of the salvation brought about by the cross is shown as a chain of cause and effect, and at the same time this salvation is rendered accessible to man's action as a moral being. The moralizing of the passion thus puts its seal on man's participation in the salvation wrought by Christ. And it is my thesis that this is just the central aim of the mystery play. The point of this utterly premodern form of theater is not a retransformation of the Gospel of salvation back into a pagan myth, but rather the activation of the promises contained therein.

Notes

1. Augustinus, *De doctrina christiana,* PL 34, c. 71–72. For the same criteria, see also c. 42: "Deinde illa [. . .] quae aperte postia sunt, vel praecepta vivendi, vel regulae credendi, solertius diligentiusque investigande sunt: quae tanto quisquie plura invenit, quanto est intelligentiae capacior. In iis enim quae aperte in Scripturis posita sunt, inveniuntur illa omnia quae continent fidem, moresque vivendi, spem scilicet atque charitatem."

2. Rainer Warning, *Funktion und Struktur. Die Ambivalenzen des geistlichen Spiels* (München 1974), p. 31. (Translation by Andreas Kablitz.)

3. Erich Auerbach, "Figura," *Archivum romanicum* 22 (1938): pp. 436–489.

4. Jan-Dirk Müller, "Mimesis und Ritual. Zum geistlichen Spiel des Mittelalters," *Mimesis und Simulation,* ed. Andreas Kablitz and Gerhard Neumann (Freiburg im Breisgau, 1998), pp. 241–272.

11 *Blinding Sight*

Some Observations on German Epics of the Thirteenth Century

Jan-Dirk Müller

Medievalists agree that the eye is the privileged sense organ in medieval culture. Intellectual knowledge is produced by visual perception. Visuality provides the metaphors for intellectual processes. Horst Wenzel emphasized the importance of visuality in the semi-oral courtly society of noble laity: courtly culture is a visual culture. The sight of a person reflects his or her inner value, the beauty of the body mirrors the beauty of the soul, corporal virtues reveal moral ones.[1] Hierarchies are represented visually: political order, contracts, feuds, defiance, and so on are expressed by visual rituals. Medieval society is represented by visual signs; understanding the signs means understanding its order.

It is true, there are examples demonstrating the opposite. Visual perception can deceive. The beauty of Ganelon in the *Chanson de Roland* is the beauty of Lucifer, an infernal beauty hiding his inner corruptness. Parzival—when he returns to the court of King Arthur at Plimizoel—seems to be an angel, but is unmasked by Kundrie as unfaithful and pitiless, for he killed his cousin Ither and failed to release king Anfortas from his pain by asking the right question.[2] On the other hand, the ugly and repugnant Kundrie *la surziere,* a creature half human being half animal, surpasses everybody in her extraordinary wisdom and moral insight. Even in a more simple sense vision is deceptive: Cunneware laughs when she first meets Parzival, because he looks like a fool. Everybody knows that she will laugh only when she meets the best of all knights. Therefore the court feels insulted by this laughter mal-à-propos, and Keie punishes her. But he is wrong in seeing only a fool; he is misled by his view, while Cunneware—against appearance—did recognize the future hero.

Visible flaws indicate invisible defects. The songs of Walther von der Vogelweide complain about the discrepancy between the appearance of the courtly society and a merciless lady.[3] The courtly society is characterized by joy (*vröide*):

> Muget ir schouwen waz dem meien
> wunders ist beschert?
> seht an pfaffen, seht an leien
> wie daz allez vert [. . .] muget ir umbesehen? (51, 13–16; 52, 19)

But for the lover all of this is meaningless: he is suffering. The trust in the visible ("Nu wol dan, welt ir die warheit schouwen," 46, 21) is confuted again and again. A song like *Herzeliebez vrouwelîn* (49, 25) considers the clash between being good and being beautiful, yet, by doing so Walther complains about the decay of courtly order: the clash means a defective state of affairs; the visible should be a mirror of virtue. So Walther insists on beauty as an indication of being worthy: "du bist schoene und hâst genuoc" (50, 9). As in dame Orgelluse in the romance of Parzival, too, the contradictory qualities have to be reconciled in the model of the perfect courtly lady.

Courtly ideology presupposes a tight link between inner and outer world, the visual and the invisible. Even if visual signs have to be supported by linguistic ones, spoken or written,[4] visuality is a guarantee of truth. The fallacy of the view—a frequent motif in heroic and courtly epics as well as in fabliaux—is always discussed on the background of its reliability, and, if this reliability is called into question, it happens by visual proof. Courtly epics invent special scenes putting to test visually what cannot be seen: the morals and secret desires of the knights and their ladies. In the so called *Tugendproben* everybody has to try a coat or to empty a goblet, and the one whom the coat fits best or who doesn't spill the wine is the most virtuous.[5] But if the coat is too short, too long, too large, or too tight or if the wine is spilled, the watching courtly society realizes that there is some flaw, some moral lapse, some forbidden thought. In Heinrich von dem Türlin's *Crône* it is the seneschal Keie—the person responsible for courtly behavior—who explains what is the inner reason of the visual defect. So, King Arthur and his knights and ladies can even see the invisible. Seeing is the privileged means to gain knowledge.

It is against this background that I will deal with visual perception in the *Trojanerkrieg* of Konrad von Würzburg.[6] Konrad was a courtly poet in the second half of the thirteenth century in southwestern Germany, who wrote for several lords, prelates, and patricians. His love songs and epics refer to "classical" courtly poetry and strive to surpass them. He is one of the most artistic writers in the German Middle Ages, a *blüemer,*[7] that is, a poet in the tradition of Latin rhetoric, displaying his rhetorical skills in detailed descriptions of persons, clothes, jewelry, arms, feasts, fights, battles. His sumptuous descriptions are *demonstrationes ad oculos,* in the sense of the rhetorical concept of *enargeia* (*evidentia*). *Enargeia* is aiming at a meticulous and vivid picture of reality. An absent object or scene that is represented linguistically is suggested to be present, in the sense that the reader or listener is made to believe that he or she can actually see them. *Ekphrasis* is the literary equivalent of sight in a culture of visuality.[8]

Konrad's descriptions of courtly life, especially courtly beauty, are not only far more detailed than in the texts of Hartmann von Aue, Wolfram von Eschenbach, or even Gottfried von Straßburg, but they also display rhetorical skills, unknown until then in German poetry, exploiting an exuberant repertory of brilliant *colors,* luxurious clothes, precious arms or jewels, and, last but not least, infinitely beautiful female and male bodies. But—this is my thesis—by surpassing his predecessors, Konrad deconstructs the basis of courtly philosophy, the apparently preestablished, only temporarily disputed harmony between exterior and interior beauty, between sight and cognition.

In the prologue of his *Trojanerkrieg*[9] Konrad is comparing the poet with other "artists" such as craftsmen, musicians, or even knights. It is impossible, he emphasizes, to learn to be a poet; the poet is gifted by God Himself; he does not need any instruments to practice his art, but speech and insight (*zunge* and *sin,* v. 135). In order to distinguish the poetaster and the true poet, Konrad returns to the usual metaphors linking cognition to sight. Bad poetry means darkness, good poetry, light, on the one hand *naht, fûle[r] spân[], vinster, dunkel, trüebe[z] herze[],* on the other *glanz, lieht, karfunkel, schîne[n]* (vv. 154–169). Exposing his matter—Troy—he claims that the true poet has to show the core, the "bottom" of things (*ergründen, boden,* 241–243); he should not cling to the surface. But the light he is talking about, which has to illuminate the immense and confusing *materia,* its branches, its turns in order to clear the nearly incomprehensible, is not the dazzling light that Konrad is effusing on his epic world. For this light does not advance cognition, but blindness.

The objects of Konrad's descriptions are either of an incredible beauty or of an incredible dread. Konrad paints the surface of the knightly world in an abundant manner. He is fascinated by visuality and at the same time aims to overcome it. Seeing, the highest sense, no longer permits one to grasp the essence of the courtly world—as it does in Hartmann or Gottfried—but is deceitful. Konrad's courtly world outshines all former courtly worlds without explicitly criticizing them. But at the same time Konrad exposes its contradictions. Surpassing his predecessors in beauty and horror is less a consequence of rhetorical *aemulatio* (even if Konrad in doing so succeeds to demonstrate his mastery as a poet), but aims at the heart of a culture based on the conviction that the invisible is mirrored by the visible.

Konrad tells a series of love stories,[10] all ending badly, and a series of brightly shining fights, all ending in disaster. The sight of the beautiful entails desire, but this desire always leads to ruin. This is not due to the usual Christian discredit of carnal love or to a clerical critique of feudal violence as, for instance, in the quest of the grail in the German *Lancelot en prose.* Konrad deals with a pagan world, but he does not criticize it from a Christian point of view. His courtly society is more beautiful and more brilliant than any before him, but this beauty and brilliance is never contested. Nevertheless the brilliance proves to be disastrous. The overwhelming beauty of women like Helen or Medea destroys everybody coming in touch with them, and the battles, seeming a symphony of colors and sounds when perceived from a distance, turn to be cruel carnage regarded from nearby.

Courtly perfection is ambiguous. This is evident in prince Paris. A prophecy predicts that his deeds will destroy Troy; so his father decides to kill him. But the beauty and the charm of the child prevent the murderers from fulfilling the task. "Courtly" virtues save his life, and his innate courtliness comes to light even in the rural world where he grows up. Linked to his courtliness is his natural sense of justice, to which he owes his name, Par-is: "daz er geheizen Pârîs / wart dur sîn gelîchez reht. / 'pâr' und 'gelîch' sind ebensleht" (662–664). So he is called to decide the strife of the goddesses about the apple of Discordia. At this occasion he is recognized by his courtly behavior as a nobleman and the son of a king. Yet, the appearance is misleading. He is a young man following his desire and therefore he gives the apple of Discordia to Venus, who promised him beforehand the most beautiful lady in the world. His judgment is fatal, for it initiates a cruel war and the destruction of his family and his city. Later on too, Paris's charms and civility cause the people of Troy to turn a deaf ear to all caution and reasonable warnings.

Konrad shows the destructive potential of courtliness, even if courtliness is nevertheless the peak of human culture, and prevents a crime, for no prophecy would justify the murder of an innocent child. Sure, Priamus is wrong when he is delighted by the charm of his unknown son and disregards the threat, but can he—noble and courtly king that he is—do otherwise? He trusts Paris's appearance, but what he sees will prove to be deceiving. Nevertheless, Konrad does not tell stories of *desengaño,* of disillusion. Nothing and nobody are unmasked. There is no *contemptus mundi,* as in medieval poems about *Frouwe Werlt,* no devaluation of the temporal world by the eternal, as in the literature of the sixteenth or seventeenth centuries. The beautiful remains beautiful even if it proves to be pernicious. In Konrad's descriptions actual perfection and future ruin are two faces of the same phenomenon. To make this evident he outdoes former courtly descriptions of beauty.

Sight dazzles the eyes,[11] for what can be seen is brilliant and radiant. The beauty and elegance of young Paris is shining, surpassing the *wunneclîche[n] schîn* of his companions (19596/19598). "Er gap [. . .] liehtebernden glast" (19615); "sîn klarheit [shining] diu dranc unde brach / in manic herze tougen" (19618f.), he is called a "spiegel, geliutert und gereinet, durliuhtec als ein engel": a "mirror, radiant as an angel" (19621, 19624, 19657). And Helen: "ein bluome glanzer wîbe / schein diu vil wunnebære"—a flower between the brilliant women of her court, shining as a miracle (19676f.); she is "die glanz[iu] künigîn" (19706), blinding all by the rays she can "mit ir clârheite blenden" (19713), extinguishing their color (*varwe,* 19717f.).

When Paris first sees Helen, he is overwhelmed by her bright, sparkling beauty (*liehte[n] schoenheit,* 19760f.). Konrad accumulates words like *brinnen, liuhten, regenboge, geverwet von der minne, glanze[],* and the corresponding expressions for seeing and being dazzled (19760–19796). The force of Helen's beauty violently penetrates his mind ("der schoene durch sîn herze brach," 19793). I give a longer quotation describing the miracle and the effects of this beauty:

> ein wildez wunder hât sîn hant
> mit vlîze an ir gebildet;
> ir schoenheit überwildet
> und überwundert allen schîn,
> der von klârheite mac gesîn
> an wîben unde an frouwen.
> Wer mac den glanz geschouwen,
> der ûz ir varwe schînet?
> Geliutert und gefînet
> Vor wandel ist ir reiner lîp. (19824–19833)

Wildez wunder (a "wild miracle") is not only hyperbolic; *wilde* is one of the crucial words in Konrad's poetry,[12] designing the extravagant, the excessive, something exceeding all limits and measure. Helen's beauty is more than *wilde* (*überwildet*) and more than a miracle (*überwundert*). Nobody can bear (*geschouwen*) its radiance (*schîn*).

Konrad gives a description of Helen's body, following the rhetorical schema *a capite ad calcem.* Nevertheless, it is impossible to imagine the shape of the body because its radiance is blinding. Konrad begins with her hair: the bright hair "schein sô liehtebære / als ez gespunnen wære / ûz golde" (19909–19911). Two curls seem threads of gold ("glizzen âne kunterfeit / reht als goldes dræte," 19914f.); the eyes are beaming like "der ôsterlîche tac" (19920), as do the eyebrows, the nose, the color of the face, the cheeks. Her mouth seems burning, is "lieht unde heiz, / der bran noch vaster unde gleiz, / denn ein rubîn durliuchtic rôt" (19961–19963). When Helen is laughing, the teeth sparkle like fresh snow ("wîz geverwet [. . .] / als ein niuvallen snê," 19972f.; cf. 19976–19982), and so forth. In short, no lady ever had such a radiant and marvelous body: "sô glanzen und sô wæhen / lîp kein frouwe nie getruoc" (20032f.). Even though Konrad uses all his rhetorical skills to visualize Helen's beauty it would be difficult to paint her. He gives neither clear contours nor too many details; the listener/reader has only a vague idea of her; instead of being able to gaze, he is overwhelmed by the effects of her shining—as are the protagonists.

It's quite an unusual example of the rhetorical *locus a corpore* and of a description *a capite ad calcem.* Look for instance at Walther von Rheinau's picture of Christ's beauty ("von Jesu schoene und von der wolgestalte sînes lîbes," 6158–6559).[13] First Walther gives a general view, then mentions details as "Wie Jêsu hût was gevar," "Von Jêsu hâre," "Von Jêsu ougen," "Von dien brân," "Von dien überbrân," "Von sîner stirnen," "Von sîner nasen," "Von Jêsu hiuveln und von sînen wangen," "Von dien lespen," "Von dien zenen," "Von der zungen," "Von dem âtme," "Von dem kinne," "Von der keln sîn," "Von dien henden," "Von den nageln," "Von dien füeczen," "Von der mâze, die Jêsu hâte an sînem gange," and finally returns to the general view ("Von der natûrlîchen zämenfüegunge Jêsu Kristes lîbes"). In Walther, even if the author tries to convey an idea of the Lord's aura, bodily details are enumerated one after the other so that one can imagine His human appearance. In Konrad's descriptions the body is dissolved in waves of light.

Visual perception is confused. Even colors become uncertain. It is impossible to determine whether in Helen's face the color red or the color white dominates. Her *glanziu varwe* (19944) is:

> z'eime wunder
> mit wîze und ouch mit rôte

vermischet sô genôte,
daz dâ weder rôt noch wîz
bewæren mohte sînen flîz
mit vollecl̂ichem schîne. (19946–19951)

Similarly her clothes. Her dress (*plyat*) changes color seven times a day; sometimes it seems to be red like a fresh rose, some times white like a lily:

daz er des tages sibenstunt
verkêrte sîne varwe.
er wart gestellet garwe
recht als ein vrischiu rôse rôt.
diu meisterschaft im daz gebôt,
diu von zouber lac dar an,
daz er in blüender roete bran
und sich verwandelte dar în.
dar nâch verkêrte er sînen schîn
in kurzer wîle, nicht ze lanc,
und wart geverwet alsô blanc,
daz nie kein lilje was sô wîz. (20072–20082)

The coat is made from the skin of a fabulous animal, an animal that shines in all colors:

sehs varwe sint ûf ez geleit,
die glîzent nâch dem wunsche dâ.
wîz, brûn, gel, rôt, grüen unde blâ
siht man von im dâ schînen. (20186–20189)

Other sensory perceptions become uncertain, too: in the coat one feels neither heat nor frost; and Helen's face seems like snow in summer, and like rosebuds in winter. In a paradoxical way the abundant visuality (and sensuality) leads to indistinctiveness.

In these descriptions we come across the core of Konrad's poetics. He himself reflects the fallacy of visual perception in a metapoetical passage, by describing the apple of discord (Discordia). The apple is as ambiguous as the beauty of Helen:

ein wunderlîch mixtûre
ûz dem rîlîchen apfel schein.
diu was verworren under ein
von aller hande glaste
sô sêre und alsô vaste,
daz keiner liehten varwe schîn

dâ vollecliche möhte sîn;
und was ir aller teil doch dâ.
wîz, brûn, rôt gel, grüen unde blâ
diu wurden elliu dâ geborn
und heten alliu doch verlorn
dâ ganzen unde vollen glanz,
sô daz ir keines was dô ganz
noch in vollecliicher kür.
ir schîn was wider unde für unde für
zerdræjet und zersprenget
und alsô gar vermenget
mit wilder wandelunge
dâ fremdeclîche lûhte
und iegelîchen dûhte
sô mæzlîch unde cleine,
als ir dô vil nâch keine
sollte schînen unde wesen. (1402–1425)

The apple is the symbol of the ambivalence of medieval courtly society, disguised in a famous story of antiquity. It is beautiful and precious, but it will be the reason, first for the strife between the goddesses, then for a cruel war which finally destroys the courtly order and the Greeks as well as the Trojans. It awakes desire and promises good fortune, but entails hatred. It confuses the eyes; it seems different seen from far away than from nearby; one time ("verre hin von der gesiht," 1431) it seems only silver and gold ("wan silbers unde goldes," 1433), and yet held before the eyes ("nâhe zuo den ougen," 1427) one can no longer distinguish any definite color. By expressions as *mixture, wilde[] temperunge, wandelunge,* and *fremde* Konrad tries to evoke ambiguity. And even scripture, which seems to fix and define the meaning of the apple, is uncertain and fluid: its purpose is written upon a green strip of emeralds—a miracle (*wunder,* 1435). The scripture is pearls; the words change their shape according to the language the reader understands:

Daz sich diu schrift verkêrte
Und jegelîchen lêrte
Dâ vinden sîne sprâche. (1478–1480)

And the magic (*zouber*) of the apple is a poisonous one (*gelüppet,* 1523).

The apple of discord is a mise en abyme of Konrad's poetics and of the world created by his poem. The qualities of the apple as a work of exquisite art—"an im lac hôher künste flîz / von meisterlîcher kûre" (1400f.)—the qualities of the epic and the qualities of the courtly world are the same. The rhetorical *colores* and the *colores* of the *ekphraseis* are sumptuous, but they do not help to distinguish objects; instead they puzzle the gaze. Even written language gets unstable; the letters of pearls are changing their shape as colors are oscillating. The apple is an allegory of the courtly world; both are of an unbelievable magnificence, fascinating and enticing, but they end in dreadful carnage.

Konrad deals with the attractiveness and the danger of courtly visuality. By doing so, he is deconstructing sight as an instrument of cognition and visuality as mirror of courtly perfection. In the case of Helen, he declares explicitly that perfect appearance coincides with destruction:

daz sich mîn zunge pînet
sêr ûf ir lop, daz tuot mir nôt,
sît daz den bitterlîchen tôt
durch si leit sô manic lîp,
daz nie durch keiner slahte wîp
verdarp sô manic hôher man. (20282–20287)

Although Paris is the perfect knight and courtier, from his birth everybody knows that he is the one who will destroy his relatives, his city, and his kingdom.

The courtly program presupposes a harmony between ethics and aesthetics. When "Joie de la curt" in Chrétien and Hartmann is achieved by the perfect knight and in a knightly manner, it is designed as the anticipation of celestial joy. The career of the *chevalier* leads to the perfection of himself and of courtly society. Fighting is the one way to overcome a frail or even hostile world, and *minne* is the impelling force behind the tireless efforts to overcome it. Konrad, after nearly a century of courtly optimism, doubts this harmony in the *Trojanerkrieg.* Fighting means cruel killing, and *minne* is a self-destructive and ruthless desire. The knights pursue their own selfish goals, unconcerned about the consequences for others. And what seems aesthetically beautiful can be morally rotten.

Yet, Konrad's objection is not based on religion, as in Walther von der Vogelweide's bitter song *Ir reinen wîp ir werden man.*[14] Walther, in the role of the old poet, near death, rejects *frou Welt* and her *lôn.* The courtly minstrel, too, was seduced by sight, the *bilde* of the beautiful *vrouwe.* Her beauty was a delusion. Thus, he has to abandon it. With *bilde* Walther uses one of Konrad's favorite terms: "Ich hât ein schoenez bilde erkorn / owê daz ich ez ie gesach" (67, 32f.). But *in hora mortis* the *bilde* lost his beauty and splendor, and its ugliness and dirty appearance infects the man who dedicated his service to her.

The result is *conversio:* "Mîn sêle müeze wol gevarn! / [. . .] lîp, lâ die minne diu dich lât, / und habe ie stæten minne wert" (67, 28f.), even if Walther expresses a vague confidence that the *bilde*—and with it courtly *werdekeit*—will not be lost forever: "daz wir ein ander vinden frô" (68, 6).

This is the Christian objection against a courtly world that claims its own hierarchy of values. This objection is associated with a devalorization of sensual perception, especially vision. To quote Karl Bertau: In the second half of the thirteenth century the devotees are replacing the refined ones ("Ersetzen der Feinen durch die Frommen"). Even if courtly romances about King Arthur and his knights are written up to the beginning of the fourteenth century, religious criticism on secular culture becomes prevalent. This can be seen in the continuations of Gottfried's *Tristan* (with their chaste morals) and the continuation of Wolfram's *Willehalm* (with its pious hatred against the enemies of Christ). It can seen in texts like Albrecht's *Jüngerer Titurel* telling how the holy grail leaves Western Christianity for India. It can seen in the German *Lancelot en prose,* where in Part 3 the Knights of the Round Table (except Galaad, Parzival, and Bohort) are excluded from the *queste du graal,* where knighthood and courtly love are interpreted as carnal sin, and where the kingdom of Arthur disappears in a battle pitting his knights against each other.

But this is not Konrad's point. Konrad is perhaps the last true courtly narrator. In his *Goldene Schmiede* he displays all the art he has at his disposal to prove that no art is able to praise the virtues of the Mother of God. In the *Trojanerkrieg* he exposes just as many rhetorical figures, metaphors, *colores rhetorici,* but with a different purpose. They are painting a seductive and dangerous world. Konrad depicts a pagan society where Christian conversion is not an option—as it is, for example, in *Willehalm*—and where courtly order cannot be replaced by a celestial one. On the other hand, this deficiency does not diminish the attraction of this world. In Troy, the cradle of knighthood, worldly beauty can be praised without any religious remorses. Behind the luring pagan world there is no other world, and Konrad displays its magnificence with brilliant colors. But as its appearance is deceptive, sight does not lead to insight, but to blindness, in contrast to the otherwise common courtly trust in the harmony of ethic and aesthetic qualities.

Notes

1. Gudrun Schleusener-Eichholz, *Das Auge im Mittelalter,* 2 Bde. (München, 1985); Horst Wenzel, *Hören und Sehen. Schrift und Bild. Kultur und Gedächtnis im*

Mittelalter (München, 1995); see *Visual Culture and the German Middle Ages* (New York, 2005), ed. Kathryn Starkey and Horst Wenzel.

2. Wolfram von Eschenbach, *Parzival,* Mittelhochdeutscher Text nach der 6. Ausgabe von Karl Lachmann; Übersetzung von Peter Knecht; Einführung zum Text von Bernd Schirok (Berlin and New York, 1998), pp. 308–318.

3. Walther von der Vogelweide, *Gedichte. Studienausgabe,* 13. Ausgabe (Berlin, 1965).

4. Jan-Dirk Müller, "Visualität, Geste, Schrift. Zu einem neuen Untersuchungsfeld der Mediävistik," in *Zeitschrift für deutsche Philologie* 122 (2003): pp. 118–132; idem, "Writing-Speech-Image: The Competition of Signs," in *Visual Culture and the German Middle Ages,* pp. 35–52.

5. Cf. the episodes in: Heinrich von dem Türlin, *Diu Crône,* zum ersten Male hg. v. Gottlieb Heinrich Friedrich Scholl, Bibliothek des Litterarischen Vereins 27 (Stuttgart, 1852); *Die Krone (Verse 1–12281). Nach der Handschrift 2779 der Österreichischen Nationalbibliothek nach Vorarbeiten von Alfred Ebenbauer, Klaus Zatloukal und Horts P. Pütz,* hg. v. Fritz Peter Knapp und Manuela Niesner, Altdeutsche Textbibiothek 112 (Tübingen, 2000); Ulrich von Zatzikhoven, *Lanzelet,* hg. v. K. A. Hahn (Frankfurt, 1845), Mit einem Nachwort und einer Bibliographie von Frederick Norman (Berlin, 1965); Heinrich von Neustadt, *Apollonius von Tyrland nach einer Gothaer Handschrift [. . .],* hg. v. S.[amuel] Singer, Deutsche Texte des Mittelalters 7 (Berlin, 1906).

6. Konrad von Würzburg, *Der Trojanische Krieg,* Nach den Vorarbeiten K. Frommanns und F. Roths zum ersten Mal hg. durch Adelbert von Keller, Bibliothek des litterarischen Vereins 44 (Stuttgart, 1858).

7. For the term, see Karl Stackmann, *Der Spruchdichter Heinrich von Mügeln. Vorstudien zu seiner Individualität,* Probleme der Dichtung 3 (Heidelberg, 1958); Johannes Kibelka, *Der ware Meister. Denkstile und Bauformen in der Dichtung Heinrichs von Mügeln,* Philologische Studien und Quellen 13 (Berlin, 1963); Kurt Nyholm, *Studien zum sogenannten geblümten Stil,* Acta Academiae Aboensis A 39, 4 (Abo, 1971); Karl Stackmann, "Redebluomen. Zu einigen Fürstenpreis-Strophen Frauenlobs und zum Problem des geblümten Stils," in *Mittelalterliche Texte als Aufgabe. Kleine Schriften I,* ed. Jens Haustein (Göttingen, 1997), pp. 298–317; Stackmann, "Rhetoricae artis practica fontalisque medulla. Zu Theorie und Praxis des Blümens bei Heinrich von Mügeln," in *Mittelalterliche Texte als Aufgabe,* pp. 318–324; and the summary in Gert Hübner, *Lobblumen: Studien zur Genese und Funktion der "Geblümten Rede"* (Tübingen and Basel, 2000), pp. 7–32.

8. Horst Wenzel, "Visualität. Sichtbarkeit und Imagination im Medienwandel," *Zeitschrift für Germanistik* N.F. 9 (1999): p. 549–556; Haiko Wandhoff, "*Velden und visieren, blüemen und florieren.* Zur Poetik der Sichtbarkeit in den höfischen Epen des Mittelalters," *Zeitschrift für Germanistik* N.F. 9 (1999): pp. 586–597; see Wandhoff, *Ekphrasis. Kunstbeschreibungen und virtuelle Räume in der Literatur des Mittelalters,* Trends in Medieval Philology 3 (Berlin and New York, 2003).

9. Cf. Trude Ehlert, "Zu Konrads von Würzburg Auffassung vom Wert der Kunst und von der Rolle des Künstlers," *Jahrbuch der Oswald von Wolkenstein Gesellschaft* 5 (1988/1989): pp. 79–94.

10. About the couples Paris and Oenone, Hercules and Deiamira, Achill and Deidamia, Paris and Helen, Jason and Medea; only the marriages of Priamus and Hecuba and of Hector and Andromache are different.

11. See Jan-Dirk Müller, "*Schîn* und Verwandtes. Zum Problem der 'Ästhetisierung' in Konrads von Würzburg 'Trojanerkrieg' (Mit einem Nachwort zu Terminologie-Problemen der Mediävistik)," in, *Im Wortfeld des Textes,* ed. Gerd Dicke, Manfred Eikelmann, and Burkhard Hasebrink (Berlin and New York, 2006), pp. 287–307.

12. Wolfgang Monecke, *Studien zur epischen Technik Konrads von Würzburg. Ad Erzählprinzip der Wildekeit,* Germanistische Abhandlungen 24 (Stuttgart, 1968).

13. *Das Marienleben Walthers von Rheinau,* [ed.] von Edit Perjus. Zweite vermehrte Auflage, Acta Academiae Aboensis, Humaniora 17, 1 (Abo, 1949), pp. 122–130.

14. Jan-Dirk Müller, "Walther von der Vogelweide: *Ir reinen wîp, ir werden man,*" in *Zeitschrift für deutsches Altertum* 124 (1995): pp. 1–25.

12 Blinded Avengers

Making Sense of Invisibility in Courtly Epic and Legal Ritual

Hildegard Elisabeth Keller

Every medium that vanquishes invisibility and heightens visibility, brings salvation to mankind.

Man is afraid of nothing more than of being touched by something for which he has no categories of experience. At the root of this fear, Elias Canetti recognizes a visual experience, given that, as he sees it, the eye is the most important sensory organ when it comes to orientation of the self in reality: "One wants to see what has one in its grip, one wants to know it, or at least be able to categorize it."[1] Given that each of us every day experiences the invisible in one form or another, Canetti's confidence in the eye's hold on reality seems unreasonably optimistic. In keeping with Volker Demuth's statement in the epigraph, confidence in things (pace Paul) seen can even become a synonym for redemption. To the contrary, however, as I will argue in this essay, this sort of faith in visible certitude, no matter how misplaced, is really only possible for those involved in an action (be it in life or in fiction), not for the outside observer, who remains out of reach.

The category of visibility, complete with its attendant connotations of salvation, functions as a central tool for the interpretation of the religious art and literature of the Middle Ages.[2] It can also be seen as operating within the literature itself. In this essay I take as my focus twelfth-century French and German courtly epic in order to show how these works self-consciously manipulate this paradigm. In the center always stands an episode narrating a fight between a visible and an invisible combatant. Whether in *Le Chevalier au Lion* by Chrétien de Troyes[3] or *Iwein* by Hartmann von Aue,[4] the protagonist kills the lord of the castle. In each work, the protagonist is then captured. While in this life-threatening situation, magic allows them to become invisible. The lord's avengers can neither see nor kill them, even though they know they are "there." Whereas the murderers end up escaping, the avengers become blinded figures, ridiculous due to their exaggerated, yet ineffective physical and psychological efforts and their ridiculous gestures. Whereas the blinded avengers experience a fundamentally frightening encounter with the uncanny, the observers embedded in the narrative, like the audience outside of the text, enjoy a sovereign cheerfulness because the narration or plot endows them with "clairvoyance." In this fashion, secular epic can be seen as using literary play with the visible and the invisible to very different ends than religious art. The existential desire for visibility reveals itself as a narrative motif that serves ideally to heighten the audience's amusement.

This essay aims to elucidate the epistemological and aesthetic premises of this pleasure in ways that require investigation of the interplay among medium, visuality, and other modes of sensory perception. Its starting point is a very unspectacular observation: whoever fights physically against an opponent depends in general on sensory perception and, more specifically, on the coherence of different modes of perception. No matter how extreme a situation, combat brings into play perceptual processes that pertain in other situations in life. As modern neurology has demonstrated, any mental construction of reality requires consistency of sensory perception.[5] For example, the inability to bring visual and tactile perception into harmony with one another causes severe cognitive confusion and makes the subject feel helpless. This is no less true of sight alone. The slightest deception of the eye can be fatal while in a battle, not least because it creates confusion that can lead to the "blinded" losing their lives. Perceptual distortion and disorientation generates a gap between those who know and see more and those who perceive less.

Within medieval narratives, no less than in the realm of science, engineered asymmetries in visual perception constitute different levels or orders of knowledge. These differences can be intensified and raised to the level of self-conscious aesthetic devices within various media, primarily through the introduction of observer figures who simultaneously stand in for the reader. These figures force reflection on the following question: which position does the text grant to its protagonists and to what end does it grant superiority to some, inferiority to others? This question in turn introduces another, of crucial importance when considering the aesthetic dimensions of a given medium: how—and with what effect—can verbal and pictorial media visualize an invisible protagonist? I will try to answer these questions in four steps.

The first part focuses on the phenomenon of invisibility, namely, on the material manipulation of visual perception that can be observed among wildlife in nature. Certain animals incorporate morphological and kinetic designs in their bodily appearance to make their victims "blind while seeing." Looking at the mimicry systems of animals in nature helps to define and critically question the terms "visibility" and "invisibility." In addition, it provides insight into the high tension inherent in this specific constellation of asymmetrically perceiving opponents. Any manipulation of visual perception by virtue of bodily shape or movement or—mutatis mutandis, by means of the magic tool of literary construction—establishes distinctions that are crucial for the argument I make in this essay.[6]

The second part—the principal part—provides a literary analysis of two closely related fictional texts both of which belong to the broadly defined genre of high medieval Arthurian epic. Both *Le Chevalier au Lion* and *Iwein* narrate a battle against an invisible opponent, ingeniously making use of a fascinating motif from the viewpoint of perception theory that makes maximum use of narrative tension. Each work stages the critical battle as an asymmetrical event—asymmetrical in that the opposing combatants and those who can identify with them are differentiated in terms of their ability to recognize and "see through" differing degrees of sensory deception. My analysis demonstrates that in not allowing everyone to see to the same extent, the narration seeks to amuse the reader in terms of mimicry of the courtly knight and his duped avengers.

The third part complements the analysis of the Iwein narrative by turning directly to the realm of the visible in the form of a pictorial example that belongs to the same epic tradition. The Ywain frescoes in the South Tyrolean castle of Rodenegg not only permit comparison across media, they also flesh out the specific appeal to vision insofar as they attempt to give visible form to an invisible protagonist. How can a scene with both visible and invisible figures be represented with material means in order to make clear who is "there," but actually not visible? And what perceptual premises ensure the observer of his sovereignty, and hence, his amusement?

The fourth part extends the argument by turning to the judicial duel at court. Embedded in a different context, we find the same motif of the battle against an invisible opponent. Why, one is forced to ask, was it of no concern that in such duels the combatant fought an invisible opponent? The *Sachsenspiegel* by Eike von Repgow, dated slightly later than the epics, describes the ritual in word and image. Both media underscore the importance of consensus when it came to the interpretation of visual perception. The example of judicial duels provides a useful point of comparison vis-à-vis the motif in courtly literature, not only with regard to the motif of invisibility and its asymmetric staging, but also in terms of its comic purpose.

There is no doubt that the medium shapes sensory experience, even as it conveys its content. Sensory perception is thus subjected to the laws of construction in several ways, not simply as a neuronal process, but also according to various media and their specific appeal to the physical and inner senses. The physical battle reveals the existential contingency of movement and visual perception to a greater extent than any other situation. In battle, the opponent has to be not merely visible to the eye of the other, he also has to be immediately identifiable as what he is. Each pertinent asymmetry is life threatening. This holds true not only for two opponents standing eye to eye in courtly epic of the Middle Ages, but also for aggression with high-tech weapons. Contemporary observations back this statement. Collective aggression at the beginning of the twenty-first century operates out of and with invisibility. An attack from invisible agents—not recognizable as aggressors—is seen as the quintessence of worldwide terrorist perfidy since 9/11. For this reason, invisibility has also turned into a developmental goal for antiterror technology.[7] Communication media have also learned how to capitalize on the invisibly present threat. They commercially use the experience of the uncanny that resides in the terrorists' invisibility. The infotainment strategies of certain TV channels, which call for increasing their audience share by demonstrating real-life battle technologies and camouflage strategies as if they were fictional, have caused a harsh outbreak of media criticism.[8] A historical perspective on the interrelation among media, visuality, and aggression, as the following pages try to open, can highlight its background.

Different media work with perspectival modes of representation in order to evoke an uncanny response on the part of the audience. Sigmund Freud is the classic scholar of the uncanny. In his essay "Das Unheimliche" (1919), he elucidates the strategies that can trigger uncanny feelings by means of artistic representation. The German word *unheimlich* is considered untranslatable; the English "uncanny" provides only a rough equivalent, and the phenomenon itself is difficult to define. The uncanny terrifies precisely because it cannot be adequately explained. Freud does not simply conceptualize the uncanny in psychoanalytical terms. Above all, he considers the aesthetic conditions of the experience insofar as they are bound to the media (in his case literary) under investigation.[9] Three of his insights are important in the context we are considering. First, the expression "uncanny" turns out to be a phenomenon involving a semantic tilt. In addition to the uncanny/unknown, the term, surprisingly, also comprehends its opposite, the known and the familiar. Second, Freud views visual experiences, and specifically, the fear of decreased powers of vision and of blindness, as central to the experience of the uncanny. Third, he is aware of literary aesthetics, meaning the contribution of the medium. In fact, he owes many of his own examples to literature: the "Unheimliche der Fiktion [the uncanny in fiction]" deserves "gesonderte Betrachtung [specific attention]" because literature grants the poet "Vorrechte [. . .] in der Hervorrufung und Hemmung des unheimlichen Gefühls [privileges in provocation and suppression of uncanny sensations]" that enables a representation which surmounts by far the everyday experience of the uncanny in complexity.[10]

The three elements identified by Freud also characterize the literary representation of combat against an invisible opponent. Some protagonists experience it as highly irritating and uncanny, whereas others experience a profound cheerfulness. This is not surprising, because, as in combat, two opposites collide: on the one hand, the most deceptive, and hence, irritating; on the other hand, the most knowledgeable and the most cheerful. Both states of mind, it turns out, take as their point of departure one and the same perceptual situation. What distinguishes one from the other is the asymmetry between those who are granted sight and those who are deceived.

When explaining how pleasure becomes recognizable to the comic hero, Hans Robert Jauss makes a point of falling back on Freud's theory on the difference of expenditure. This theory operates on the opposition between physical and psychological expenditure, which is exercised by a protagonist before our eyes; if he engages in a supreme physical effort (compared to the psychological expenditure), he then appears funny to the audience because they can feel superior to him.[11] This psychogenesis of the comic can further illuminate the aforementioned asymmetry. He who is made "seeing" by the text can feel superior. He experiences neither the invisible opponent nor his wildly gesticulating avengers as frightening and uncanny, but rather as amusing and funny. Wolfgang Iser adds a dynamic to the relationship of opposition, which in turn makes the comic possible. The binary patterns, which also characterize Freud's definition, are destabilized. For that reason, Iser designates the comic to be a true tilt-phenomenon.[12] Thus, he circumscribes an event, which turns around the expectations of those involved. This is precisely what can be observed in the battle scenes which will be analyzed in the second part of this chapter: a captured knight, doomed to die, escapes without having touched a weapon, and a group of armed and angered avengers have to retreat despite their not having accomplished their mission after having twice spent their rage to no avail in an absolutely involuntary comic situation. This perspective, however, is granted only to those who have been informed by the narration. Only they can smile with sovereignty.

Fallacy of the Eye: Wild Life

> *Where the law of eating and being eaten holds way, camouflage, deception, lying and cheating are indispensable rules of life.*[13]

The uncanny invisible is not solely bound to the human world and its cultural artifacts. It simply influences communication in animal and human societies because camouflage techniques, or more general, the techniques of influencing one's visibility for others, ensures survival in the *struggle for life.* Animals as well as humans fall back upon sensory patterns of camouflage and deception, which not only challenge those involved in the deception but also the external observers on a perception-theoretical level. According to Volker Sommer, human and animal techniques of disguise are comparable from a cultural-anthropological perspective. He, therefore, includes human tactics of perceptual deception in the bioevolutionary and neuromedical analysis of animal mimicry.[14]

A true battle situation for animals and humans makes readily apparent how activity and passivity go hand in hand in the actual process of perception. Viewed functionally, the neurological processes in animals and humans define visual perception as an active process, that is, as the result of a process that seeks to give the best possible interpretation to sensory signals.[15] By the same token, however, sensory perception also consists of moments of receptivity, even passivity, when viewed from the point of its being done. Media philosopher Dieter Mersch introduces the German term *Ereignis* (an event) into media-aesthetics, accentuating the receptive moment that is especially attached to the performance of visual perception.[16] Although Mersch is aware of the etymology of the term, his concept could lean much more heavily on the historical semantics of the term "event" than it does. The expression *ereignen* (to take place) does not stem from *eigen* (own), respectively *proprium*,[17] but instead derives from the Old High German *irougen* "to show (oneself), to make (oneself) visible."[18] It can therefore be said that this earliest Old High German verb and the noun derived from the verb grant an active part to that which is perceived by the seeing human being.

For Mersch visual perception thus entails a process in which the taking in of signals comes first. An *Ereignis* (event) is insofar an *Eräugnis* (a situation of visual perception) when, within it, something is *revealed* to the eye that could conceivably and incalculably be withdrawn from the active influence of the perceiving subject.[19] As a result, the role of the subject appears to be nonintentional, passive in the sense of "receiving" the signals of presence of what "happens" or "manifests itself" (*was sich ereignet/eräugnet*).[20] What might seem a mere act of receptivity also has a reverse, productive side. The activity of the human being consists in bringing forth the "reality" inherent in the received sensory perceptions. This perspective on sight, complementary and also, to a certain extent, reversed, is the determining parameter to the media-aesthetics postulated by Mersch. Later in my argumentation, it will help as a critical concept to explain the narrative importance of sensory traps in medieval fiction.

The next step, however, draws attention to the still-unmediated situation of asymmetry of perception. Wildlife mimicry systems lay many cunning traps for the eye to allow one animal to overcome the other in order that the first can survive. If the asymmetries of perception determine the outcome of a confrontation between two opponents, then the techniques of sensory deception will represent the most primary of all attack and defense strategies. This holds true for an attacker that wants to capture its victim unseen, as well as for the potential victim, which wants to escape possible attacks by using camouflage. It is so much more surprising that the seriousness of the situation is countered by seemingly playful body and movement mechanisms.

Mimicry: Traps for the Animal Eye

Whoever camouflages himself pretends "not to be there." To be precise: he pretends not to be the person he actually is. Strangely enough, this pretending not to be there can play in important role in the survival of a species. Camouflage mimicry ensures existence; it connects the sender and the receiver of perception signals in a highly complex manner. Today, theses systems of mimicry belong to the most carefully and extensively analyzed systems of communication.[21] In principle, mimicry targets a semiotic triangular relationship between at least three members, who do not necessarily, but often, belong to different species: a so-called *mimet* tries to imitate as perfectly as possible the visual appearance of its *role model,* including shape, color, and kinesis (movement as well as the renunciation of movement) in order to divert the perception of the *signal's receiver* in a specific direction. It should react to the falsified appearance instead of recognizing what lies behind this appearance. Depending on the point of the view, the aim of camouflage is either self-camouflage or the deception of the other. If the signal's receiver is an aggressor, then the *protective mimicry* should protect the mimet from the aggressor. If the deceptive signal is directed toward the eyes of the prey, then the predator tries to approach or lure its prey with aggressive mimicry (which is why this type is also called luring mimicry). Extremely artful signal systems that are difficult to decipher combine protective and luring mimicry. I will only briefly touch upon protective mimicry.

The Ghanaian *Myrmarachne formicaria* serves as illustration for this protective mimicry (fig. 12.1).[22] Anatomically and kinetically, the leaping spider pretends to be an ant. The corseted, brown, and hairless front part of the spider imitates the ant's head and thorax and lifts its front pair of legs into the air like an ant lifts its feelers. This visual deception is foremost directed to the female spider wasp (*Pison xanthopus*), the preferred prey of leaping spiders. A sting paralyzes the prey, and then it is brought as living bait to the nest burrow where the larva feed on it. This ant-camouflage ensures the survival of the leaping spider. Surprisingly the South American *Aphantochilus rogersi* operates morphologically and kinetically in a similar way, but it combines protective and aggressive mimicry. This spider specializes in ant hunting; it imitates the silhouette of its prey, copies its zigzag walk, and further mimics its feelers with its front pair of legs. Visually, the predator is barely distinguishable from its prey, which it approaches, attacks from behind, and immediately lifts over its body. This is kinetic camouflage as well; for this is the way ants carry dead members of their species. The spider, however, uses the dead ant as protective shield and sucks it out in the middle of "enemy territory."[23]

Mimicry—this observation will be relevant for the textual analysis—is a system of visualization which is foremost oriented toward perspective. Mimicry demands the dissolution of the peculiarities of one's own form and movements in favor of a different, camouflaging appearance. This disintegration of one's own appearance (Morpho- or Somatolysis),[24] and of one's own pattern of motion, calls for the renunciation of differentiation from the environment. That this does not solely mean immobility is shown by the South Australian *Phycodurus eques,* a mimet belonging to the family of sea horses.[25] *Phycodurus eques* camouflages its body with an alga that is typical of its habitat and that naturally moves with water (fig. 12.2).[26] Only the extinction of difference enables the necessary sensory deception of the other and to selectively redirect

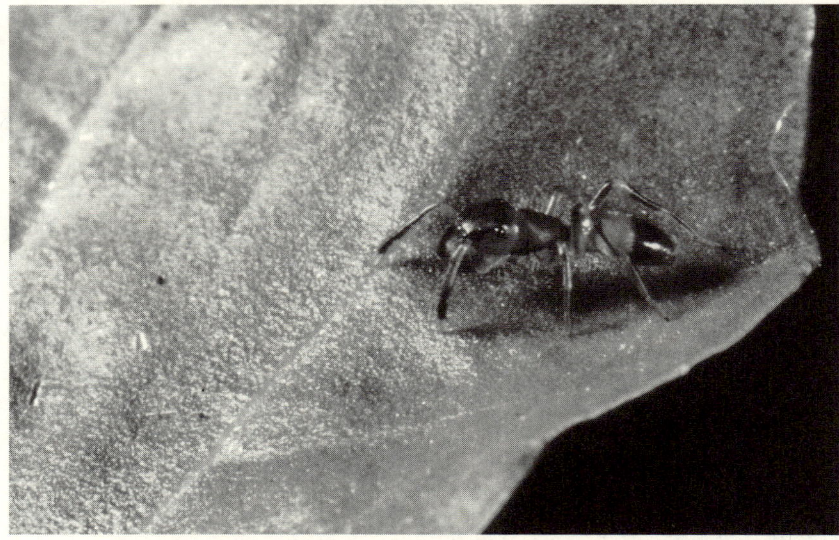

Figure 12.1. *Myrmarachne formicaria,* Ghanaian leaping spider. Courtesy Klaus Lunau.

individual signals. As a consequence, the prey does not "see" the mimet as a whole, which means it cannot identify the mimet's own, personal value.

Like all ambush hunters, the alligator snapping turtle *Macroclemys temminckii* refers back to this strategy. Weighing up to ninety kilograms, the turtle lies motionless with a wide open mouth at the bottom of the sea like an algae-covered rock. Only the red, worm-like tongue projections constantly twitch to draw curious fish. Compared to the total body size of the turtle, the part which actually catches the attention of the fish is the tiny worm-like attractor (fig. 12.3).[27] The mimicry systems of animals illuminate how strongly the eye is fixed on differential identification. The eye can only distinguish something and identify it as an object in its own right when it can be differentiated from the environment. The intentions for the masking of one's own appearance, but not of one's own being, vary—speaking of "intentions" means putting it anthropocentrically[28]—according to the profile of prey and predator. They converge in the motif of survival by appearing to be non-identical-to-self in order to create the necessary asymmetry of perception: eye to eye but yet "invisible."

Let's now include the function of media in this line of thought. As far as we know, there are no animal observers in the wild who chuckle while observing other living beings winning or losing a battle for survival. If there is anywhere an observer, it is the human being who is fascinated by these processes, which are presented to us in zoological reference books and films. The perceptual processing of counterfeited signals creates an amused wonder in which uncanny and comic aspects are permanently intertwined. In order to enjoy this spectacle, we (or at any rate the nonexperts, who themselves do not do fieldwork) have to rely on the medialization of mimicry. Scientific articles and (static or moving) images of the visual media lure us to the sensual trap in which the prey falls due to being "blind" or due to signal deception. Thus, media make us "see"; it is through media that we recognize the trap in which the miming animal directs the eye of its prey.

This is the decisive function of media, as far as our fictional texts are concerned: they can open up mental display rooms and intensify the perspectives of different observers. This contrasts with the paintings, which are based on courtly narratives (see the discussion of the Ywain frescoes in the third part of this chapter). The texts analyzed in this study use their aesthetic difference for the empirical observation of animal mimicry. They play with several levels of observation, which are either inside or outside of the text. They let certain protagonists enter the sensory trap—just like the miming animal's prey—and privilege the eyes by letting them see more than they actually could. The narrator grants them mental insight to the successful or failed perceptions of others; they hear their own and other people's comments on the visually deceived and so they become observers of second-degree observers.[29] This differentiation of perspectives increases foremost the complexity of the succeeding passage, and greatly enhances its visuality in surprising ways. At this point, the media-aesthetic question joins to the courtly epic: which asymmetry of perception is developed amongst the protagonists in the two Iwein epics, the French and the German versions? And what possibilities are offered to the audience outside of the text?

Fallacy of the Eye: Courtly Epic

Invisibility quite simply means someone's "not being there."[30]

The courtly Arthurian world demands visible presence and transparent actions from its members. Everything that happens perceptively in public at court before eye- and earwitnesses is therefore not to be doubted.[31] Secret actions already represent a first form of invisibility. This is a rather conven-

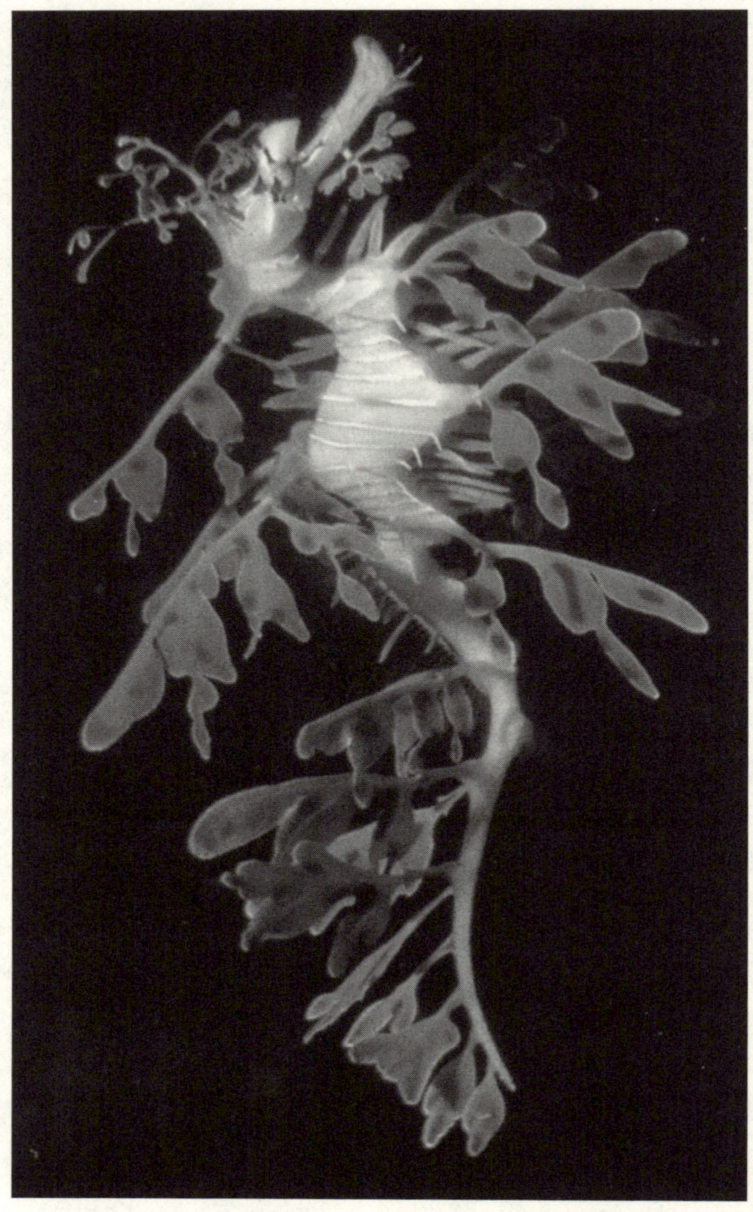

Figure 12.2. *Phycodurus eques,* leafy sea dragon, belonging to the family of sea horses. Photo: John G. Shedd Aquarium, Chicago.

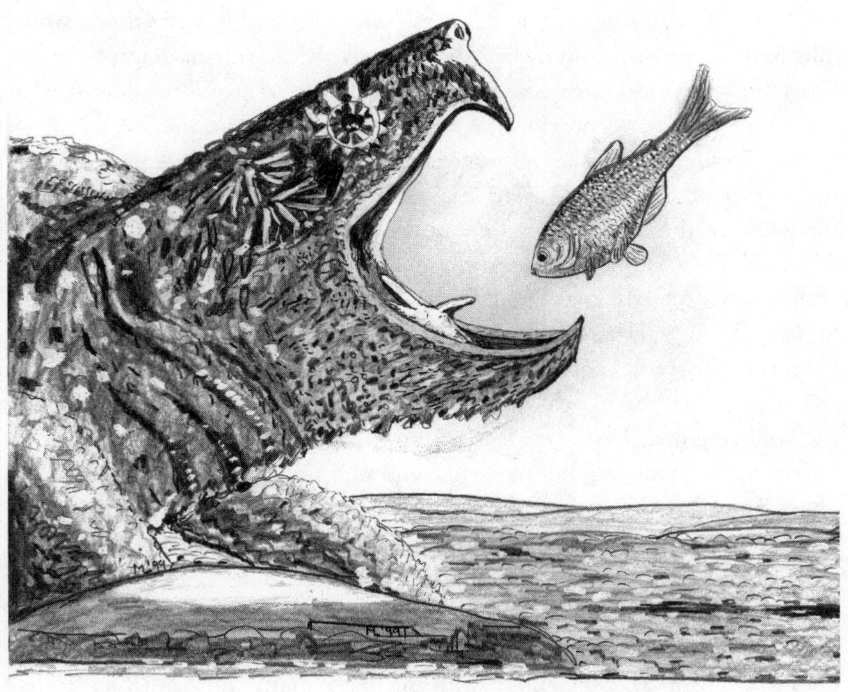

Figure 12.3. *Macroclemys temminckii,* alligator snapping turtle. Courtesy Klaus Lunau.

tional narrative motif and need not be explored further in this epistemological context. Invisibility created through magic, however, is another matter. In line with the mimicry of animals, magical invisibility makes us believe that somebody is "not there." Visual perception, however, is only misled either by a falsification of visible signals or by the creation of a fallacy (as in *Iwein*). This invisibility has no sensory consequences other than bioevolutionary camouflage. Magical invisibility manipulates the eye, and as secret action in court society, it is viewed as fraud in front of eyewitnesses. For that reason, magical invisibility violates court etiquette in two ways.

The fictional texts from the world of the heroic and the Arthurian epic document this breech. They offer different narrative perspectives; but they also differ in the way the fraud is socially sanctioned, if it is sanctioned at all. The mimicry of Siegfried, when wearing his magical camouflaging cloak, enables him to be invisible and yet physically present as someone superficially not identical with himself. He fights as "Gunther" and wrestles down Brünhild both in athletics and in bed. It is exactly this fallacy of perception that turns out to be the "Sprengsatz für die höfische Welt von Worms [detonation charge for the courtly world of Worms]"[32] in the catastrophic continuation of the *Nibelungenlied.* The camouflage techniques of Laurin are placed under the verdict of treacherous dwarf tricks and are completely obliterated from the world of the Dietrich epic in a quickly told elimination of the dwarves. Strangely, only Yvain and Iwein, the heroes of the French and the German versions, respectively, manage to rescue themselves without sanction thanks to a magic ring. The constraint which forces them to prove their worth as knights in the second course and thus be worthy of marrying Laudine has—at least from a narrative logic point of view—a different motivation than the trick of being invisible.

The scene involving the trap at the entrance, in which both Chrétien and Hartmann stage the fight of the avengers against the invisible Iwein, groups the internal figures of the text and the audience into two layers of observation. Each layer can be differentiated still further.[33] The inner layer includes both opposing parties: on the one hand, the lady of the castle, Laudine, with her slain husband Askalon and her servants, and on the other hand Iwein, the murderer of Askalon. Apart from the anonymous court inhabitants and mourners, the trickster figure Lunete is also part of Laudine's entourage. She, however, is a threshold figure because she secretly watches the scene and is aware of the special visual circumstances.[34] Moreover, we—in short, the everlasting narrators and listeners—need to be considered too, as we also know the reasons for the invisibility. The concurring information stems from the autopsy of the internal figures of the text and from the narrator. This information renders us "seeing" showed by no other internal figure of the text. Hartmann takes this aesthetics of operating with different perspectives in the battle against the invisible further than any other Arthurian or heroic epic text.

The Knight in the Portcullis Prison

As we know, Yvain and Iwein are taken captive in the castle of the slain Askalon. How does this happen, and what happens as a result of the narrative's strategy of "blinding" almost all the figures internal to the text by means of magic? In a gregarious round of storytelling at Pentecost, Iwein hears the knight Kalogrenant tell a story about an unsuccessful *aventiure* (adventure). Several years before, he had been forced to flee from Askalon's castle after having lost battle near a mysterious source that causes thunderstorms. Iwein, who is mobilized by this information, secretly leaves the court and starts the *aventiure* and thus his involvement in a life-threatening action. At the source, he triggers a storm and again, the source guardian, Askalon, comes galloping. A fight and a chase scene follow, in which Iwein pursues the severely wounded Askalon and tries to follow him into the castle. While reaching out for the final sword thrust, the deadly portcullis of the castle's entrance falls, just missing Iwein's back with such precision that he manages to survive (as opposed to his horse and Askalon, who both die). He, however, is now trapped in the closed-off entrance. It would be highly surprising if he survived.

Lunete, the lady-in-waiting to the now widowed lady of the castle, and a very important trickster figure for this whole passage, enters the scene. She secretly visits the trapped Iwein to announce his certain death. She says the servants of the Lady Laudine were experiencing "awful anger" (*grimmeclichen zorn,* 1163). The protagonist wants to face the battle in as manly a fashion as possible, in keeping with the laws of the genre, an aspect that Hartmann accentuates even more in his rewrite. Hartmann's Iwein underscores the hero's readiness to fight with a directness that makes the ensuing episode (in which, by lying invisibly on a bed, he does anything but put up a fight!) that much more ironic: "Be that as it may," he declares, "I do not intend to forfeit my life like a woman, no one catches me off guard" (*so ensol ich doch den lîp / niht verliesen als ein wîp: / michn vindet nieman âne wer*).[35]

Iwein's determination to fight an obviously hopeless battle also motivates Lunete's wish to help him more effectively, since she speaks of wanting to honor Iwein's indisputable courage. Nonetheless, Lunete's wish to redeem a debt is only barely constructed in the narration. Lunete immediately "recognizes" Iwein and calls him by name because she had met him earlier in Britain, an encounter not narrated in the text. At that time, he was the only one to have greeted her at court. She now wants to thank him for this gesture of honor.[36] In order to save him, she cunningly reaches for the magic ring, a pendant to the different models of invisibility cloaks worn by protagonists in fiction from the Middle Ages up to Harry Potter. If worn correctly—and Lunete instructs Iwein on just how to do that—the ring will hide its wearer "like wood under the bark."[37] The ring protects its wearer with magical invisibility,[38] making it impossible to either "see or find" him. This magic tool not only makes possible the physical fallacy of perception, it also enables second-order observers to reflect on its meaning. In the French text, the perceptual paradox initiated by the magic ring is emphasized through repetition: nobody could see the wearer of the ring, no matter how wide they had opened their eyes (*tant aix les iex ouvers,* 1035).

After ensuring Iwein's invisibility, Lunete acts the good hostess under the circumstances. She entertains Iwein by asking him to sit in the entrance—in a courtly, decorated room with a richly covered bed—and serves him *guoter gâchspîse gnuoc* ("a variety of tasty snacks").[39] The French text discusses in depth the architecture and technical details of the castle: both portcullises, the courtly decoration of the room, and the menu served at the banquet.[40] Hartmann, though, radically shortens this description. This streamlining accentuates the following events. As the loudly approaching avengers are heard after the light meal, Lunete augurs a visual spectacle to the murderer (and hence also to the readers of the text). The avengers of Laudine will not be able to kill the murderer of their master because of the fallacy of perception. Their pitiful failure should turn into an entertaining event for Iwein, providing he remains on the bed with the gem clasped in his hand. Thus, he will be able to see the threatening gestures of his "blinded" avengers. The pun is that they will seek his life unsuccessfully, even though he is sitting amongst them:

nû wâ mite möht iu wesen baz,
dazs iu alle sint gehaz,
und ir sî seht bî iu stân
unde drônde umbe iuch gân,
und sî doch sô erblindent
daz si iuwer niene vindent,
und sît doch rehte under in.[41]

Lunete's rhetorical question grasps the essence of the possibly experienced paradox in this scene: Iwein will be absolutely "meant," that is, he is the target of his killers and gets therefore the full attention of all figures in the text, yet he nevertheless finds himself comfortably invisible in the midst of the action. Iwein, that much is predictable, cannot be held accountable for his murder due to the extraordinary conditions for sensory perception in this scene. This is a status not normally granted to humans, a fact of which Iwein is also aware. Chrétien emphasizes the frivolousness of the old French maid here even more. The maid announces the scene clearly as a visual spectacle, but only for the one who need not fear anything. Objectively, this can only apply to the observers outside of the text. For them, the strange movements of the blinded fumbling pack and their blazing anger are especially amusing: *soulas et delis* (or according to the modern translation: "un sujet de joie et de divertissement [an object of joy and amusement]").

> Che seroit soulas et delis
> A homme qui paour n'aroit,
> Quant gent si avoele verroit,
> Qu'il seront tuit si avoelé,
> Si desconfit et si maté,
> Quë il errageront tuit d'ire.[42]

At this point, the parameters that determine the visual perception among the circles of bystanders and establish different orders of observation have been clarified. A fundamental asymmetry of perception characterizes the battle. Even though Laudine's followers, the avengers, are superior in number and weapons and emotionally far more passionately involved, to the point of all-consuming anger, than the camouflaged victim on the bed, they succumb to the fallacy of perception in an unpredictable way. The victim—or, viewed from a different perspective, the murderer—does not only escape deadly revenge. He is even allowed to enjoy this adventure and be a figure of identification for the audience. Together with the listeners and readers who have been informed by the narrative, he is visually confronted with the seeing-blind who are almost being fooled into desperation (see my discussion, to follow, of the South Tyrolean wall paintings of the Iwein narrative). Their gestures, mimicry, and fighting would have to be interpreted as insanity and looming self-loss, were it not for the narrated omniscience. One can even ask oneself if the wild gesticulation of Laudine's angry followers, which resembles the depictions of dancers, angered, crazy, or possessed people in medieval iconography, contrasts with the order imposed on the courtly body in medieval aesthetics.[43] In addition, the same scene sheds light on the extensively described, very expressive mourning of Laudine. Despite her many topical elements drawn from the body language of mourning, the desperate widow seems to be depicted as a parallel to her enraged followers, whose first and second chases frame her entrance into the scene. She enters the focal point of attention by clawing, scratching, and tearing at her entirely strange yet beautiful appearance.[44] Her behavior appears to be motivated not only by her loss, but also by the murderer's invisibility, which has induced her fury. Chrétien explicitly associates the behavior of Laudine with that of the insane.

It is precisely at this point that a close comparison of the French and the German texts provides deeper insights about the perceptual asymmetry. Let us therefore go back to the very beginning of the encounter between the invisible murderer and his avengers. What occurs after Iwein's light meal and to whom? The consideration of perspective is imperative here. Iwein's situation is quickly outlined. He lies quietly on the bed and, abiding by the rules, clasps the ring with the magic stone in his palm, making him invisible. As the informed audience outside of the text, we lend the narrator great credibility concerning the magic effect of the ring, also because the reactions of the noninformed, perplexed figures in the text authenticate its concealing power. The immobile Iwein sees and hears the followers of Laudine approaching as they search for the murderer. Chrétien describes these events explicitly and—in contrast to Hartmann's more sober description—highlights the escalation of affect among the avengers: *Et ils le veoit erragier, / Et forsener et couroichier.*[45] Undoubtedly, the displayed passivity of an uninvolved observer is a rather odd and therefore somewhat comic attitude for a knight who wants to survive a personal attack.

Pouring in from both sides of the castle's entrance, Askalon's furious avengers now see things that they can immediately interpret: *in front of* the entranceway trap lies the *hindquarters* of the horse and inside the trap they see *forequarters* of the horse with its saddle. Their conclusions are not exceptional. Every human being with normal visual perceptive and interpretative competence would conclude that the rider of the bisected horse would also be in between the two gates, and, further, that he would be immediately visible to the eye. This interpretation no doubt stems from a basic human confidence in one's senses (nobody expects to encounter cognitive "blind spots" in their daily lives, and certainly not magically induced ones). In addition, it manifests the processing of perception as conceptualized by Mersch. The sensory stimulus is assimilated passively, but is processed as part of an active, productive process—productive in that the process of perception creates the object out of the expectation awakened by the received sensory signals.[46] The avengers experience such a turning point, but magic prevents them from reaching cognitive closure: they see, yet simultaneously fail to see. With their eyes, they take in both halves of the horse, which both authors are at pains to describe in great detail, but not the knight.

Both Chrétien and Hartmann elucidate the perception-influencing function, describing as if in slow motion the falling of the razor-sharp portcullis, the leaning position of Iwein as he reaches for Askalon, which saves him by a hair's breadth, as well as the evidence of the horse, and (albeit only in Chrétien), spurs, which are visible from the inside and outside of the entranceway prison.[47] These are signals—according to Mersch—that invite the production of the sought-after object as if they were saying: "There is more to see in this entranceway trap than just us." But this "more"—the invisible Iwein—remains concealed from their eyes. The narrative plays with the premises of perception. The visible awakens visual expectations in the eye, but these then are duped by the invisible. As I will show, the deceived are aware of their own faulty perception. The fact that the audience can knowingly follow these events turns them into second-order observers.

We should first consider more closely the scene to which Chrétien, in the French original, grants more narrative space than Hartmann. Chrétien's version depicts the step-by-step interplay of the correct perception of signals, the false processing of signals, and, in addition, the inappropriate actions of the avengers. In contrast, Hartmann's abbreviated account of perceptions appears rather abrupt.[48] The enraged avengers in the French version call out: "we see it [half of the saddle] well, but we see nothing of him [Yvain]" (*che veons bien, / ne de lui ne veommes rien,* 1123–1124). In addition, their furious self-commentary is more explicit and, in the individual enumeration of the visually perceived signals, more repetitive. How is it, they ask themselves, that they cannot see him, because at most only a little bird, a squirrel, a little marmoset, or a comparatively tiny animal could escape the window- and doorless room, that is, through the iron bars of the portcullis. They also evoke the additional evidence that proves Yvain's presence (the position of the bisected horse, the spurs cut off exactly at the heel).[49] The more their outrage grows, the more desperately they reassure themselves of their own visual faculties. It appears as if they did this tactilely, an act which would practically label them as "blind." Like "a blind person who tentatively looks for something" (*comme aveule qui a tastons / va aucune chose querant,* 1142–1143), "the angered strike at the air with senseless movements" (*ainsi trestuit d'ire escaufé,* 1132); desperate, they strike the walls with their clubs, causing pandemonium.[50] The text mentions explicitly that the bed—and, as a result, the protagonist too—is still spared the blows: *Mais des caus fu quites et frans / Li lis ou il s'estoit couchiés, / Qu'il n'i fu ferus ne touchiés,* 1136–1139).

These sentences grant the reader a rare visual privilege: the reader is permitted to "see" what the avengers themselves cannot see, insofar as the text informs him or her what Yvain is doing, despite his invisibility. Reading itself becomes tantamount to seeing and, at a certain level, understanding. This, at least for the "seeing" audience, is a comparatively exclusive spectacle. In addition, the audience sees in its imagination people whose perceptual fallacies put them in a rage while, amidst the turmoil, the invisible protagonist lies comfortably on a bed in the blind spot. The scene must have been just as bizarre as it was comic, due also to the complete lack of physical expenditure on the knight's part. The bed is still excluded from the blows, creating again a situation of suspense only for the audience outside of the text. We—the readers—already know that even though Yvain is visually deleted, he is materially "there," his invisible body tactilely present, which means that it could be injured. These discrepancies in the tactile and visual perceptibility of Yvain actually offer an additional narrative opportunity to irritate the avengers further, for instance, by letting them catch a piece of him. There is no question that such a tactile experience would have intensified the visual aporia with the fragments of the horse! Yet neither Chrétien nor Hartmann does more than make the audience aware of this possibility. Their solutions differ insofar as Yvain remains motionless on the bed even though he is fiercely beaten, whereas Iwein nimbly evades the beatings.[51]

This difference between the French and the Middle High German versions in staging the hero's perceptibility contrasts with the camouflage scenes in the *Nibelungenlied.* Siegfried, acting as a replacement for Gunther wearing a camouflage cape, must appear as a corporeal but invisible fighter. The text stages a different, but analogous, aporia of perception for Brünhild, just as Iwein and Yvain do for their avengers. Brünhild believes that the man who touches her, wrestles with her at the competition, and finally, also defeats her in bed is the same one whom she sees: Gunther. Instead, Gunther's fraud lies precisely in the discrepancy between seeing and touching. In contrast to the fraud perpetrated in the Iwein narratives, that in the *Nibelungenlied* is much more belated. Moreover, its exposure has—for reasons that cannot be discussed here—far more profound implications than for Yvain and Iwein, primarily because it serves as the catalyst for the subsequent chain of revenge.

Turning back to Yvain, we can ask how his avengers in the French original interpret their fallacy of perception. It seems as if their slowly making their way through the entranceway trap entails not only a corporeal, but also a cognitive, groping and grasping, due to the mysteriousness of the experience. Clearly, it is a threshold experience for them. For that reason, they cloak themselves with the terms available for the liminal; especially with terms for the uncanny and the base. They are convinced the devil is involved in this trick of the senses, that he has duped, jinxed, or demonized their eyes.[52] Which role does the devil or—in Laudine's speech of anger (1208–1243; see below)—the demons play? They serve as a tool allowing interpretation of the fallacy of perception. According to ontological concepts of demons stemming from Late Antiquity that survived into the Middle Ages, demons were considered creatures of the air that lived on the threshold between heaven and earth, between the spiritual nature of the gods and the material body of human beings. The ethereal body of these princes of the air was thought to permeate every solid body, possess them, and commit every sort of perceptual fraud with them.[53] Two of the many qualities ascribed to them concern the sensory perceptibility of the body: the one, mobility, is shared by demons and humans alike, and the second, airy embodiment, is purely demonic.[54] The combination of both leads to a distortion of what is seen, since under demonic influence the visible is never what it seems to be. The reliability of the human *aisthesis,* especially of visual perception, is questioned as well as the authenticity of the visible objects in the outside world. From these two directions, then, people's control over their perception of the world and its interpretation slips from their hands.

Let's now turn to the Middle High German version of the first chase scene. In summary, the avengers experience similar things in *Iwein.* Moreover, their failures of perception also receive metaphysical explanation. They struggle with God and curse the devil, speak about the *zouberliste* of the wanted person and ask each other who could have taken their senses from them:

sî sprâchen,warst der man komen,
ode wer hât uns benomen
diu ougen und die sinne?
er ist benamen hinne:
wir sîn mit gesehenden ougen blint.
ez sehent wol alle die hinnen sint:
ezn wær dan cleine als ein mûs,
unz daz beslozzen wær diz hûs,
sone möht niht lebendes drûz komen:
wie ist uns dirre man benomen?
swie lange er sich doch vriste
mit sînem zouberliste,
wir vinden in noch hiute.
suochent, guote liute,

in winkeln und under benken.
erne mag des niht entwenken
erne müeze her vür.[55]

When struggling with the fallacy of perception, they summarize their self-perception with a paraphrase of Matthew (13:13–14), commonly applied to Jews: "We are blind with seeing eyes." Not only does this represent an addition compared with Chrétien's text, it also rhymes with the verse *ez sehent wol alle die hinnen sint.* It can be read not only as a self-referential comment asserting the avengers' ability to see (see McConeghy's translation: "not one of us here is blind"), but also as a second-order observation ("all in this room can see well" that the avengers cannot see). Understanding the verse in this fashion implies that the avengers know that their eyes have been deceived and that others possibly could see what they, the avengers, cannot. But this insight does not prevent them from being furious. On the contrary, their self-reflection intensifies their irritation. It was "not to be prevented" (*ungewärlich*) that they too strike at nothing as if they are out of their minds, stab the air, and fumble about like blind people. Without a doubt, they present a comic scene to the uninvolved observers.

Chrétien doubles the narrative motif by letting the avengers attempt to find Yvain, not once, but twice; Hartmann adheres both to this structure and the asymmetrical conditions of perception. The second attempt is infused with an element that stems from legal discourse: the conventional evidence for a murderer's physical presence. As the servants try to carry Askalon's corpse to the nearby palace, the wounds of the slain reopen. The fresh blood now takes on the same functions as the two horse halves and the spurs in the first scene; it provides proof that someone is present, but, in fact, invisible. The fresh blood of the corpse suggests that the murderer is "there," that he is in the same room as the dead body. Again, perception is misled by visible and even judicially coded circumstantial evidence. Hartmann appeals to this general understanding because the judicial institution of the medieval bier test is conclusive:

Nû ist uns ein dinc geseit
vil dicke vür die wârheit,
swer den andern habe erslagen,
und wurder vür in getragen,
swie langer dâ vor wære wunt,
er begunde bluoten anderstunt.
nû seht, alsô begunden

im bluoten sîne wunden,
dô man in in daz palas truoc:
wan er was bî im der in sluoc.[56]

Both authors stage the truth of the bier test in their own way, but both stay within Mersch's understanding of an event: Hartmann appeals directly to the eyes of his audience (*nû seht,* 1361), and Chrétien describes the observers standing around the bier, staring at the oozing blood (1178–1181; 1195–1198). Both evoke the performative quality of this visualization of a hidden truth by means of the fresh blood. The blood's visibility embodies law and would allow the murderer to be convicted—were he to find himself in the room. Folkloristic sources give evidence for such rituals of legal performance. Several records from the old Swiss confederation that stretch into the sixteenth century highlight this meaning of the bier test for the finding of justice. Actual stagings were organized. A suspect had to approach the corpse slowly, and if more blood gradually appeared, then the blood visualized the perpetration of the crime itself.[57] This incident exposes the principle of evidence, which, into early modern times, fulfilled its epistemological function of authenticity: "Faith is not the evidence of things not seen. No, faith is earned by the evidence that certain things have been seen—and touched [even if by someone else]."[58]

Further, during the second chase scene, the deceived react as if they were berserks, harassed by the increased pressure to succeed. But their swords still attack nothing because their eyes are deceived. This time, however, they also strike the bed on which Yvain/Iwein lies. In the French version, Yvain endures the apparently harmless blows. Hartmann, in contrast, has just the bed become *vil dicke wunt* ("hacked to shreds").[59] In terms of narrative logic, he seems to take the sword strokes more seriously since he has Iwein dodge the blows and stabbings continually (*ouch muoser dicke wenken,* 1375). This detail can be interpreted as the genre-specific irony of the narrator, who expands the comic moment of the avengers' gestures and motions to those of the invisible "fighter" as well.

After the second attempt, which forces the avengers to capitulate, the angry widow speaks up. She does this as expressively as when she was earlier mourning through mime and gestures. There are, however, significant differences in her speech in the versions of Chrétien and Hartmann. Hartmann lets Laudine have the last word of the whole passage; she emphasizes that he who is really present has cast a *zouber* on the *sinne* and accuses God, but *only* Him.[60] On the whole, Hartmann cuts her angry speech (1382–1402), not only shortening it, but also diminishing that dimension that characterizes the struggle against the invisible subject in Chrétien. He eliminates the uncanny invisible and lessens its demonic qualities by having Laudine alone address God. In the French version, this invisible being is rendered highly present through Laudine's intense emotional words, and by her channeling her anger directly against Him. First, the despairing, screaming widow accuses God (*crioit comme hors de sens,* 1205) of acting unjustly were He to let the murderer escape. Further still, God would even commit a grave injustice by not permitting her to see the one invisibly present (*que veoir mie ne me lais / Chelui qui est si pres de moi,* 1216–1217). Then, in an abrupt change of mind, Laudine argues that the invisibility points toward a ghost or a demon who has cast a spell on her (*qu'entre nous chi s'est chaiens mis / ou fantosmes ou anemis, / s'en sui enfantosmee toute,* 1219–1221). Her angered speech, directed toward the devilish demon (see *diablie,* 1202) that killed her husband, is unique and found only in Chrétien:

> Ha! fantosme, couarde chose,
> Pour quoi es si acouardie,
> Quant vers mon seigneur fus hardie?
> Chose vaine, chose faillie,
> Que ne t'ai jë en ma baillie!
> Que ne te puis ore tenir!
> Mais comment puet che avenir
> Que tu mon seigneur ad ochis,
> S'en traïson ne le feïs?
> Ja voir par toi conquis ne fust
> Me sire, se veü t'eüst,
> Qu'el monde son pareil n'avoit,
> Ne Dix ne hom ne l'i savoit,
> N'il n'en y a mais nul de tix.
> Chertes, se tu fusses mortix,
> N'osaisses mon seignor atendre,
> Qu'a li ne se pooit nus prendre.[61]

This lengthy invective demonizes the invisible. The metaphysical caricature of the knight nonetheless has a narrative function. The desperate widow develops the unique rhetoric of a lamentation for the dead that exaggerates the invincibility of a combatant. The fact that the battle happened under such apparent asymmetrical conditions of perception leads her to the plausible, albeit false, conclusion: her husband must have been killed by an "immortal."

For both texts, the end of the scene can be narrated quickly. The protagonist stays hidden in the castle, still in the immediate vicinity of his victim's widow, whom he observes in the subsequent mourning ceremony. He falls in love with her. Acting as a matchmaker, Lunete again does serious work: only a thousand verses later, Yvain (or Iwein) is engaged to Laudine amid courtly acclamations. Without a doubt, one can state that a protagonist of a courtly epic seldom escapes death so comfortably. It is even more seldom that he can ensure himself the glorious succession as protector of the source and of its mistress in such an adventurous manner.[62] Faced with the way the story continues and the way Iwein camouflages himself, one is reminded of the leaping spiders. Their actions seem to be more intentional than those of the fictional hero. In the end, his apparently random survival is due to a logic of narration and action which strictly focuses on the turbulent development of a knightly hero. For this reason, his fate is organized by this logic as long as the epic has not been told to its end.

Medium and Material: The Ywain frescoes of Castle Rodenegg

We have seen how blind spots in visual perception play an important thematic role in the Iwein narratives. These blind spots work within and without the text to establish distinctions in knowledge, be it among the protagonists or between them and the audience for the narrative. When it comes to the issue of visibility, pictorial sources, or, more precisely, visual media, inherently raise a different set of questions. By his nature, the invisible combatant presents author and reader with all sorts of problems. He also, however, presents a possibility: by making the invisible protagonist visible to his audience, the author grants it the privilege of sharing in special knowledge as well as the feeling of exclusiveness that comes with the denial to others of such sensory and cognitive advantages.

By virtue of a fortunate survival, we are in position to pursue our analysis of invisibility, not only in works of literature, but in a set of murals that take the Iwein narratives as their point of departure. Before turning to these images, however, it must first be observed, if only in passing, that the pictorial depiction of the invisible by no means represented an unfamiliar challenge for medieval artists. Consider the various ways in which the visualization of the invisible arises in a very different, yet nonetheless very relevant context, that dictated by the doctrine of the Incarnation.[63] The question of how to make the invisible visible was central to Christianity from its inception, as was the notion of making the blind see. Moreover, from Late Antiquity and throughout the Middle Ages, the theology of the *imago Dei* had a manifest impact on visualizations of the deity, playing an important role in the development of image theory. During the High and later Middle Ages, it also became increasingly important in relationship to another body of texts, the visualizations of the hidden God attributed to charismatic visionaries.[64]

The Iwein narratives serve as the source for a series of South Tyrolean wall paintings that have survived to the present day at the castle of Rodenegg in Southern Tyrol. The frescoes were painted shortly after the composition of Hartmann's novel. I will focus on scene 10 in the middle of the south wall of the Ywain room (figs. 12.4 and 12.5).[65] First though, a word about the topography of the castle: the wall paintings are located in a room that is only accessible over long wooden bridges and several gateways, one of which could be closed with a portcullis, a protective mechanism which is exceedingly rare in Tyrolean castles, even in the late Middle Ages and, in fact, at first totally unknown in Southern Tyrol (fig. 12.6).[66] Whoever recited the story could have made use of this architectural parallel between the place of the frescoes (the castle of Rodenegg) and the site of the narrative action (the castle of Laudine) in a performance involving two media. He could build upon the concrete spatial experience of the audience and explicitly refer to the extraordinary portcullis in the castle—the device which turns it into Iwein's prison. There is no evidence for a dual-media presentation of the Iwein narratives at Rodenegg, but in view of the evidence from other South Tyrolean castles, one may reckon with such a possibility. For example, at Runkelstein, the most famous South Tyrolean castle, there is solid evidence for certain customs in performance. Here it can be shown that Niklaus Vintler employed a speaker in addition to other entertainers, especially musicians (their pay for the year 1401 is registered in the Schlandersberg book of accounts); such performance artists probably performed mostly in rooms with frescoes or wall paintings decorated with literary motifs.[67]

Central to our investigation is the question: how to portray someone invisible? In modernism, attempts to convey images of invisibility using the eye often result in the self-referential showing of the showing, or, for that matter, the showing of not being able to show. Scene 10 in the Ywain frescoes solves this representational problem by referring back to a perspective established within narration, one involving the initiated circle of observers. The reconstruction of the illustration's design, however, remains an open question due to partial damage to this segment of the painting. Nonetheless, a fragment of a hand and a forehead are recognizable as most likely belonging to Iwein,

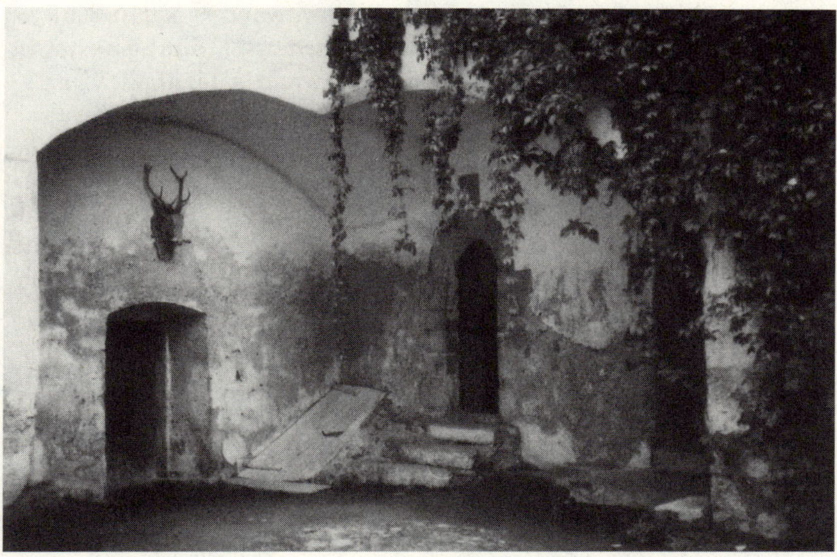

Figure 12.4. Schloss Rodenegg, entrance to room with frescoes. Reproduced from Volker Schupp and Hans Szklenar, *Ywain auf Schloß Rodenegg. Eine Bildergeschichte nach dem "Iwein" Hartmanns von Aue* (Sigmaringen: Jan Thorbecke Verlag, 1996), by permission of the publisher.

who appears lying on the patterned bed-covers (fig. 12.7). If this hypothesis is correct, then the invisible Iwein was depicted visibly as a figure. In this case, the conception of the image does not represent the experienced perception of the deceived, who swing their weapons throughout the room and point their fingers at their own eyes and at the eyes of others. Instead, the fresco tries to transpose the omniscience of the novel's audience to its medial equivalent; it tries to create a sort of "omnivisuality" of the frescoes, which wrap around the room.

The experience of the invisibly visible protagonist necessarily relies on both media: "The 'ironic story' represents . . . a productive and extremely self-conscious engagement with literary narration."[68] As has been demonstrated, the latter opens an inner-mental space of visuality, in which all figures are shown before the inner eye by the narration. More than any other scene, the segment depicting the visible-invisible Iwein depends strongly on its medial opposite in a performative situation—the oral presentation supported by mimicry and the gestures of a possibly professional recitator. How else would the audience

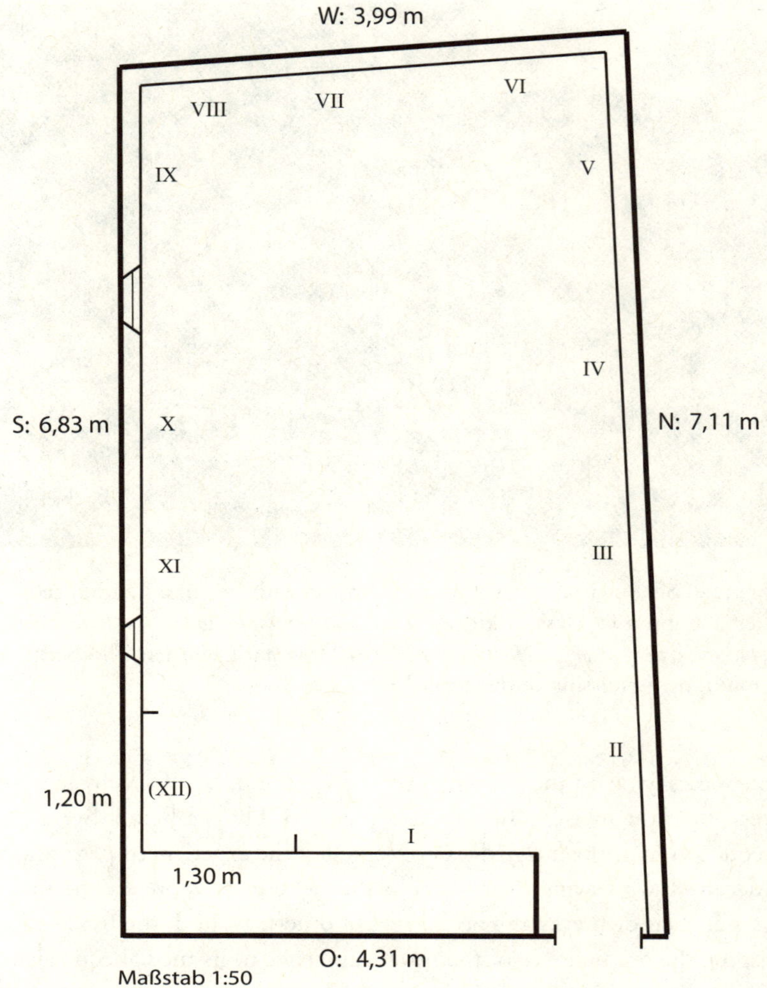

Figure 12.5. Division of scenes in the Ywain frescoes at Schloss Rodenegg. Reproduced from Volker Schupp and Hans Szklenar, *Ywain auf Schloß Rodenegg. Eine Bildergeschichte nach dem "Iwein" Hartmanns von Aue* (Sigmaringen: Jan Thorbecke Verlag, 1996), by permission of the publisher.

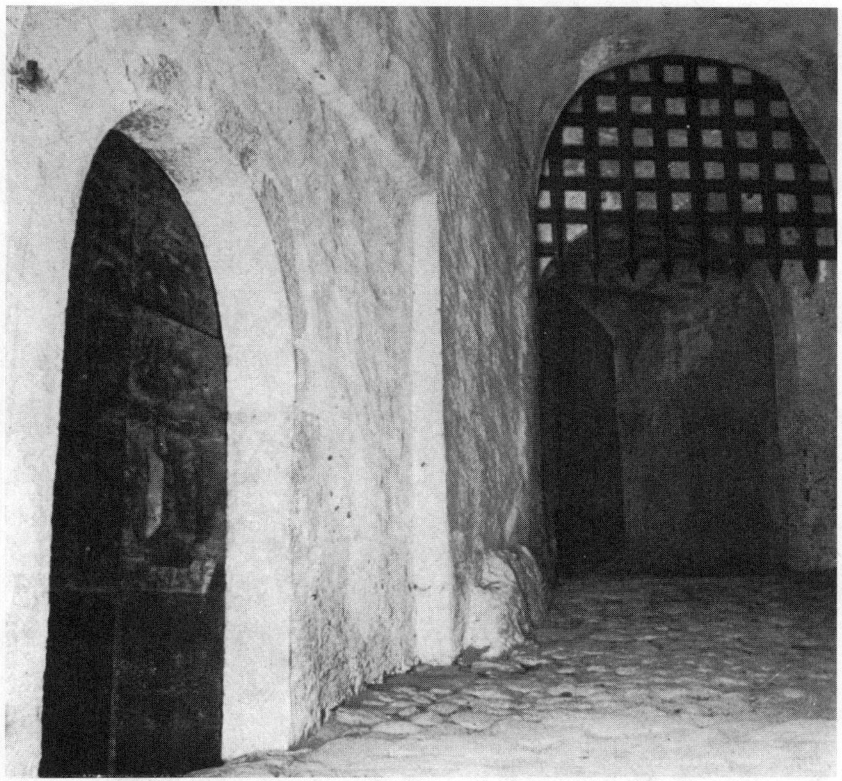

Figure 12.6. Portcullis at Schloss Rodenegg

have "seen" that the pictorially visible Iwein was actually invisible on the level of action? How else would the audience have recognized that this explains why the avengers grapple with their weapons and point at their eyes? Thus, both media generate a visual event for their audience. Through the courtly epic, the narrative intervention on its own conveys the perspectival complexity. Only it can distinguish between the informed and the deceived.

Today, we no longer can see the frescoes of Rodenegg as they would have been perceived by their original audience. Time has defaced scene 10, causing a performance failure. Apart from the above-mentioned fragments, the formerly visible-invisible Iwein has vanished from the colored layer of chalk and has been replaced with a white area of restoration.[69] This act of replacement lifts the medium as well as the portrayed motif (invisibility) into consciousness; an act which could not be more suitable even though it is only a coin-

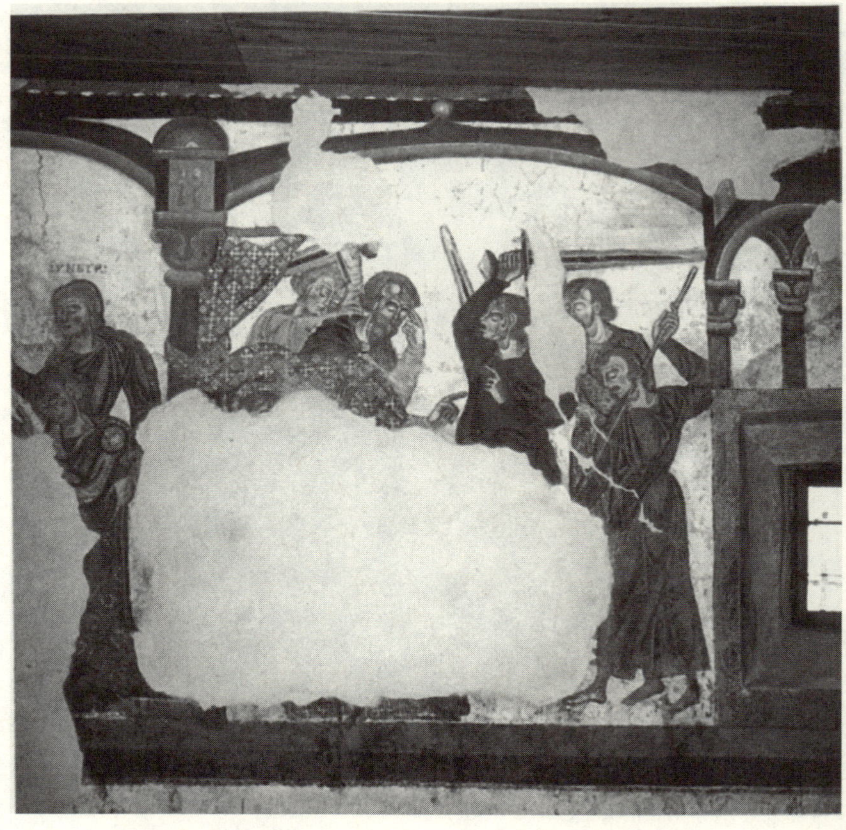

Figure 12.7. Ywain frescoes at Schloss Rodenegg, scene 10. Reproduced from Volker Schupp and Hans Szklenar, *Ywain auf Schloß Rodenegg. Eine Bildergeschichte nach dem "Iwein" Hartmanns von Aue* (Sigmaringen: Jan Thorbecke Verlag, 1996), by permission of the publisher.

cidental media-aesthetic trick of time. It is the substantiality of the medium itself that now obviously compensates for the meagerness of the representation.[70]

The Fight against the Invisible as a Ritual of Law: Sachsenspiegel

I now return to my starting point, to the battle against an invisible opponent narrated from a specific perspective. In the courtly epic, this asymmetric confrontation actually occurred, even though one of the principle participants remained invisible to his opponent, both "there" and "not there." The same could be said of the animal mimicry traps presented earlier. The legal ritual I wish to introduce here, however, represents a case apart, even though it too involves a battle against an opponent who is invisible because, quite simply, he is not present to take part in the duel. The actual absence of one of the two participants underscores the ritualized and, hence, controlled character of the ceremonial battle. The battle in question is a particular type of duel at court, an instrument of judgment that was used in lieu of a trial. The duel at court has to be viewed in the context of medieval strategies for resolving conflicts. It later became an independent method of establishing evidence at trial, a means of rule-oriented conflict management that evolved into less violent verbal processes still in use in courts.[71] Under special circumstances, the duel could also take place as a fight against someone invisible without seeming to be irritating or funny. If the opponent—namely, the accused—did not appear in the arena and did not take his place opposite the accuser, then the fight was staged publicly with a single fighter according to strict, ritualized rules of movement.

The regulations governing this late-medieval trial process, both the equipment and the personnel, are described in minute detail in Eike von Repgow's *Sachsenspiegel* (written between 1209 and 1233), which is one of the oldest and most influential law books written in the German language.[72] The five paragraphs of the *Landrecht* I 63 contain extensive descriptions of the *iudicium pugnae,*[73] which are illustrated in three of the four available manuscripts (see below). Eike drew up his law writings between 1225 and 1235. At this time, the court duel had already been subjected to clear restrictions due to its damnation at the Fourth Lateran Council (1215).[74] In his writings, the author supports his statements with common law (*Gewohnheitsrecht*; see the preamble in verse, vv. 151–158), which had been practiced for generations. The elaborateness of his rules documents a long-established tradition of court battles. These rules also structure combat against an accused who did not appear at court—a highly ritualized performance. Such a fight executed an as-if-action against the other combatant, who was considered to be present in absentia. The final *sentence* (*Landrecht* I 63 §5) makes this explicit by affirming that the performance (concretely, the strictly monitored course of movements) justifies the judgment in favor of the present fighter: "With this, the accused was convicted of whatever it was of which he stood accused, on account of which he had been challenged to a duel. And the judge was then to judge the accused as if he had been defeated in combat."[75] The visual perception of the performance was transparent for everyone involved. The accused who failed to appear was nonetheless invisibly present, due not to magic but rather to an agreement inherent in the ritual. It was the only way to carry out the ritual and to resolve the conflict.

At first, the text describes the circumstances under which a plaintiff could demand a duel with the defendant.[76] Only the last paragraph (*Landrecht* I 63 §5) discusses the exception that is of interest here: if the accused does not appear in the arena, then the court bailiff, accompanied by two lay assessors, should summon him once, and if necessary, twice more, to fight. If he still defaults, the trial takes an extraordinary course:

> En kumt her [der Beklagte] zu der dritten ladunge nicht vor, der kleger sal uf sten unde sich zu kamphe erbiten, unde sal zwene slege unde einen stich ton wider den wint.[77]

This description exemplifies the underlying rules of battle, consisting of an actual choreography of movement—apart from the rules for equipment and personnel (eyewitnesses must be present!). The plaintiff has to rise from the battle chair, consent to the fight and execute two blows and one stab against the wind. These clearly regulated elements of body language visualize law—a performative feature which strongly characterizes the Germanic-German concept of law: "The bodies of the persons participating in the legal process functioned to a certain extent as concrete embodiments of abstract concepts, of the law itself."[78]

This function of gestures raises a methodological problem, namely, how to abstract the law-performing gesture from signs that had other functions, for example, communicative or referential gestures. Norbert Ott argues that "their actual use in the judicial process" has hardly ever been described. In our case, however, it seems to be unmistakably encoded. The ritualized physical procedure imparts a clear function to invisibility. Contrary to the examples that have been presented thus far, invisibility does not represent an insidious threat and attack by an invisible aggressor (as, for example, in the wild or in the *Nibelungenlied,* when Siegfried acts under the invisibility cloak. The legal ritual also does not entail for any of the participants a fallacy in perception or a loss of control. It is, as it were, the exact opposite: the result of an agreement by all persons involved. The invisibility of the accused stands for his virtual presence in the duel and provides the legal basis for the performance of a battle with two fighters of whom only one is visible. As a result, the interpretation of all visual signals follows this joint convention.

As previously mentioned, the extensive textual description of the duel with the invisible opponent is illustrated in three of the four extant manuscripts with pictures (it is omitted in the manuscript from Heidelberg). How do the illustrated manuscripts, which have a common model, visualize the conflict-solving ritual in this special case? I will focus on the relevant folio in the latest illuminated codex (W, fol. 26^r, picture register 3).[79] The Wolfenbüttel Codex is essentially an exact copy of the pictorial manuscript of Dresden and was written no later than 1375. It differs only minutely from the illustration in the Dresden manuscript (the "head of the wind" has a slightly more coarse physiognomy and he rests on a house of clouds). The comparable illustration in the Oldenburg manuscript is laterally inverted. The "head of the wind" is in the upper right corner, whereas the judge sits on the left, enthroned over the plaintiff, who is on the right. Contrary to the other two judges, he is shouldering a sword on his left and is executing a demonstrative and commanding gesture toward the "head of the wind."

The Wolfenbüttel Codex represents the scene as a whole. As far as our special case is concerned, its illustrations remain true to the text, which is located in the right column of the same folio, to which the illuminations in the registers are anchored by rubricated initials. The miniaturist adheres precisely to the legal prescriptions (fig. 12.8).[80] The same approach also holds true in those instances in which the illumination at first seems abstract or not very close to the text, for example, as with the two duels depicted at the edge of the picture.[81] The sun shines on both opponents and watches over them because this is the way in which the image is anchored to the text: the sun and the shadow, respectively, need to be distributed equally over both figures (fig. 12.9).[82] At first glance, the blue, blowing face in the upper left-hand corner of the illustration of the fight against the invisible opponent also seems to represent an abstraction. Here again, however, the text provides an explanation: the face personifies the wind against which the plaintiff has to fight (fig. 12.10).[83] In addition, the blue face functions as a real substitute for the combatant who has, as it were, vanished into thin air. He loses the case as soon as the blows and the stab against the wind have been executed.

The Wolfenbüttel Codex demonstrates in exemplary fashion the relevance of the bond between the two media (word and image). It also offers insights into the meaning of invisibility. Text and picture remain bound to each other both in the *Sachsenspiegel* and, as has already been shown, in the Ywain frescoes at the castle of Rodenegg. The descriptive text of the legal ritual—as well as the narrative of the magic fighter—adds to the transparency of the image.

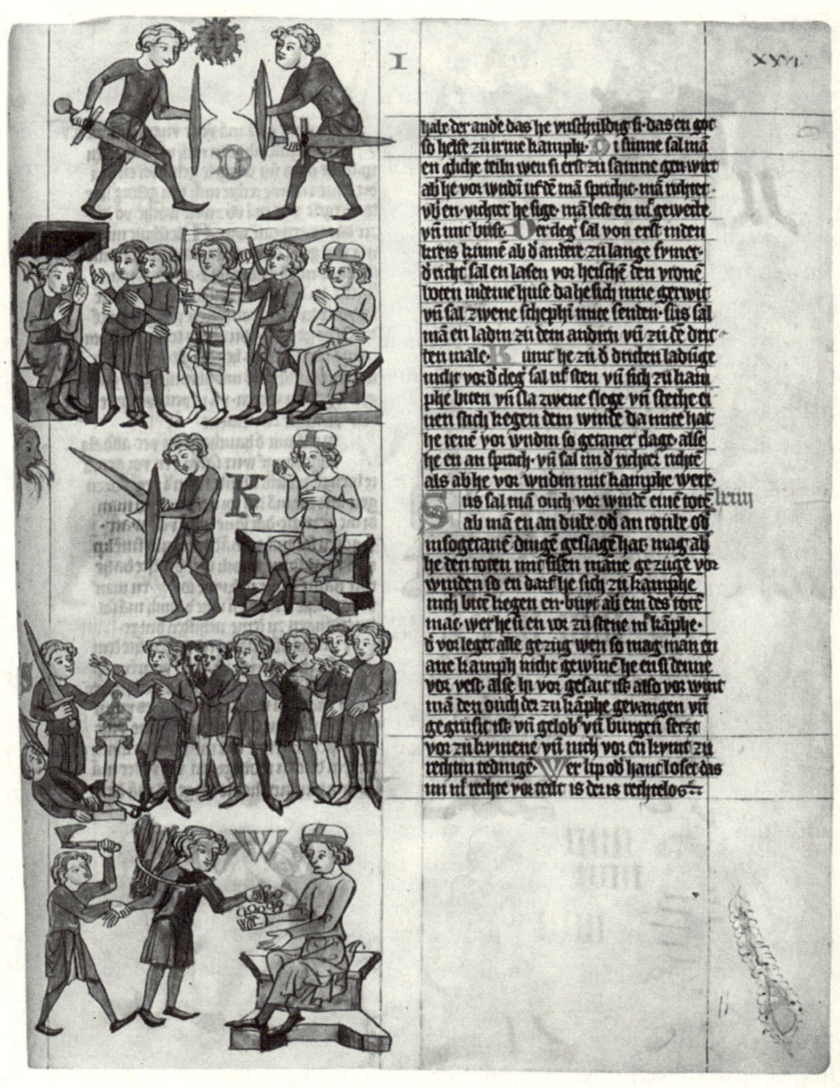

Figure 12.8. Eike von Repgow, *Der Sachsenspiegel, Landrecht* I 63 §4–5, after: Wolfenbüttel, Herzog-August-Bibliothek, Cod. Guelf. 3.1. Aug. 2°, fol. 26ʳ.

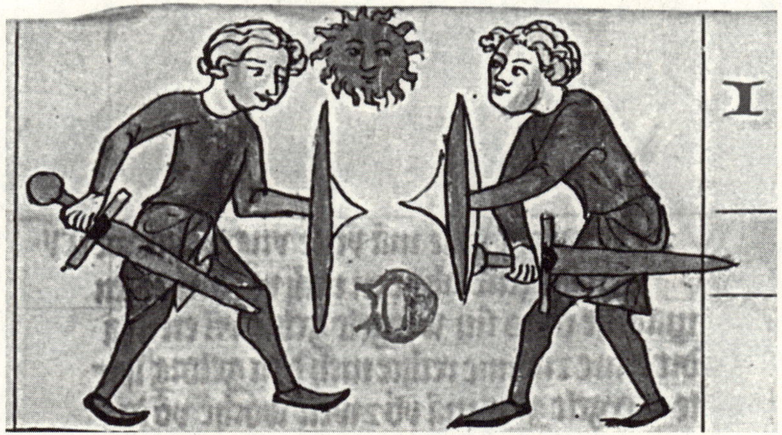

Figure 12.9. Eike von Repgow, *Der Sachsenspiegel, Landrecht* I 63 §4–5, after: Wolfenbüttel, Herzog-August-Bibliothek, Cod. Guelf. 3.1. Aug. 2°, fol. 26^{r}, image register 1.

In the first instance, they express the consensual basis for the visual perception of the battle. In the second case, they shape the audience's perception of the visualized invisibility—precisely that element that is interpreted so differently in the sources discussed in this essay.

Conclusion

> *The alternate reality of the Middle Ages was a slippery and dangerous world of motion.*[84]

Whoever orients himself in this world with the help of his eyes is exposed to an invisible aggressor; whoever wants to avenge himself against an invisible opponent and physically attack him, runs the great risk of ridiculing himself—at least in front of the informed observers of the battle. This is probably true for all historically possible worlds. Whereas under the omen of terrorism, late modernism is forced to accustom itself to such uncanny opponents, the Middle Ages never seemed to have lost sight of them. Moreover, literature and the arts seemed to have suggested such visual images to their audiences in order to explore the inner-mental liminal grounds in which the eyes cannot add any knowledge. These literary fictions did not only offer amusing visual spaces to the audiences for epic. They also have enabled cautious fumbling

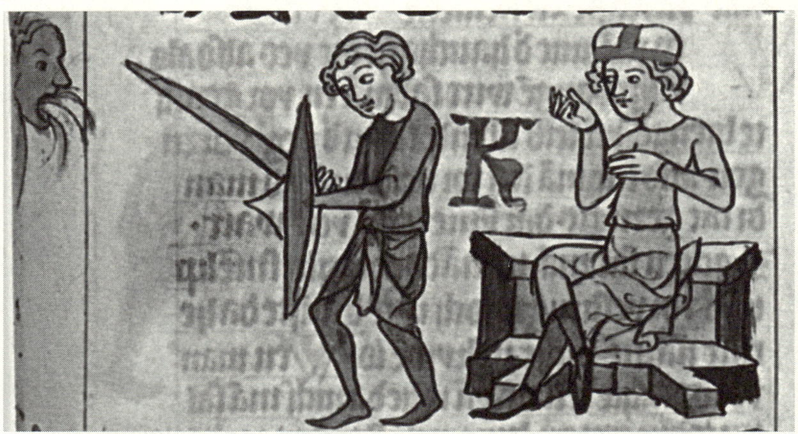

Figure 12.10. Eike von Repgow, *Der Sachsenspiegel, Landrecht* I 63 §4–5, after: Wolfenbüttel, Herzog-August-Bibliothek, Cod. Guelf. 3.1. Aug. 2°, fol. 26r, image register 3.

in a world that causes disorientation. Visually observing the outside world meant to secure one's self as much as possible in an obscurely ordered world. Not knowing how to orient oneself in that world was tantamount to being lost. Perhaps it was so much more reassuring to be told stories in such a way that one could open one's inner eye and then be amused with sovereignty by those who had been visually deceived.

Whoever exposes the invisible endangers its *telos* in the battle for survival. Wild animals and knights battling for courtly honor avoid this in order to ensure their own lives. He who in paradoxical fashion makes the invisible present to the physical eye, however, creates opportunities for deepened theoretical insight into the nature of perception. In this *telos,* the courtly epic does not differ from the visionary literature of the Middle Ages. Both the courtly narrators Chrétien de Troyes and Hartmann von Aue use the narrative's power of exclusion to this end. They build on a selective transparency that favors their audience in a special way. Using the characteristic irony of the narrator, they honor their audience with a wink by letting it participate in a liminal experience that forces open every restriction in human perspective. This ironic point of view also serves as an amusing didactic commentary on visuality, even as it remains a source of severe distress for both the avengers and Laudine. Chrétien and Hartmann grant the narration its best and most powerful opportunity. This chance can be termed an "art of distinction." But what does distinction mean within the context of seeing or not-seeing? The narrative assigns to some participants aporias of perception, and as a result, they remain furious. To others, however, namely, the readers, it offers the possibility of presence and sovereign, reflective amusement.

Notes

Epigraph: "Jedes Medium, das Unsichtbarkeit aufhebt und Sichtbarkeit erhöht, bringt den Menschen Erlösung." Volker Demuth, "Ästhetik des Unsichtbaren. Camouflage, Blendung, Verdunkelungsgefahren," *Lettre international* (2000): pp. 90–96, here p. 92. My thanks to Caroline Domenghino (Johns Hopkins University), the initial translator of this article, and to Jeffrey F. Hamburger (Harvard University), who helped me enormously with his finishing touches. This paper presents a revised and elaborated version of the following article: Hildegard Elisabeth Keller, "Vom Kampf gegen einen Unsichtbaren. Freie Wildbahn—höfisches Epos—mittelalterliches Rechtsritual," in *Kunst der Bewegung. Kinästhetische Wahrnehmung und Probehandeln in virtuellen Welten,* ed. Christina Lechtermann and Carsten Morsch, Publikationen zur Zeitschrift für Germanistik. Neue Folge 8 (Bern, 2004), pp. 103–136.

1. Elias Canetti, *Masse und Macht* (Frankfurt am Main, 1991), p. 13.

2. As Jeffrey Hamburger points out, medievalists have, on the whole, come late to the debate over visuality. See his review of Suzannah Biernoff, *Sight and Embodiment in the Middle Ages* (Houndmills and New York, 2002) in *Speculum* 71 (2004): pp. 133–136; Jeffrey F. Hamburger and Anne-Marie Bouché, eds., *The Mind's Eye: Art and Theological Argument in the Middle Ages* (Princeton, 2005).

3. Chrétien de Troyes, *Le Chevalier au Lion,* in *Romans suivis des Chansons,* avec, en appendice, Philomena, sous la direction de Michel Zink (Paris, 1994), pp. 705–936; idem, *The Knight with the Lion, or Yvain (Le Chevalier au Lion),* ed. and trans. William W. Kibler, Garland Library of Medieval Literature, Series A 48 (New York and London, 1985). All Old French quotations and English translations follow these editions.

4. Hartmann von Aue, *Iwein,* ed. Max Wehrli (Zürich, 1988); an English translation in *Hartmann von Aue, Iwein,* ed. and trans. Patrick M. McConeghy, Garland Library of Medieval Literature, Series A 19 (New York and London, 1984). All Middle High German quotations and English translations follow these editions.

5. Wolf Singer, *Der Beobachter im Gehirn. Essays zur Hirnforschung* (Frankfurt am Main, 2002); idem, "Conditio humana aus neurobiologischer Perspektive," in *Die Rolle der Seele in der Kognitions- und Neurowissenschaft,* ed. Markus F. Peschl (Würzburg, 2005), pp. 41–61.

6. See Niklas Luhmann's statement about the distinctive function of magic: "Die Magie beruht auf der einfachen Unterscheidung sichtbarer und unsichtbarer

Dinge in ein und derselben Welt. [Magic depends on the simple distinction between visible and invisible things in one and the same world.]" Niklas Luhmann, *Die Religion der Gesellschaft,* ed. André Kieserling (Frankfurt am Main, 2000), p. 85.

7. E.g., the RQ-1 (predator), a type of miniature airplane which is used by the United States in its fight against terror. It destroys its victim without having once been seen with the eye. See Siegesmund von Ilsemann, "Tödliches Auge," in *Spiegel* 46 (2002): p. 222.

8. See: "Auch eine Schlacht um Bilder. Wie sich Fernsehsender auf den Ernstfall Vorbereiten" (by: tpg); "Die Rakete als strafender Blitz Gottes. Recht und Rache im Hightech-Zeitalter" (by: H.Sf), both articles can be found in *Neue Zürcher Zeitung* 31, 7.2 (2003): p. 73; further Sieglinde Geisel, "Unsichtbare Mächte. Terrorismus und die Furien des Verschwindens," *Neue Zürcher Zeitung* 263 (2001): p. 25.

9. Sigmund Freud, "Das Unheimliche" (1919), in idem, *Der Moses des Michelangelo. Schriften über Kunst und Künstler,* intro. by Peter Gay (Frankfurt am Main, 1993), pp. 137–172; idem, "The Uncanny," in *The Standard Edition of the Complete Psychological Works of Sigmund Freud,* vol. XVII, ed. and trans. James Strachey, (London, 1953), pp. 219–252.

10. Freud, "Das Unheimliche," pp. 150–152; Freud, "The Uncanny," pp. 231–232. As to be expected, he connects the first observation (the semantic ambivalence of the term) with the suppressed (the uncanny as the suppression of original knowledge) and the second observation (fear of blindness) with the fear of castration. The third observation manifests Freud's awareness of the artist's ability to trigger uncanny feelings via literary or imaginative representation.

11. Hans Robert Jauss, "Über den Grund des Vergnügens am komischen Helden," in *Das Komische,* ed. Wolfgang Preisendanz and Rainer Warning, Poetik und Hermeneutik 7 (München, 1976), pp. 398–402. Jauss refers back to Sigmund Freud, *Der Witz und seine Beziehung zum Unbewussten* (1905). See *Jokes and Their Relation to the Unconscious,* trans. James Strachey (New York, 1963).

12. Wolfgang Iser, "Das Komische: Ein Kipp-Phänomen," in Preisendanz and Warning, *Das Komische,* pp. 398–402.

13. "Wo das Gesetz von Fressen und Gefressenwerden regiert, sind Tarnung, Täuschung, Lug und Trug unverzichtbare Lebensmaximen." See Volker Sommer, *Lob der Lüge. Täuschung und Selbstbetrug bei Tier und Mensch* (München, 1992), p. 46.

14. Ibid.; for a liminal discussion of human and animal societies, consider the analyses on the primates, pp. 66–160, and esp. "Bruder Affe. Was die enge Verwandtschaft von Mensch und Affe bedeutet," *NZZ Folio. Die Zeitschrift der Neuen Zürcher Zeitung* 8 (2003): pp. 14–18.

15. Ingo Rentschler, "Weltbilder der Kunst-Erscheinungsformen der Wirklichkeit," in *Geist und Natur,* ed. Hans-Peter Dürr and Walther Ch. Zimmerli (Bern, 1989), p. 116, cited after Gottfried Boehm, "Sehen. Hermeneutische Reflexionen,"

in *Kritik des Sehens,* ed. Ralf Konersmann (Leipzig, 1999), pp. 272–298, here p. 284.

16. See Dieter Mersch, *Ereignis und Aura. Untersuchung zu einer Ästhetik des Performativen* (Frankfurt am Main, 2002), and idem, *Was sich zeigt. Materialität, Präsenz, Ereignis* (München, 2002).

17. The Grimm article expresses irritation about the semantic warping and distortion (*entstellung; verwirrung*) of the word; see Jacob and Wilhelm Grimm, *Deutsches Wörterbuch* (Leipzig, 1885–1984), vol. 3, col. 785.

18. The oldest word forms are the Old High German expressions *irougen, irougnissa, irougnessi, irougida,* which are all part of the semantic field *(sich) zeigen, offenbaren, zu erkennen geben, ans Licht bringen, erweisen, beweisen* (to show [oneself], to reveal, to make understood, to bring to light, to show or indicate, to demonstrate). *Althochdeutsches Wörterbuch,* ed. Rudolf Große (Berlin, 1997–), vol. 4, col. 1715, which mentions the lexical root for the first time; Rudolf Schützeichel, *Althochdeutsches Wörterbuch* (Tübingen, 1995), p. 231. Middle High German has the following word formations *ougen/erougen/eröugen* (possibly *erougenen*) "vor Augen stellen, zeigen, offenbaren." *Mittelhochdeutsches Wörterbuch,* ed. Georg Friedrich Benecke, Wilhelm Müller, and Friedrich Zarncke (Leipzig, 1854–1861), vol. 2, p. 453; Matthias Lexer, *Mittelhochdeutsches Handwörterbuch* (Stuttgart, 1992), vol. 1, col. 662). Older New High German forms of the verb such as *eräugnen*, make the etymological connection between "event" and visual sense apparent. See Jacob and Wilhelm Grimm, *Deutsches Wörterbuch,* Neubearbeitung (Leipzig and Stuttgart, 1983–), vol. 8, col. 1691–1693; Friedrich Kluge, *Etymologisches Wörterbuch der deutschen Sprache,* ed. Elmar Seebold (Berlin and New York, 1995), p. 229; and *Etymologisches Wörterbuch des Deutschen,* ed. Wolfgang Pfeifer (München, 2000), p. 293.

19. See Grimm, *Deutsches Wörterbuch,* vol. 8, col. 1691–1693.

20. This play with the expression *ereignen,* its etymology and its (misleading) similarity to other German words such as *eigen* (own) or *aneignen* (to appropriate) is one of the main parameters which determine the *aisthetic* of Mersch. He claims to find support in the early history of the German word.

21. According to the aims of this essay I concentrate on the morphological and kinetic aspects of *visual* mimicry. Deceptions of the other senses through chemical, electric, acoustic, and tactile signals have to be ignored. See Klaus Lunau, *Warnen, Tarnen, Täuschen. Mimikry und andere Überlebensstrategien in der Natur* (Darmstadt, 2002), and Sommer, *Lob der Lüge;* from a terminological point of view, he makes use of the established mimicry concept of Wolfgang Wickler, *Mimikry. Nachahmung und Täuschung in der Natur* (Frankfurt am Main, 1973). This is supplemented by the analysis of Volker Sommer, which is not considered by Lunau, *Warnen, Tarnen, Täuschen,* pp. 37–45, which discusses the "classical" mimetic fallacy between hunter and prey; as well as findings on interspecies fallacy (pp. 46–65) and the tactical patterns of deceptions amongst primates, which are especially interesting for behavioral science (pp. 66–91).

22. Klaus Lunau, *Warnen, Tarnen, Täuschen,* image 4, p. 19 (photographed by Klaus Lunau). I thank Prof. Klaus Lunau, University of Düsseldorf, for letting me use and reprint his images. Lunau also offers a summary on the state of art for this highly intricate system of mimicry; see pp. 18–19 in the same work.

23. Ibid., p. 20.

24. Sommer, *Lob der Lüge,* pp. 30–33; Lunau, *Warnen, Tarnen, Täuschen,* pp. 32–40. *Krypsis* is the disguising *color adaptation* to the background, *Mimese* is considered to be the disguising *shape adaptation* to indifferent elements of the natural environment.

25. See also the same strategy in the mantis *Empusa pennata,* Lunau, *Warnen, Tarnen, Täuschen,* image 13, p. 32.

26. The leafy sea dragon can be viewed online at the John G. Shedd Aquarium Chicago (www.sheddaquarium.org), at the Australian Museum (www.amonline.net.au/fishes/fishfacts/fish/peques.htm) and in several, good shots on the Web page www.dragonsearch.asn.au/photolib/photolib.html (viewed 10 January 2006).

27. See Klaus Lunau, *Warnen, Tarnen, Täuschen,* p. 35.

28. See Sommer, *Lob der Lüge,* p. 45.

29. Concerning the term "observation" (first-order and any subsequent level), I refer to Claudio Baraldi, Giancarlo Corsi, and Elena Esposito, *GLU. Glossar zu Niklas Luhmanns Theorie sozialer Systeme,* Suhrkamp Taschenbuch Wissenschaft 1226 (Frankfurt am Main, 1999), pp. 123–128; to Niklas Luhmann, *Soziale Systeme. Grundriß einer allgemeinen Theorie,* Suhrkamp Taschenbuch Wissenschaft 666 (Frankfurt am Main, 1999); as well as to William Rasch, *Niklas Luhmann's Modernity: The Paradoxes of Differentiation* (Stanford, 2000).

30. "Unsichtbarkeit ist entscheidend dafür, dass jemand 'nicht da ist.'" See Jan-Dirk Müller, *Spielregeln für den Untergang. Die Welt des Nibelungenliedes* (Tübingen, 1998), p. 259.

31. For a differentiated analysis of the reverse condition, refer to Rüdiger Brandt, *Enklaven-Exklaven. Zur literarischen Darstellung von Öffentlichkeit und Nichtöffentlichkeit im Mittelalter,* Forschungen zur Geschichte der älteren deutschen Literatur 15 (München, 1993).

32. Jan-Dirk Müller, *Spielregeln für den Untergang,* p. 248.

33. I am adapting the approach of Jan-Dirk Müller, who speaks of "'Ringe[n]' von Betrachtern [circles of observers]." Ibid., p. 250.

34. After Lunete says good-bye to Iwein (1257), she is not mentioned again. Only when she reappears the text states: *diu juncvrouwe sich dô stal/von dem gesinde dan* (1414–1415). From this statement it can be deducted that she was present amongst the people surrounding her mourning mistress Laudine.

35. *Iwein,* 1169–1171.

36. *Iwein,* 1181–1200; *Le Chevalier au Lion,* 1005–1020. In the Old French text the question concerning Lunete's latent conflict of loyalty stays completely open, the Middle High German adaptation signals in one sentence that Lunete weighs her loyalty obligations (see 1178–1179).

37. *Iwein,* 1208–1209.

38. According to Hartmut Semmler in his phenomenology of courtly cunning, Hartmann von Aue is discrete in using "Schutzzauber in handlungstragender Funktion." Hartmut Semmler, *Listmotive in der mittelhochdeutschen Epik. Zum Wandel ethischer Normen im Spiegel der Literatur,* Philologische Studien und Quellen 122 (Berlin, 1991), p. 65. The observable shift of magic in the high-courtly epic into spheres within the human, thus turning magical forces into processes of the soul can be seen within this context. Semmler also recognizes that the portcullis episode has a self-referential dimension influenced by perception theory; he sees Hartmann's interest in the episode based in the dilemma in which Laudine and her servants find themselves: to acknowledge that perception (of the hidden Iwein) is not possible knowing simultaneously that their senses are deceived.

39. *Iwein,* 1222.

40. For the portcullis, see 905–929, for the courtly decoration of the room, see 960–965, and for the meal, see 1048–1054.

41. "Now how could you be better served / Than to have all those who hate you / Standing right next to you, / Menacing encircling you, / And yet so blinded / That they will never discover you, / Though you are right in their midst?" *Iwein,* 1239–1245.

42. "It will be an amusing sport / to a man who is unafraid / to see people so blinded; / for they'll be beside themselves with rage." *Le Chevalier au Lion,* 1074–1079.

43. See Umberto Eco, *Art and Beauty in the Middle Ages,* trans. Hugh Bredlin (New Haven, 2002). For high medieval culture, see C. Stephen Jaeger, *The Origins of Courtliness: Civilizing Trends and the Formation of Courtly Ideals, 939–1210* (Philadelphia, 1985); Joachim Bumke, "Höfischer Körper-höfische Kultur," in *Modernes Mittelalter. Neue Bilder einer populären Epoche,* ed. Joachim Heinzle (Frankfurt am Main, 1994), pp. 67–102. For a visualization of such a body order and its moral implications, see, e.g., the iconography of the Spanish *Beatus* manuscripts in the early Middle Ages, which impressively demonstrates that the status of redemption and, respectively, the condemnation of humans at the end of time is expressed in terms of disparate or harmoniously presented body parts. François Garnier discusses body movements and positions influenced by the Christian value system: *Le langage de l'image au Moyen Âge. Signification et symbolique,* 2 vols. (Paris, 1982), and Jean-Claude Schmitt, *La raison des gestes dans l'occident médiéval* (Paris, 1990).

44. *Iwein,* 1307–1349; for the topical arrangement of the mourning gestures, see Dietmar Peil, *Die Gebärde bei Chrétien, Hartmann und Wolfram. Erec-Iwein-Parzival,* Medium Aevum 28 (München, 1975); Martin J. Schubert, *Zur Theorie des Gebarens im Mittelalter. Analyse von nichtsprachlicher Äußerung in mittelhochdeutscher Epik. Rolandslied, Eneasroman, Tristan,* Kölner germanistische Studien 31 (Köln et al., 1991).

45. *Le Chevalier au Lion,* 1088–1099, here 1109–1110.

46. See Mersch, *Ereignis und Aura,* p. 36: "Die Wahrnehmung nimmt von der Sache, den bestehenden Tatsachen der Außenwelt, ihren Ausgang, und zwar so, dass sie zunächst ein 'Nehmen' bedeutet, das im Vollzug des Wahrnehmens gewendet wird, um es als Wahrgenommenes allererst hervorzubringen."

47. *Iwein,* 1108–1118, 1268–1270; *Le Chevalier au Lion,* 932–951 (*C'au res du dos li vint raiant,* 948), 1093–1105.

48. *Le Chevalier au Lion,* 1088–1099; *Iwein,* 1258–1262.

49. *Le Chevalier au Lion,* 1111–1131.

50. Ibid., 1132–1143.

51. *Si fu mout ferus et boutés / Mesire Yvains la ou il jut, / Mais ains pour che ne se remut:* "My lord Yvain was constantly / struck and jostled there where he lay." *Le Chevalier au Lion,* 1192–1194: see below, during the second chase.

52. The speech mentions the devil three times: *Le Chevalier au Lion,* 1130–1131, 1200–1202, 1218–1242 (Laudine on the devilish phantom).

53. This is one of the main causes of theological speculation on the subject, e.g., in Augustine, *De divinatione daemonum,* CSEL 41, 597–618; Hrabanus Maurus, *De magicis artibus,* MPL 110, 1095–1110. See Walter Stephens, *Demon Lovers: Witchcraft, Sex, and the Crisis of Belief* (Chicago, 2001); Jean-Claude Schmitt, "Le corps des fantômes," in *Micrologus. Natura, scienze e società medievali. I discorsi dei corpi,* ed. Véronique Pasche et al., Micrologus. Natura, scienza e società medievali: Nature, Sciences and Medieval Societies 1 (Paris and Turnhout, 1993), pp. 19–25; idem, *Les revenants. Les vivants et les morts dans la société médiévale,* Bibliothèque des histoires (Paris, 1994).

54. *Daemones sunt genere animalia, [. . .] corpore aëria.* Lucius Apuleius, *De Deo Socratis,* in Apulée, *Opuscules philosophiques et fragments,* ed. Jean Beaujeu (Paris, 1973), ch. 13, §148, S. 33, quoted and discussed in Stephen G. Nichols, "Melusine between Myth and History: Profile of a Female Demon," in *Mittelalter. Neue Wege durch einen alten Kontinent,* ed. Jan-Dirk Müller and Horst Wenzel (Stuttgart and Leipzig, 1999), pp. 217–240, here pp. 220–222.

55. "'Where did he go,' they said / 'Have we been robbed of / Our sight and our senses? / The man must be here! / We are wide awake, but cannot see! / Not one of us here is blind, / And since this room was secured, / No living thing could have escaped, / Unless it were as small as a mouse. / How has this man eluded us? / But no matter how long he is kept alive / By his sorcery / We will still find him today. / Search well, good people, / In the corners and under the benches. / There is no way he can keep us / From flushing him out.'" *Iwein,* 1273–1289.

56. "Now there is a saying / And many believe it, / That if a man has been killed / And is carried past his murderer, / No matter how long he has been dead / He will begin to bleed again. / And sure enough, when the lord was carried / into the great hall / his wounds began / to bleed anew, / Since he was near the man who killed him." *Iwein,* 1355–1364 (similar wording is used in *Le Chevalier au Lion,* 1177–1191).

57. See Leo Zehnder, *Volkskundliches in der älteren schweizerischen Chronistik,*

Schriften der Schweizerischen Gesellschaft für Volkskunde 60 (Basel, 1976), pp. 392–394, and n. 21 (with further literature). For further literature on the ordeal to which the bier test belongs, refer to n. 71.

58. Stephens, *Demon Lovers,* p. 174.

59. *Iwein,* 1372–1374.

60. *Iwein,* 1367–1369 (Hartmann gives parts of the speech of the avengers to Laudine); on the accusation, see 1382–1402.

61. "'Ah! Phantom, cowardly creature, / why are you afraid of me / when you were so bold before my husband? Empty and elusive creature, / if only I had you in my power! Why can't I get you in my grasp? / Yet how could you ever / kill my husband, / unless you did it through deceit? / Truly my husband would never have been / defeated by you, had he been able to see you, / for there was no one in the world his like, / neither God nor man knew his like, / and never was there another his match. / Indeed, if you had been a mortal man, / you would never have dared attack my husband, / for no one could capture him.'" *Le Chevalier au Lion,* 1226–1243.

62. In this context it is interesting to note the study on historical traditions by Sandra Hindman, who, starting from the images of the French collective manuscript with the Arthur epic (Bibliothèque Nationale, MS 1433), does a sociohistorical reconstruction of Yvain's function for the audience of his time; see Sandra Hindman, "King Arthur, His Knights and the French Aristocracy in Picardy," in *Contexts: Style and Values in Medieval Art and Literature,* ed. Daniel Poiron and N. Freeman Regalado, Yale French Studies, Special Issue (New Haven, 1991), pp. 133–144; idem, *Sealed in Parchment: Rereadings of Knighthood in the Illuminated Manuscripts of Chrétien de Troyes* (Chicago, 1994).

63. The possibility of a connection between the Ywain frescoes and sacral mural programs and art in South Tyrol is a topic that heretofore has only been broached by Michael Curschmann, who inquires into the intellectual climate and whatever other considerations might have motivated the Rodeneggs and the artists they commissioned to undertake such a novel and ambitious program of decoration. Curschmann considers it beyond doubt that only a prestigious and well-established workshop, such as might have been available in nearby Brixen, could have undertaken the task. In support of his thesis, Curschmann argues (in ways comparable with Hindman's analysis of Paris, BN MS 1433—see n. 62) for the visualization of a didactic agenda, aimed at the nobility, especially its youth, and based in part on theological traditions, specifically, the early medieval Gregorian dictum that images were the Bible of the illiterate (*pictura liber laicorum*). He demonstrates that the world of knightly *aventiuren* had to be visualized according to certain theological models (and by artists of corresponding background or experience); see Michael Curschmann, "*Der aventiure bilde nemen:* The Intellectual and Social Environment of the Iwein Murals at Rodenegg Castle," in *Chrétien de Troyes and the German Middle Ages: Papers from an International Symposium,* ed. with intro. by Martin H. Jones and Roy Wisbey, Arthurian Studies 26 (Cambridge and London, 1993), pp. 219–227.

64. See Jeffrey F. Hamburger, "Rewriting History: The Visual and the Vernacular in Late Medieval History Bibles," in *Retextualisierung in der mittelalterlichen Literatur,* ed. Ursula Peters and Joachim Bumke, Sonderheft der Zeitschrift für deutsche Philologie (Berlin, 2005), pp. 259–307; Jeffrey F. Hamburger and Anne-Marie Bouché, eds., *The Mind's Eye: Art and Theological Argument in the Middle Ages* (Princeton, 2005); Herbert L. Kessler, *Spiritual Seeing: Picturing God's Invisibility in Medieval Art,* The Middle Ages Series (Philadelphia, 2000); idem, "Real Absence: Early Medieval Art and the Metamorphosis of Vision," in *Morfologie sociali e culturali in Europa fra tarda antichità e alto medioevo, 3–9 Aprile 1997,* Settimane di Studio del Centro Italiano di Studi Sull'Alto Medioevo 45 (Spoleto, 1998), pp. 1157–1211; idem, "'Facies Bibliothecae Revelata': Carolingian Art as Spiritual Seeing," in *Testo e immagine nell'alto medioevo, 15–21 aprile 1993,* Settimane di Studio del Centro Italiano di Studi Sull'Alto Medioevo 41 (Spoleto, 1994), vol. 2, pp. 533–594; idem, *Spiritual Seeing: Picturing God's Invisibility in Medieval Art,* The Middle Ages Series (Philadelphia, 2000). See also Moshe Barasch, "Das Gottesbild: Studien zur Darstellung des Unsichtbaren" (München, 1998), in idem, *Blindness: The History of a Mental Image in Western Thought* (New York and London, 2001); Alois M. Haas, "Bildresistenz des Göttlichen und der menschliche Versuch, Unsichtbares sichtbar zu machen. Feindschaft und Bild in der Geschichte der Mystik," in *Homo Pictor,* ed. Gottfried Böhm, Colloquium Rauricum 7 (München and Leipzig, 2001), pp. 283–301.

65. To the (partially contradictory) dating propositions, see Volker Schupp and Hans Szklenar, *Ywain auf Schloß Rodenegg. Eine Bildergeschichte nach dem "Iwein" Hartmanns von Aue* (Sigmaringen, 1996), pp. 105–112. On the Ywain cycle, refer additionally to Michael Curschmann, *Vom Wandel im bildlichen Umgang mit literarischen Gegenständen. Rodenegg, Wildenstein und das Flaarsche Haus in Stein am Rhein,* Wolfgang Stammler Gastprofessur für Germanische Philologie. Vorträge 6 (Freiburg [Schweiz], 1997); Achim Masser, *Die Iwein-Fresken von Burg Rodenegg in Südtirol und der zeitgenössische Ritterhelm* (Innsbruck, 1993); Norbert H. Ott, "Rodenegg revisited oder Zur Veränderung von Struktur und Gebrauchssituation literarischer Bilderzeugnisse im historischen Prozess," in *Helle döne schöne. Versammelte Arbeiten zur älteren und neueren deutschen Literatur. Festschrift für Wolfgang Walliczek,* ed. Horst Brunner et al., GAG 668 (Göppingen, 1999), pp. 61–86, and on the choice of scenes, esp. pp. 65–68.

66. See Schupp and Szklenar, *Ywain auf Schloß Rodenegg,* pp. 39–40 and n. 125.

67. See Ott, "Rodenegg revisited," pp. 69–71; René Wetzel, "Quis dicet originis annos? Die Runkelsteiner Vintler-Konstruktion einer adligen Identität," in *Schloss Runkelstein. Die Bilderburg,* edited by the city of Bozen with the help of the Southern Tyrol Institute of Culture (Bozen, 2000), pp. 291–310, esp. p. 303; and idem, "L'image du monde dans un monde d'images. Les fresques littéraires et courtoises de Castelroncolo dans leur contexte socioculturel et historique (Haute

Adige, XIV–XVe siècles)," in *L'histoire dans la littérature,* ed. Laurent Adert and Eric Eigenmann (Genf, 2000), pp. 139–150.

68. Ott, "Rodenegg revisited," p. 70: "Die 'ikonische Erzählung' repräsentiert [. . .] eine höchst bewusste, weil produktive Auseinandersetzung mit der literarischen Erzählung."

69. Concerning the painting technique, I refer again to the investigation at Runkelstein, which can, with provisos, also be applied to Rodenegg; see Christine Kenner, "Maltechniken und Arbeitsprozesse bei der Ausführung der Wandmalereien," in *Schloss Runkelstein,* pp. 217–233.

70. Mersch, *Ereignis und Aura,* p. 63: "Materialitäten werden insonderheit auffällig, wo Störungen eintreten oder Geräte versagen. Sie drängen sich auf, wo sie irritieren: in 'Dysfunktionalitäten' wo die Strategien der Mediatisierung scheitern oder Programme abstürzen, wo sich ein Nichtwiederholbares in den Wiederholungen einschreibt oder die Lektüren verwischen": "Material things now become especially noticeable insofar as disturbances occur or devices fail. They obtrude as they irritate: in disfunctional moments in which various media-based strategies fail or programs crash, in which things that can't be repeated inscribe themselves in repetitions or various readings interfere with one another." For the context (of the "duplicity of the medium"), refer to ibid., pp. 54–66.

71. See Gerd Althoff, *Spielregeln der Politik im Mittelalter. Kommunikation in Frieden und Fehde* (Darmstadt, 1997); Thomas W. Gallant, "Honor, Masculinity, and Ritual Knife Fighting in Nineteenth-Century Greece," *American Historical Review* 105 (2000): pp. 358–382. For the duel in court and its genesis out of the church ordeal, refer to Adalbert Erler, "Gottesurteil," in *Handwörterbuch zur deutschen Rechtsgeschichte* (quoted hereafter as HRG), 5 vols., ed. Adalbert Erler and Ekkehard Kaufmann (Berlin, 1971–1998), vol. 1, col. 1769–1773, esp. col. 1770ff.; Karl Demeter, "Duell," in HRG, vol. 1, col. 789–790; D. Brennecke, "Kempfe," in HRG, vol. 2, col. 700–701; idem, "Lohnkämpfer," in HRG, vol. 3, col. 31–32; Dagmar Hüpper-Dröge, "Der gerichtliche Zweikampf im Spiegel der Bezeichnungen für 'Kampf,' 'Kämpfer,' 'Waffen,'" *Frühmittelalterliche Studien* 18 (1984): pp. 607–661, on the *Sachsenspiegel,* esp. pp. 659–661.

72. Eike von Repgow. *Der Sachsenspiegel,* ed. Clausdieter Schott, Manesse Bibliothek der Weltliteratur (Zürich, 1991), municipal law I 63, pp. 84–88; idem, *Sachsenspiegel. Landrecht und Lehnrecht,* ed. Friedrich Ebel, RUB 3355 (Stuttgart, 1999), pp. 66–68.

73. Ulrike Lade-Messerschmied, "Die Gebärdensprache der Wolfenbütteler Bilderhandschrift des Sachsenspiegels," in *Die Wolfenbütteler Bilderhandschrift des Sachsenspiegels,* commentary volume to the facsimile edition, ed. Ruth Schmidt-Wiegand (Berlin, 1993), pp. 185–200, here p. 198.

74. See Hüpper-Dröge, "Der gerichtliche Zweikampf," p. 660.

75. Eike von Repgow, *Der Sachsenspiegel, Ldr.* I 63 §5, ed. Schott, p. 88: "Damit hat er jenen solcher Klage überführt, derentwegen er ihn zum Zweikampf heraus-

gefordert hat. Und so soll denn der Richter den Angeklagten richten, als ob er im Zweikampf überwunden worden wäre."

76. Eike von Repgow: *Der Sachsenspiegel, Ldr.* I 63 §1–4, ed. Schott, pp. 84–88.

77. Eike von Repgow, *Der Sachsenspiegel, Ldr.* I 63 §5, ed. Ebel, p. 68. "If the accused does not present himself after having been invited a third time, the plaintiff shall rise and begin the fight, executing two blows and one stab against the wind."

78. Norbert H. Ott, "Der Körper als konkrete Hülle des Abstrakten. Zum Wandel der Rechtsgebärde im Spätmittelalter," in *Gepeinigt, begehrt, vergessen. Symbolik und Sozialbezug des Körpers im späten Mittelalter und in der frühen Neuzeit,* ed. Klaus Schreiner and Norbert Schnitzler (München, 1992), pp. 223–241, here pp. 226–227: "Der Körper der am Rechtshandeln beteiligten Personen fungiert gewissermaßen als konkrete Hülle des Abstrakten, des Rechts selbst."

79. Wolfenbüttel, Herzog-August-Bibliothek, Cod. Guelf. 3.1. Aug. 2°; facsimile: Eike von Repgow, *Sachsenspiegel,* the Wolfenbüttel pictorial manuscript of the *Sachsenspiegel.* 3 vols., facsimile-volume, ed. Ruth Schmidt-Wiegand (Berlin, 1993).

80. Eike von Repgow, *Der Sachsenspiegel, Ldr.* I 63 §4, ed. Schott, p. 87 (Cod. W, fol. 26[r]); see the introductory remarks to the iconography of gestures by Lade-Messerschmied, "Die Gebärdensprache," pp. 185–188.

81. See Clausdieter Schott, "Zur bildlichen Wiedergabe abstrakter Textstellen im Sachsenspiegel," in *Text-Bild-Interpretation. Untersuchungen zu den Bilderhandschriften des Sachsenspiegels,* ed. Ruth Schmidt-Wiegand, Münstersche Mittelalter-Schriften 55/1 (München, 1986), S. 11–58; and also, in the same volume, Ruth Schmidt-Wiegand, "Text und Bild in den Codices picturati des 'Sachsenspiegels.' Überlegungen zur Funktion der Illustration," pp. 189–203; for the iconography of law and, more concretely, the modes of visualization in lawtexts, see Colette Brunschwig, *Visualisierung von Rechtsnormen. Legal Design,* Zürcher Studien zur Rechtsgeschichte 45 (Zürich, 2000), on the iconography of the *Sachsenspiegel,* see pp. 116–216.

82. Eike von Repgow, *Der Sachsenspiegel, Ldr.* I 63 §4, ed. Schott, p. 87 (Cod. W, fol. 26[r], picture rail 1).

83. Eike von Repgow: *Der Sachsenspiegel, Ldr.* I 63 §4, ed. Schott, p. 87 (Cod. W, fol. 26[r], picture rail 3).

84. Stephen G. Nichols. "The New Medievalism: Tradition and Discontinuity in Medieval Culture," in *The New Medievalism,* ed. Marina S. Brownlee, Kevin Brownlee, and Stephen G. Nichols (Baltimore and London, 1991), pp. 1–26, here p. 23.

PART FOUR
Frames

13 Cardiosensory Impulses in Late Medieval Spirituality

HEATHER WEBB

Medical evidence is not always adequate to dispel certain deeply held convictions.[1] One would imagine that the example of patients who had sustained a brain or spinal cord injury might have offered ample visible proof to permanently refute Aristotle's notion that the heart ruled motion and sensation. But many late medieval philosophers, theologians, and even physicians found ways to insist that the heart ruled the brain, even if they accepted the idea that the brain ruled the nervous system. Generally, we have dealt with the coexistence of apparently conflicting sense perception systems in the thirteenth and fourteenth centuries by suggesting that Aristotle's heart-centered system appealed to philosophers, while physicians subscribed to the Galenic brain-centered system. This would lead us to assume that the Galenic system was understood as the medical explanation of the perception of objects while the Aristotelian system was employed in metaphysical or philosophical contexts.[2]

I intend to show that these common assumptions are misleading. Today, terms such as "spiritual," "physical," "philosophical," "medical," "mind," and "body" define themselves by the distinctions between the realms that they describe. But late medieval usage of the same terms did not correspond to the same distinctions. The term "spiritual" had such an extension that many entities or processes called by that name would today be described as "physical." The complex systems for spiritual sense perception that developed in this period seamlessly integrated older systems that might, from a modern perspective, seem to blatantly contradict each other, or at the very least to belong to entirely distinct and distant spheres of concern. This integration was made possible by a different conception of the physiological, the psychological, and the spiritual, not as three separate realms, but as three continuous aspects of a single life-process.

I will examine some articulations of this integrated life-process in the writings of a Dominican preacher who studied physiology (Giovanni da San Gimignano, c. 1260–1333), a physician who published an eschatological treatise (Arnau de Vilanova, d. 1311), and a poet who claimed an anagogic level of meaning for his verses (Dante Alighieri, 1265–1321), among others. I show that each of these scholars believed the body to be capable of perceiving the world through a *cardiosensory* process. By this I mean a process centered in the heart, understood as both the physical organ *and* as seat of the soul, and carried out by means of the heart-based spirit, understood as both a physiological entity *and* as the immortal soul itself.[3] The cardiosensory was therefore a continuum of organic and spiritual processes, accounting for the full range of human sensory experience, from encounters with the supernatural to everyday interactions. It responded to both philosophical and medical concepts of the human and of corporeal sensation, envisioning an intimate cohabitation of body and soul.

Interest in issues of the nature of the spirit and its relationship to the body arose following the diffusion of twelfth-century Latin translations of Arabic medical texts by Avicenna (980–1037) and Costa ben Luca (864–923), among others.[4] These works held that the spirit was no abstract or intangible concept, but was rather a substantial material entity operating through traceable physiological systems centered in the heart. Presenting a neat synthesis of the frequently conflicting medical knowledge available to them at that point, the works proposed to settle the long-standing debate between Aristotelian and Galenic theories of bodily function.

Aristotle (384–322 BCE) believed that the heart was the center and source of all life-processes, including procreation.[5] His *De generatione animalium* identified *pneuma* (*spiritus* for late medieval scholars) as the substance that rendered sperm fertile. Galen (c. 129–c. 216) disputed many of Aristotle's theories, maintaining that the heart was much less important than previously estimated. *Pneuma,* according to Galen, was formed in the brain, not the heart, and traveled around the body via the arteries. Galen further explained that *pneuma* was engendered in concert with the body, from a combination of exhalations of the blood and inhaled air.

Avicenna and Costa ben Luca integrated Galen's insights regarding the formation and distribution of *pneuma* into a cardiocentric system. Albertus

Magnus (1206–1280) cites Avicenna's positioning between Galen and Aristotle as follows:

> Non oportet verum dixisse Galienum . . . dicta autem magistri primi probabimus supponendo quod anima quidem, secundem se est una virtus, a qua fluunt omnes virtutes membrorum. Cum enim ipsa sit organica, oportebit unum esse membrum in quo sita omnes effluat a se virtutes: et sicut ipsa est principium virtutum, ita necessario erti illud membrum principium organorum. Constat autem animam secundum actum vitae et potestatem esse in corde. Oportet igitur cor esse principium omnium nervorum et venarum per quos anima in membris perficit suas operationes.

> Galen must have been mistaken . . . we will prove the words of the First Master [Aristotle] by setting forth the supposition that the soul is one power in and of itself, from which flows all the powers of the members. Since it is organic, there will necessarily be one member in which it is located and from which it causes all powers to flow. And just as it is the principle of the powers, so will that member necessarily be the point of origin of the organs. Now it is agreed that the soul, with respect to the act and power of life is in the heart. It is therefore necessary that the heart be the point of origin of all the nerves and the veins through which the soul accomplishes its operations in the members.[6]

This move from a Galenic model, in which "powers" were divided between the heart, the liver, and the brain, to an Aristotelian, centralized model provided medieval thinkers with an entirely integrated system through which they could understand virtually every aspect of human life. The rarefied blood-based spirit was continually produced in the heart and pushed through the arteries to all extremities, where it took on different functions according to location. The vital spirit, or windy spirit, regulated the heartbeat and respiration, the natural spirit maintained digestion, and the animal spirit controlled intellectual responses. These spirits also acted as intermediaries with the external world, carrying sensory perceptions into the body and bringing internal substances out into the world, in the forms of breath, semen, and voice.

Western scholars began to explore this new physiology of the spirit as a central issue in both theology and medicine. *De spiritu et anima,* a text written in the 1160s but mistakenly attributed to Augustine and thus widely read, was one of many to utilize Avicenna's synthesis in order to create unitary systems in which the heart and its spirit established a common basis not only for all the structures of life but also for salvation. In short, for the brief duration of this cardiocentric culture, scholars looked to the workings of the heart to understand both body and soul.[7] The implications of these theories for the present study are the following: the heart acted as the organ of continuity between the human body and the cosmos, continually mixing external air and internal blood, receiving perceptions from outside and giving forth that which was created inside. It thus contained the space of fusion between body and soul and, on another level, between the body and everything that lay outside that body.

It is important to note that while Avicenna's rendition of the problem of origins and principles in the human body as stated above alludes to the resolution of a true conflict of opinion ("Galen must have been mistaken"), the two sides of the debate were not as starkly opposed as one might imagine. Galen himself explains that when a man is spurred to love by means of one of the five senses, the heart is strongly shaken and gives birth to two spirits. One goes directly to the member while the other goes first to the brain and, from there, to the testicles.[8] In this particular example, sense perceptions do effectively travel to the heart and spur reactions there. Furthermore, we may already see a possible model by which to mitigate the conflict about the importance of the brain versus the heart: the spirit, born of the heart, moves to the brain before completing its function. In this particular case, that of the love-reaction, the center of circulatory sense perception is the heart. Galen was, after all, deeply invested in philosophy and drew extensively on Aristotle for the concepts upon which to base his physiology. The supposed debate, then, between the Aristotelian philosophers and the Galenic physicians, is already considerably clouded.[9]

In fact, the reception history of ostensibly conflicting Aristotelian and Galenic models for sense perception presents a series of models for integrating the two authorities rather than choosing between them. The first of these models lies in Galen's own works, as we have seen, while the second, and perhaps the most compelling of these, was Avicenna's delicately balanced reconciliation. In Avicenna's works and in the myriad of subsequent syntheses, a generally Aristotelian epistemology was supplemented by physiological details from Galen's writings. Theologians of the thirteenth through the fifteenth centuries had a strong interest in physiology and furthered the integration of the two authorities. Not content to simply cite the information available to them, they added their own interpretations and conclusions to debates on the precise role of the heart, or the workings of the soul and spirit within the body.[10] Giovanni da San Gimignano, a Dominican preacher, demonstrates the tendencies of his time as he blends Galen and Aristotle within one single example, a detailed description of embryology.[11] Arnau de Vilanova, a Galenic physician who also wrote spiritual texts, echoes Aristotle when speaking of the heart: "nam sicut cor est principium motus corporalis sic desiderium est principium motus spiritualis" (the heart is the origin of corporeal motion just as desire is the origin of spiritual motion).[12] A physician following Galen's teachings ought not believe that the heart is the origin of corporeal motion and yet that assertion serves as the "concrete example" portion of Arnau's analogy about desire.

As Nancy Siraisi points out, physiological subject matter is treated in a similar fashion in medical, natural philosophical, and theological works from this period. Authors asked the same questions, used the same scholastic apparatus of arguments, objections, and solutions, and employed many of the same citations of authorities. Of course, medical authors had practical ends to their investigations as physiological theory served to explain illness and prescribe treatment.[13] I would add, however, that theologians, preachers, and others described their aims in similar terms of practicality. Sin was intimately correlated with illness and had sometimes detectable and often dangerous physical effects on the body.[14] The preacher, for instance, had to understand bodily function in order to know how to recognize and heal the suffering spirit, as we shall see in greater detail below.

The relevance of bodily function to salvation depended greatly on the vision of the soul and its relationship to the body. *De spiritu et anima* explained that:

> the soul is an intellectual, rational spirit, always living, always in motion, capable of good or evil will. . . . It is known by various names according to its works. It is called soul when it vivifies; spirit, when it contemplates; a sense, when it senses; consciousness [*animus*], when it knows; when it understands, mind; when it discerns, reason; when it remembers, memory; when it consents, will. These are not, however, differences of substance, but of names, for all these things are a single soul: diverse properties, but one essence.[15]

In short, it is the same entity that senses, gives life, knows, understands, and so on. The spirits that carry out sense perceptions were often, in fact, thought to be an extension of, or part of, the soul. According to widely held opinion, the mist-like vital spirit moved from the heart toward the brain, passing through the *rete mirabile,* where it was purified, rarefied, and renamed the animal spirit. The animal spirit was believed to relay sense perceptions and transmit them, via the nerves, throughout the body. Despite its diverse functions as it circulated throughout various parts of the body, the spirit was thus conceived of as unitary and heart-centered.[16] Giovanni da San Gimignano balanced the roles of brain and heart as follows:

> Nam ad alios tres sensus derivat virtus sensitiva, ex corde mediante cerebro, ita quod a corde primo venit ad cerebrum, & a cerebro postea ad ipsos sensus.
>
> The three other senses derive the sensitive virtue from the heart through the mediation of the brain, as from the heart first it passes to the brain, and from the brain then to those senses.[17]

As the formative matrix of the spirits that carry out sensory perceptions, the heart is the natural locus of origination for the senses. The brain functions entirely in the capacity of mediator, essentially a processing and distribution center.

In the words of William of Auvergne (d. 1249), "the senses are like gates into the body through which ingressions and egressions . . . are made."[18] Every instance of sense perception, then, was a potential opening to spirit possession. As Nancy Caciola's *Discerning Spirits: Divine and Demonic Possession in the Middle Ages* points out, spirit possession was thought to involve a literal entry into the body, usually through the senses. Tracing the pathways of the foreign spirits within the body was one method of discerning the nature of those spirits. Vincent of Beauvais's (c. 1190–1264) *Speculum Naturale* states that God can pour himself into the human soul and unite with it, essentially replacing the vital spirit. A demon or devil cannot, however, enter the heart precisely because the soul is there. Manifestations of the spirit within the heart, therefore, were judged to be of divine origin, while supernatural movement in the area of the bowels clearly indicated a demonic possession.[19]

Fourteenth-century texts such as Henry of Freimar's (1245–1340) *The Four Inspirations* and Venturino of Bergamo's (1304–1346) *Treatise on the Holy Spirit* and *Remedies for Spiritual Temptation* offered advice on opening the heart to God by guarding the senses.[20] Processes were prescribed for closing the senses to demonic forces and making way for the divine. Reading Scripture, for instance, was one way of properly opening the body to God. Arnau de Vilanova explains that understanding of Scripture is a physical process in which stiffness and heaviness are removed from the mind and the coagulated heart, opening them to the sensory penetration of the divine Word.[21]

In the stilnovist lyric, poets celebrated an extreme openness or vulnerability to their beloveds. In Dante's (1265–1321) *Vita Nuova,* we may note the ways in which the aforementioned theories of sense perception were mapped out by a scholar familiar with a range of natural philosophical and spiritual works:[22]

> In quello punto dico veracemente che lo spirito de la vita, lo quale dimora ne la secretissima camera de lo cuore, cominciò a tremare sì fortemente che apparia ne li menimi polsi orribilmente; e tremando disse queste parole: *Ecce deus fortior me, qui veniens dominabitur michi.* In quello punto lo spirito animale, lo quale dimora ne l'alta camera ne la quale tutti li spiriti sensitivi portano le loro percezioni, si cominciò a maravigliare molto, e parlando spezialmente a li spiriti del viso, sì disse queste parole: *Apparuit iam beatitudo vestra.* In quello punto lo spirito naturale, lo quale dimora in quella parte ove si ministra lo nutrimento nostro, cominciò a piangere, e piangendo disse queste parole: *Heu miser, quia frequenter impeditus ero deinceps!*
>
> At that moment I say truly that the spirit of life, which dwells in the most secret chamber of the heart, began to tremble so strongly that it appeared terrifying in its smallest veins; and trembling it said these words: "Behold a god more powerful than I, who comes to rule over me." At that point the animal spirit, which dwells in the upper chamber to which all the spirits of the senses carry their perceptions, began to marvel greatly, and speaking especially to the spirits of sight, it said these words: "Now has appeared your beatitude." At that point the natural spirit, which dwells in that part that ministers to our nourishment, began to weep, and weeping said these words: "Wretched me, for often hereafter shall I be impeded!"[23]

The three loquacious spirits in this passage demonstrate Dante's interest in making use of medical knowledge to describe Beatrice's effects. The first "verbal" respondent to the stimulus of the encounter is, in fact, the heart. The other two spirits that speak, the animal and the natural spirit, only perceive this new and disrupting stimulus by way of transmission through the heart's vital spirit. The heart remains, throughout the *Vita Nuova* and beyond, the first receptor of Beatrice's presence.[24] Even when Dante has not yet seen her, his heart has already perceived her: "mi parve sentire uno mirabile tremore incominciare nel mio pecto dalla sinistra parte e distendersi di subito per tutte le parti del mio corpo. . . . levai li occhi, e . . . vidi la gentilissima Beatrice" (I seemed to feel a wondrous tremor commence in my breast's left side and quickly spread throughout my body. . . . I raised my eyes and . . . saw . . . the most gentle Beatrice),[25] or later: "io mi sentio cominciare un tremuoto nel cuore, così come se io fosse stato presente a questa donna. . . . vidi venire la mirabile Beatrice" (I felt the beginning of a tremor in my heart, as if I were in the presence of this lady. . . . I saw approaching the wondrous Beatrice).[26]

This careful, physiologically informed mapping of the perception of Beatrice may be read as a kind of discernment strategy to demonstrate the worth of the beloved. We may read her access to Dante's heart as a sign of divinity, physically manifested within the poet's body. Dante stresses not only Beatrice's power to inhabit his heart, but his own openness to that spiritual inhabitation. For both poets and theologians, sense perceptions that were routed to the heart indicated experiences of a privileged order, mediations of God's divine power to meld with the vital spirit filling the heart.

I'd like to turn now to late medieval mappings of spiritual experiences as manifested in relationship to the specific sensory portals of the human body. A fifteenth-century exorcism manual scripts the healer's tour through the spirit pathways of the possessed human body. The instructions begin as follows:

> *Ad oculos, dic:* Domine Pater omnipotens eterne Deus, qui cuncta creasti et per unigenitum filium tuum Dominum nostrum Ihesum Christum caecum illuminasti, ut tua manifestaretur Gloria. Nam luto quod fecisti ex sputo tuo linisti oculos suos; lini oculos famule tue N. . . . ut te oculis exterioribus ac mentis posit intueri et ab obsidione dyaboli et cuctis infestationibus suis te solum intelligat . . . et te collaudat.

> To the eyes, say: Lord Father omnipotent eternal God, who created everything and who, through your only begotten son Jesus Christ, made a blind man see in order to manifest your glory. For you daubed his eyes with muck made from your spit. Daub the eyes of your maidservant N. . . . so that she may look at you with her exterior eyes and mind; and so that, once healed from the obsession of the devil and all his infestations, she may understand you . . . and praise you alone.[27]

The woman must be able to look upon God with her "exterior eyes," not some internal or metaphorical eye of the mind. The connection between the external, corporeal eyes and the mind is the true focus of the exorcist's concern. Presumably, the demon is blocking the conduits between eye and mind, preventing perception and therefore understanding. The "obsession [and infestations] of the devil" have physically sealed off the woman's mind. As Arnau de Vilanova stresses, stiffness or blockage of the mind must be removed to permit understanding or the sense perception of divine truth. For the demonic spirit, only the mind is accessible and corruptible, while the heart is utterly beyond its reach.

The exorcism manual is borrowing heavily from accepted medical ideas of vision. While there was an intense debate raging at this time over whether vision worked by extramission, as argued in Plato and Galen, or by intromission, as argued in Aristotle, Avicenna, Averroës, and Alhacen, it was generally accepted that animal spirits carried the power of vision from the brain through the hollow optic nerve to the eye.[28] Blindness and blocked vision could thus be signs of a breakdown in this connection and consequently indicative of sin or possession. Frequently, sins manifested externally by blindness were thought to be of an obsessive nature and to reveal a mind enclosed within itself, not permitting access to the outside world through the eyes.

Giordano da Pisa (d. 1310) employed the following example of sinful, obsessional blindness:

> Uno invaghí d'una saracina, ed era nera come carbone, sozzissima, ed avea la moglie sua ch'era bella, e poteasene passare molto: e lasciava la donna sua, e stava con colei. Vedi, come accieca il peccato non solamente degli occhi della mente, ma degli occhi del corpo!
>
> One man became filled with desire for a Saracen, and she was black as coal and foul. And he had a wife that was beautiful, with whom he could pass the time well. And he left his wife and got together with the other one. See, sin blinds not only the eyes of the mind, but also the eyes of the body![29]

Again, as in the exorcist's handbook, the "eyes of the body" are stressed. Sin has actual physical manifestations, blocking the normal pathways of sense perception. It thus may be recognized by the trained professional. In this case, the abandonment of a beautiful wife for a Saracen reveals corporeal blindness as both a consequence of sin and as the means by which that sin propagates itself.

In his *rime petrose* and later his *Inferno,* Dante employs images of blindness and obsessed, blocked minds to illustrate the deepest forms of sin. The symptoms of the poet of the *petrose* are explained as: "la mente mia, ch'è più dura che petra / in tener forte imagine di petra" (my mind is harder than stone, in tightly holding an image of stone).[30] Here, the normal cycle within the body, in which external perceptions are constantly relayed to the brain, has been halted. The mind fixates on the contemplation of one particular image in an obsessive manner, rejecting any new input. In the ice of Cocytus, Fra Alberigo addresses the pilgrim and his guide with a description of his own similar symptoms:

O anime crudeli
tanto che data v'è l'ultima posta
levatemi dal viso i duri veli,
sì ch'io sfoghi 'l duol che 'l cor m'impregna
un poco, pria che 'l pianto si raggeli.

Oh cruel souls,
so cruel that you have been given the last place,
remove the hard veils from my face,
so that I may relieve the pain that gathers in my heart
a little, before the tears freeze again.[31]

In this realm of damnation, where the heart is no longer the provenance of a blessed soul, even that organ is susceptible to the blockage of sin. The cold, self-obsessed heart is mirrored by the image of the sinner's eyes, covered with a veil of frozen tears. This is no possession that can be exorcised, no sin that can be confessed. The "sweet light" of the outside world will never strike the eyes of the sinners in this realm. They are permanently enclosed within themselves. In the case of the eyes then, sin may be discerned by the disconnection of normal sensory pathways to the brain. The brain of itself is a cold organ, and prone to freezing in isolation. A failure of visual perception thus demonstrates that the brain has become cut off both from external influence and from the interior warmth of the vital spirit and soul in the heart.

The possessed woman, as we are beginning to note, essentially has a general problem of sense perception. The exorcist proceeds to the nose:

> *Ad nares:* Domine sancta Domine sancta Pater omnipotens eterne Deus, qui per quinque sensus exteriors tuam dedisti percipere maiestatem . . . da, quaesumus, propter ipsam benignitatem et misericordiam tuam ut haec famula tua N. odorem suavitatis tue sano percipiat corpore atque mente, et expulsa nequita spirituum malignorum, tibi plena serviat libertate.
>
> Lord, holy Lord, holy Father omnipotent eternal God, who bestowed five exterior senses to perceive your majesty . . . grant, we beg, through your goodness and mercy, that this your maidservant N. might perceive the scent of your sweetness and be healthy in mind and body, and let the wickedness of evil spirits be expelled so that she might serve you in full freedom.[32]

Once again, the exorcist insists that humans must perceive the Lord with our "exterior senses." Here, he seeks to open the possessed woman's nostrils to the scent of divine sweetness, an action that would create health in mind and body, expelling the blockage of evil spirits.

As the demonically possessed suffer from the inability to detect sweet scents, the divinely possessed suffer from their enhanced powers of olfactory sin detection. Raymond of Capua's *Legenda maior,* written between 1385 and 1395, recounts Catherine of Siena's acquisition of the power to discern the spiritual value of those around her. Catherine apparently asked Christ for this gift and was granted it due to her virtue. In the subsequent stories that Raymond relates as proof of her abilities, it becomes clear that a portion of this supernatural power was located in Catherine's nose. One example is that of the prelate's concubine:

> Invenimus semel quamdam mulierem, quae, proh dolor! Cujusdam magni Praelati Ecclesiae erat continua concubina. Haec dum cum ea, praesente me, loqueretur, et apparentiam ostenderet tam in actibus quam in vestibus honestatis; numquam tamen faciem virginis ex opposito prospicere potuit, quia semper avertebat vultum ab ea. . . . Quod cum postmodum ei retulissem secrete respondit mihi: Si vos sensissetis foetorem, quem ego sentiebam dum loqueretur mihi, evomuissetis.

> Once we met a woman who, painful to relate, was a concubine of a high prelate of the Church. She spoke with Catherine in my presence and seemed in her actions as well as in her clothing to be honest. But she could not see the face of the virgin, as Catherine kept it always turned away in the opposite direction. . . . I mentioned it to the virgin, and she responded to me in private: "If you had smelled the stench that I smelled while I spoke with her, you would have vomited."[33]

In addition to the charming details about Catherine's tact, the anecdote reveals numerous points of interest. The stench of sin is detectable only to Catherine, but is by no means a metaphysical intuition. Catherine's body reacts to the smell, causing her to turn her head away while she speaks, presumably in an effort to avoid vomiting. The concubine's scent triggers effects in the stomach, effects that are echoed in a different context in one of the next stories Raymond tells:

> Et primo ab ipsa sacra virgine incipiens, quadam die, dum, detecto per ipsam languentis ulcere, foetor nimius exhalaret, voluntatem ejus in Christo petra fundatam movere non valens carnis ejus stomachum movit: unde coepit stomachus ejus ex foetore illo nimium turbari, et quasi ad vomitum provocari.

> One day, as she exposed the wound of the sick woman, a stench more asphyxiating than usual came forth. The demon, unable to move her will that was founded in the rock of Christ, assaulted her stomach. Because of

> the terrible stench, her stomach began to be agitated and to move toward vomiting.[34]

Here, as Catherine is tending a woman with a rotting wound, a demon attempts to turn her from her righteous task. Raymond notes that the demon could not touch her will, traditionally located in the heart, but he could, by means of this terrible odor, assault her stomach. While this is not the stench of sin, but the fetid exhalations of an innocent woman's wound, the effects on Catherine's body are the same: she experiences nausea. However, in the case of the sick woman, the reaction is demonically provoked and therefore improper. Catherine subsequently attempts to train her senses to accept innocent stench, thrusting her face into the wound until the demon departs.

Again, tracing the sensory perceptions of odors allows for judgments about the quality of the receiving body and the quality of the odor being produced. In the case of the possessed woman, the body is not capable of receiving the presence of God through the sweet odor of the divine because, as we have seen in the description of her blindness, the woman's obsessed mind has isolated itself and cannot receive external olfactory stimuli. In Catherine's case, the receiving body has achieved what I would like to call a hypernatural sensitivity to odor. It is not a supernatural power, as the smell of sin enacts entirely natural, nauseating effects on the body just as the odor of a rotting wound does. The smell exuding from the priest's concubine went directly to Catherine's stomach, the sign of a lower order of spiritual being. While the odor of the innocent woman's wound ought not to have traced such a pathway according to discernment schemas, it disturbed Catherine's stomach because of demonic intervention. This was a sort of demonic bypass of the proper channels of Catherine's olfactory powers of discernment, a bypass to be overcome through training and discipline.

The mouth and the tongue of the possessed woman are, as the other sensory gateways have been, hindered or blocked by the devil: "emunda os et linguam huius famule N." (cleanse the mouth and tongue of this maidservant N.) the exorcist asks "ut libere laudem tuam proferre posit absque Sathane impedimento" (so that she may freely offer you praise without any hindrance from Satan).[35] The mouth was a particularly important entrance into the body, potentially opening the way to two different systems, the spiritual system in the heart and the digestive system in the stomach and intestines.[36] The sensation of taste was a means of judging those substances entering by that gateway.

Mary of Oignies, for instance, "felt all delectation and all savor of sweetness in receiving [the Host] . . . sometimes she happily accepted her Lord . . . as a taste of honey, sometimes a sweet smell, and sometimes in the pure and gorgeously embellished marriage bed of the heart." In fact, "the holy bread strengthened her heart."[37] The sweetness of the Host is a sign of its holiness, an indication that this substance is routed to the heart. It was believed that the Host passed directly into the heart, bypassing the digestive system (and a number of unpleasant questions).

Taste was frequently thought to be closely associated with the heart. Of course, numerous Galenic physicians limited themselves to stating that the tongue was the organ of taste and was endowed with this power by the cerebral nerves running to the tongue.[38] But medieval thinkers with an interest in physiology, like Giovanni da San Gimignano, managed to integrate the heart-centered process described in Aristotle's *De anima* and *De sensu et sensato* with Galenic accounts that centered on the tongue.

It is important to note that Giovanni's long discussion of the physiology of taste is by no means an introductory citation employed to set up a series of moral admonitions. He instead combines Aristotle's theory with Constantinus Africanus's (c. 1010–1087) Galenic theory by means of careful reasoning, adding his own interpretation of the material. Joseph Ziegler's recent study of Arnau de Vilanova and Giovanni da San Gimignano divides up Giovanni's *Summa de exemplis et rerum similitudinibus* into a chart of "medical analogies." Ziegler lines up two separate categories: signifier, for the medical content, and signified, for the religious content.[39] While Ziegler's study is a welcome foray into this important but neglected work, I believe he proposes a rather rigid partition of Giovanni's text. The *Summa de exemplis* does not delve so deeply into medical theory simply to set up an analogy that will deliver the same biblical messages in an unaltered form. Upon close examination, the text does not map smoothly onto the categories of signifier and signified. Physiology and morality, proper conduct and perfect physical health merge entirely. Giovanni's audience is meant to understand his or her own complete being more perfectly, a being that is revealed to be a seamless union of body and spirit.

Let us examine Giovanni's passage on taste:

> Organum enim & instrumentum gustus, (ut Philosophus dicit) est aliquot intrinsecum circa cor, & similiter, organum tactus. Nam ad alios tres sensus derivat virtus sensitiva, ex corde mediante cerebro, ita quod a corde primo venit ad cerebrum, & a cerebro postea ad ipsos sensus. Tactus autem, &

gustus referunt ad ipsum cor per medium coniunctum, quod est caro. Sed Constantinus dicit, quod proximum, & manifestum instrumentum gustus provut est diferentuus saporum, est lingua, quae spiritum animalem ad perfectionem virtutis gustabilis defert. Fit enim gustus, sicut ipse dicit, hoc modo: quia duo nervi linguae medio infigunt, quia in multos ramos in extremis lateribus linguae disperguntur, & per eos (ut dictum est) spiritus animalis ad linguam defertur. Cum ergo res gustando subintrat lingua, spiritus animalis, quod ibi est immutatur secundum proprietates eius, quas postea iudicio animae repraesentat. Sicut ergo circa cor est primum gustus instrumentum, ita in corde dicitur esse primum sapientiae habitaculum, secundum illud Prove. In corde requiescit sapientia prudentis: sed proprium instrumentum sapientiae quo aliis manifestatur, est lingua, Psal. Os iusti meditabitur sapientiam & lingua eius & c. sed duo nervi infixi, sunt due cautelae, quae debent esse in lingua sapientis: una ad loquendum & alia ad tacendum.

The organ and instrument of taste (as the Philosopher says) is internal, in the area of the heart, and the same is true of the organ of touch. Indeed the three other senses derive the sensitive virtue from the heart through the mediation of the brain, as from the heart first, it passes to the brain and from the brain then to those senses. Touch and taste bring their sensations to the heart by means of the connective medium, the flesh. And yet Constantine says that the closest and most evident instrument of taste, as far as the difference of flavors is concerned, is the tongue, which leads the animal spirit to the fullness of taste virtues. Taste, as he says, happens in this way: two nerves are fixed in the middle of the tongue and are dispersed by many branches to the extreme edges of the tongue, and through them (as it is said), the animal spirit is brought to the tongue. Thus when something tasted penetrates the tongue, the animal spirit is there transformed according to the properties of that thing, which it then re-presents to the judgment of the soul. Thus as the heart is the first instrument of taste, so the heart is said to be the first lodging of *sapientia,* according to the Proverbs. In the heart rests the *sapientia* of the prudent man: and yet the instrument of proper wisdom by which it is manifested to others is the tongue. The mouth of the just man will consider *sapientia* and the tongue and the two nerves fixed in it are two cautions that must be in the tongue of the wise man, one to speak and the other to be silent.[40]

In short, Giovanni sets up a complex spiritual and physiological system for taste and *sapientia,* which may be understood as wisdom, discernment, discretion, or good taste. Taste and *sapientia,* as terms and as they are brought together in Giovanni's example, are closely interrelated. In his own vernacular as in Latin, the words for taste and knowledge were one and the same.

The process of taste sensation is described as circulation, moving from the heart to the brain to the tongue and then back to the heart. This process is one of discernment. The individual must taste or judge that which enters his body and manifest that judgment or *sapientia* by means of that same access point to the body, the mouth. Speech or praise must then be the result of an inner circulation and heart-centered discernment within the body. The possibilities of giving forth speech or withholding it and keeping silence are linked to the organ of discernment by the two nerves within the tongue that connect it to the center of wisdom and taste within the body. The tongue will then taste of, or understand the world, when it is properly connected to the heart. The exorcist's command: "cleanse the mouth and tongue so that she may freely offer you praise without any hindrance" is then a desire that this portal to the body be reopened to the circulation that would allow the possessed woman to judge the world properly, bringing forth praise for the divine to which she is newly available.

There was no particular gateway to the body that the exorcist might address as far as touch was concerned. The text examined above seems to indicate that the sensory process for touch was considered to work much as the process for taste did. Giordano da Pisa explains how touch was associated with the other senses, and thought of as the basis, in some way, of all the natural senses:

> Questo senno del toccamento dicono i savi ch'è il primo senno del corpo, e nel quale si fondano tutti gli altri senni naturali; onde il primo senno che l'uomo hae della cosa è il toccamento, e ogni animale ha questo senno. Che dovete sapere che ogni animale nonn-ha tutti i senni: la talpa, ben sapete, non ha il vedere.
>
> This sense of touch, according to the wise ones, is the first sense of the body, and the one in which all of the other natural senses are melded. Thus the first sense that man has of a thing is touch, and every animal has this sense. And you must know that not every animal has every sense. The mole, as you know, does not have the sense of sight.[41]

So by this account, every sense and thus every process of discernment might be considered to require a kind of touching. But how exactly was the process for the sense of touch described? Giovanni explains as follows:

> Nam organum tactus (sicut dicit Philosophus) non est caro, quia in nullo sensu potest fieri sensatio si tangatur organum, ut si qui aliquod corpus ponat album in superficie oculi non videtur: sed tactus sentit sensibilia pos-

ita supra carnem & ideo caro non est organum tactus: & idcirco (sicut Arist. dicit) organum sensus tactus, est aliquod intrinsecum circa cor: organum enim tactus, & si non possit esse a qualitatibus tangibilibus totaliter denudatum, propterea, quod a huiusmodi qualitates sunt elementorum ex quibus ipsum organum componitur: ut oportet ipsum esse medium temperatum, ut sit in potentia ad obiecta tangibilia, sicut medium ab anima. Unde quanto animal habet complexionem magis reductam ad medium, tanto est melioris tactus oportet ergo, quod organum tactus sit multum terrestre, quia terra minus inter elementa habet de virtute activa: & oportet, quod si positum in loco calidissimo circa cor ex cuius caliditate terrae frigiditas ad temperiem reducat. Sicut ergo organum & principium tactus, non est caro, sed aliquid circa cor, cuius signum est, quia si laesio accidat in locis circa cor est, maxime dolorosa. Sic et amor charitatis non est amor carnalis, sed spiritualis in corde radicatus, secundum illud, Diliges dominum Deum tuum ex toto corde tuo. Unde circa cor videtur esse proprium organum charitatis: propter quod dicit. Apostolus quod charitas Dei diffusa est in cordibus nostris, per Spiritum sanctum qui datus est nobis. Augustinus. Non autem carnalis, sed spiritualis inter vos debet esse dilectio: ergo organum spiritualis amoris non caro est, sed cor.

The organ of touch, as the Philosopher tells us, is not the flesh, as there is no sensation when an organ is touched, and if a white object is placed on the surface of the eye, it cannot be seen. But when something is placed on the flesh it is perceived and therefore the flesh is not the organ of touch. And thus, as Aristotle says, the organ of the sense of touch is something internal in the area of the heart. Indeed the organ of touch, even though it cannot be completely stripped of its tangible qualities for the reason that this organ is made up of elements that contain these qualities: it is necessary that it must be a balanced medium so that it may be receptive to tangible objects, just as befits a medium functioning for the soul. . . . The organ of touch must therefore be very earthly because among the elements the earth has the least active virtue, and it is necessary that if something is placed in the very hot area around the heart, the coldness of the earth is brought to tepidity owing to the heat of that place. Thus the organ and principle of touch is not the flesh but is something in the area of the heart. The proof of this is that when a wound occurs in the area of the heart, it is more painful. In the same way love that is *caritas* is not carnal love, but a spiritual love rooted in the heart, according to that verse: "love your lord God with all of your heart." Thus it seems that the very organ of *caritas* is in the area of the heart. As the Apostle says, the *caritas* of God is diffused in our hearts by the Holy Spirit, who was given to us. Augustine says that the love between you must not be carnal but must be spiritual; thus the organ of spiritual love is not the flesh, but the heart.[42]

According to Giovanni's rendition, the sensation of touch must be routed to the heart for two reasons; first, only in this way can it be comparable to the other senses (and this is Aristotle's argument), and second, if the sense of touch is not routed to the heart and not processed properly, it is a moral malfunction, a carnal love or an erotic sensation. Giovanni's reasoning is based in physiological and philosophical knowledge, following rational arguments and referring, at the same time, to Scripture as another source of proof that may be added to the mix. Again, the physiological and the spiritual blend in the search for the "organ of spiritual love."

The ears are the final sensory portal the exorcist must address:

> Domine sancte Pater omnipotens eterne Deus. Quia percipiendum verbum filii tui Domini nostri Ihesu Christi, aures hominibus dedisti. . . . Da, quaesumus, propter misericordiam maiestatis tue, ut huius famule tue N. sine impedimento Sathane aures sint aperte, et exclusa ab ipsa malignitate demonum, liberata percipiat verba tua in laudem et honorem.
>
> Lord Father omnipotent eternal God. You gave ears to men for receiving the Word of your Son, Our Lord Jesus Christ. . . . Grant, we beg, that the ears of this, your maidservant N., might be open without any blockage from Satan and that she may be freed, with the evil of demons cast out from her, and might receive your words with honor and praise you.[43]

As we have come to expect, the ears are blocked openings to the body. Once opened, the possessed woman may be freed to receive the words of God with honor, and to understand them as good.

The above texts reveal that the sensory pathways within the body are variable. They may be blocked off entirely or they may lead to the brain, to the stomach, or to the heart. "Spiritual" texts (and by that I mean any of those texts that take *spiritus* for their subject matter) that route sense perceptions to the heart are not, then, committing themselves to an anachronistic Aristotelian view of the world. The authors of these texts are not thinking metaphysically or ignoring Galenic medical physicality. The description of sensory pathways leading to the heart can indicate a privileged situation: a hypernatural sensitivity or openness on the part of the perceiving body and a divine aspect to the perceived object or force. Divine aspects of the perceived object do not prevent it from being understood as acting physiologically by alternate, but no less "real," systems within the body.

In short, we are not dealing here with a simple conflict between two systems for describing sense perception, the Galenic and the Aristotelian. Nor can we designate specific roles (medical versus philosophical or spiritual) to each of those systems. We find, rather, that these systems can coexist and converge, as they are of an equivalent ontological status. Late medieval notions of the integration of body and spirit and the desire to centralize and synchronize physiological and spiritual function created the concept of a totalizing cardiosensory circulation.

Each sense perception offered the possibility of spiritual discernment to the perceiving body or to the astute observer. Privileged experiences set into motion one system of sense perception, ordinary experiences another, and suspect experiences yet another. In those cases where the individual was somehow unhealthy, by reason of sin or possession, an observer would be able to discern the nature of the problem by means of the unhealthy individual's sensory interaction, or lack of sensory interaction, with the outside world. Usually, the healthy and perceptive individual could monitor his interactions with the outside world and discern the quality of those objects and forces he or she came into contact with by means of the senses. In a state of heightened sensory function, a spiritual circulation brought the world into the mysterious cavity of the heart, discerned its divine qualities, and brought forth divinely sanctioned speech.

The impulse to account for spiritual and physical sensory phenomena within a unified cardiosensory system seems to be quite specifically located in the thirteenth and fourteenth centuries. Beginning with the profusion of texts responding to Avicenna and Costa ben Luca's Aristotelian unifications of body and spirit, these impulses thrived, despite significant controversy, until they were eventually largely suppressed by the beginning of the fifteenth century. During the Great Schism, theologians claimed that the Church had been led into crisis under the leadership of falsely inspired women such as Catherine of Siena and Brigid of Sweden. These theologians described new models of sanctity to counteract the influence of the two charismatic women, stressing a metaphysical relationship with the divine in order to oppose such examples of sensory, somatic union with Christ. Bodily manifestations of spirit possession were, as historians have shown, increasingly interpreted as demonic, rather than divine, possessions.[44] As a consequence of this censure, human experiences were progressively divided into two categories: a metaphysical extrasensory process of religious experience and a physical, sensorial process of everyday (or potentially demonic) perceptions of physical matter.

The brain was understood to enact the operations of physiological sensation, a process from which the soul was utterly detached. As a consequence of this drive to impose boundaries on the bodily, the concept of an all-encompassing cardiosensory system was gradually diminished to the status of a spiritual metaphor.

Notes

1. I am indebted to Philippe Buc, Hans Ulrich Gumbrecht, Robert Harrison, and Miguel Tamen for their comments on this essay. I am also very grateful to the organizers and participants at the Medieval Senses Colloquium for their extremely generous and valuable feedback.

2. See Nancy Siraisi, *Medieval and Early Renaissance Medicine* (Chicago: University of Chicago Press, 1990), 81, for a summary of this dispute between "the philosophers and the physicians." Siraisi also points out that there is, however, no "radical or unambiguous separation" between the two approaches to physiology.

3. While many thinkers conflated notions of spirit and soul, some, like Albert the Great and Thomas Aquinas, took pains to make distinctions between spirit and soul, describing the spirit as an intermediary between body and soul. On the multiple meanings of *spirites,* see James J. Bono, "Medical Spirits and the Medieval Language of Life," *Traditio* 40 (1984): 91–130.

4. Nancy Caciola's *Discerning Spirits: Divine and Demonic Possession in the Middle Ages* (Ithaca: Cornell University Press, 2003) provides a fascinating analysis of late medieval theological uses of the theories of spirit physiology. For an extensive bibliography of theological and medical approaches to the physiology of the spirit, see Caciola chapter 3, n. 20, 140 and chapter 4, n. 5, 179–180.

5. The 2003 issue of *Micrologus* is dedicated to the heart and contains numerous essays on different aspects of the heart's metaphorical and organic importance: *Micrologus: Rivista della Società Internazionale per lo Studio del Medioevo Latino,* ed. Agostino Paravicini Bagliani, Nature, Sciences and Medieval Societies (Belgium: Sismel, 2003).

6. Albertus Magnus, *De animalibus,* ed. Hermann Stadler (Munich: Aschendoffsche Verlagsbuchhandlung, 1916) 3.1.5, par. 41, 294. Trans. Kenneth F. Kitchell, Jr., & Irven Michael Resnick (Baltimore: Johns Hopkins University Press, 1999), 363.

7. Giorgio Agamben speaks of a "pneumatic culture" in *Stanze* (Turin: Einaudi, 1977), 118.

8. *Galeno ascriptus liber de compagine membrorum* in *Operum Hippocratis Coi et Galeni pergameni medicorum omnium principium* (Lutetiae, 1679), c. 11. See Agamben, *Stanze,* 129.

9. Siraisi, *Medieval and Early Renaissance Medicine,* 81.

10. Ibid., 79.

11. See Joseph Ziegler, *Medicine and Religion c. 1300: The Case of Arnau de Vilanova* (Oxford: Oxford University Press, 1998), 66.

12. In W. Burger, "Beiträge zur Geschichte der Katechese im Mittelalter," *Römische Quartalschrift* (Geschichte) 21/4 (1907): 182. Trans. Ziegler, *Medicine and Religion,* 72.

13. Siraisi, *Medieval and Early Renaissance Medicine,* 79.

14. At least since Gregory the Great's *Book of Pastoral Rule* c. 590. See Frederic Austin Ogg, ed., *A Source Book of Mediaeval History: Documents Illustrative of European Life and Institutions from the German Invasions to the Renaissance* (New York: Cooper Square Publishers, 1972), 91–96.

15. Alcher of Clairvaux, *De spiritu et anima* in *Patrologia latina,* ed. J. P. Migne (1st ed., 1844–1855), vol. 40, 784. Spirit and soul were not always conflated in this manner. However, even for those who distinguished between the two, the heart-based spirit was nonetheless understood as a material extension of the soul into the body. For a more complete view of this relationship between spirit and soul, see Nancy Caciola, *Discerning Spirits,* 180–183. Trans. ibid., 181–182.

16. Agamben, *Stanze,* 114.

17. Joannes de Sancto Geminiano (Giovanni da San Gimignano), *Summa de exemplis et rerum similitudinibus locupletissima* (Venice: Apud Dominicum Farreum, 1548), 194. All translations of Giovanni da San Gimignano are my own.

18. William of Auvergne, *De universo,* in *Guillelmi Alverni Opera Omnia,* 2 vols. (Paris, 1674; reprint, Frankfurt-am-Main, 1963), vol. 1, 1042. Trans. Caciola, *Discerning Spirits,* 189.

19. See Caciola, *Discerning Spirits,* for a close analysis of these issues, especially chapter 3. For Vincent of Beauvais in Caciola's argument, see particularly 196.

20. Ibid., 216–218.

21. Ziegler, *Medicine and Religion,* 71.

22. Bruno Nardi has established the significance of Albert the Great, among others, for Dante in *Saggi di filosofia dantesca,* 2nd ed. (Florence: La Nuova Italia, 1967).

23. *Vita Nova,* ed. Guglielmo Gorni (Turin: Einaudi, 1996), 1.6. Trans. Dino S. Cervigni and Edward Vasta (Notre Dame: University of Notre Dame Press, 1995), 47–48.

24. Robert Harrison's *Body of Beatrice* makes a crucial distinction between Beatrice's presence and her appearance (Baltimore: Johns Hopkins University Press, 1988), 48.

25. *Vita Nova,* 7.4.

26. *Vita Nova,* 15.1–3.

27. Bäyerische Staatsbibliotek, Munich, ms. Clm. 23325, 24r–25v. Trans. Caciola, *Discerning Spirits,* 259–261.

28. Siraisi, *Medieval and Early Renaissance Medicine,* 108.

29. Giordano da Pisa, *Esempi,* in *Racconti Esemplari di Predicatori del Due e*

Trecento, ed. Giorgio Varanini and Guido Baldassarri (Rome: Salerno Editrice, 1993), 343. The translation is my own.

30. *Rime,* ed. Domenico De Robertis (Florence: Le Lettere, 2002), vol. 9, 12–13. The translation is my own.

31. *La "Commedia" secondo l'antica vulgata,* ed. Giorgio Petrocchi, 7 vols. (Florence: Casa Editrice Le Lettere, 1994), *Inf.* 33:110–114. The translation is my own.

32. Bäyerische Staatsbibliotek, Munich, ms. Clm. 23325, 24r–25v. Cit. and trans. Caciola, *Discerning Spirits,* 259–261.

33. Raymond of Capua, *Legenda maior,* in J. Bollandus and G. Henschenius, *Acta sanctorum . . . editio novissima,* ed. J. Carnandet et al. (Paris, 1863–), April, vol. 3, 900, par. 153. The translation is my own.

34. Ibid., 901, par. 155.

35. Bäyerische Staatsbibliotek, Munich, ms. Clm. 23325, 24r–25v. Cit. and trans. Caciola, *Discerning Spirits,* 259–261.

36. Caciola, *Discerning Spirits,* 191.

37. James of Vitry, *Life of Mary of Oignies,* in *Acta sanctorum,* June, vol. 5, 568. See Caroline Walker Bynum, *Holy Feast and Holy Fast* (Berkeley: University of California Press, 1987), 59.

38. *La medicina medioevale,* ed. Giuseppe Penso (Parma: Edizioni Essebiemme, 2002), 175.

39. Ziegler, *Medicine and Religion,* 277ff. Very little has been written about Giovanni, despite the immense popularity of his *Summa de exemplis,* a popularity that lasted into the sixteenth century. There is no modern edition of the *Summa de exemplis.* For an additional call to further study of Giovanni's works, see Massimo Oldoni, "Giovanni da San Gimignano," in *L'enciclopedismo medievale* (Ravenna: Longo Editore, 1994), 213–228.

40. Giovanni da San Gimignano, *Summa de exemplis,* 194. Book 6, c. LXV.

41. Giordano da Pisa, *Esempi,* 388. The translation is my own.

42. Giovanni da San Gimignano, *Summa de exemplis,* 167. Book 6, c. XIII.

43. Bäyerische Staatsbibliotek, Munich, ms. Clm. 23325, 24r–25v. Cit. and trans. Caciola, *Discerning Spirits,* 259–261.

44. See Nancy Caciola and Dyan Elliott, *Proving Women* (Princeton: Princeton University Press, 2004).

14 "The Pupil of Your Eye"

Vision, Language, and Poetry in Thirteenth-Century Paris

Stephen G. Nichols

In a previous paper, "Rethinking Texts through Contexts: The Case of *Le Roman de la Rose,*" I urged that material philology be construed as the dialectical exchange between history and literature by means of cross-disciplinary study of manuscript versions of medieval vernacular literature in historical context. I suggested that with manuscript versions of a work like the *Roman de la Rose,* we could pursue this goal by focusing on the phenomenology of the manuscripts, on the one hand, and on the historical specificity of the linguistic context of the thirteenth century, on the other. The *Rose* offers an excellent subject for studying vernacular attitudes toward language, because of its linguistic self-consciousness, particularly in the second part, although Guillaume de Lorris has his share of what Wittgenstein calls "language games." Indeed, it seems to me that one of the more fascinating aspects of the *Rose*'s historical alterity may well be what it has to tell us about a very different "linguistic turn" from that of our own time taken by speculative grammarians of the period.

These thinkers believed in a close relationship between language and the world that it postulates. Rather than equating itself to reality, the linguistic turn of the thirteenth century conceived language dialectically, as a means of perceiving and describing a reality lying beyond and, often, in conflict with social conventions out of tune with its self-consciously scientific worldview. After exploring some key themes of their philosophy of language, I ventured to suggest some practices by which the *Rose* might be seen to illustrate, explore, and extend this linguistic turn in imaginative ways. This was plausible, it seemed to me, because the *Rose* repeatedly calls itself a treatise or *art,* in the manner of the grammarians, a designation obsessively echoed by manuscript rubrics: "Cy commence li Romans de la Rose / ou tout l'art d'amour est enclose."

If the *Rose* styles itself a treatise, it also fractures its characters and their psyches into ever more discrete units and subunits, the better to analyze how the emotions and vicissitudes of love shape the lovers' affect and intellect. This is not dissimilar to the method of speculative philosophers who focused on the logic of meaning—the ways and reasons by which language signifies—and did so by analyzing into ever more discrete units and subunits syntax and parts of speech. Since Jean de Meun, at least, was active in Parisian intellectual circles frequented by many speculative logicians or *modistes,* we cannot doubt his familiarity—and, as the *Rose* bears witness, his sympathy—with this innovative movement. The *Rose*'s penchant for language games, for highlighting the ambiguities and ambivalence of linguistic signification situates it squarely within the linguistic turn of the thirteenth century.

This essay focuses on another aspect of the work: its preoccupation with and—in its manuscripts—proliferation of images. The *Rose*'s preoccupation with seeing—in the Greek sense of *theôria*—propels the work toward specularity, toward a compulsive recourse to mirroring as a way of multiplying perspectives, particularly of splitting into ever greater numbers the complex of elements that define humans and their interactions, above all the emotional entanglements precipitated by love (or hate or fear). The multiplicity of reflections on and of human interactions—above all the insistence on the indeterminacy of what we see—render the *Rose* at once a highly visual work, but also a profoundly confusing one, since the reader can discern no especially privileged perspective or viewpoint among the plethora of perspectives introduced.

This trend marks the texts and manuscripts of the *Rose* in a manner that sets it apart from vernacular literature of the period in its obsessive iteration of the perils and fascination of optical perception. If it differs from most vernacular literature in its fascination with optics, however, the *Rose* finds itself very much in the mainstream of the thought and practice of thirteenth-century philosophy and science. For this was the era when Arabic and Greek treatises on optics were translated and commented on with fervor. Among the most important were: Alkindi's *De aspectibus* (*On Vision*), Ibn Mu'adh's *De crepusculis* (*On Twilight*), Euclid's *De speculis* (*On Mirrors*), *De visu* (*On Vision*), Witelo's *Perspectiva,* and Ibn al-Haytham or Alhacen's *De aspectibus* (*On Vision*) and *De speculis comburentibus* (*On Burning Mirrors*).

Alhacen had discredited ancient theories of vision by demonstrating the intromission theory of vision, according to which we perceive thanks to the eye's ability to process light rays that reach it via reflection from objects within our field of vision. A Syrian mathematician, Alhacen (Ibn al-Haytham) used mathematics to arrive at his hypothesis, which he then demonstrated by experiments with light rays which he explained and illustrated by scientific diagrams.

The physical analysis of Arabic philosophers like Alkindi and Alhacen made use of mathematics, particularly geometry, to demonstrate the visual cones or "pyramids" and the various physical properties of light rays, particularly their behavior when they encounter various objects that bend, distort, or reflect them. If the Arabic philosophers bequeathed to Latin Europe an abiding sense of the role of mathematics in understanding visual perception, and an appreciation for the necessity of practical experimentation to verify hypotheses along with an appreciation of the necessity of diagrams for illustrating abstract principles, "this complex heritage embodied strong, opposing tendencies."[1] While agreeing, more or less, on the topics to be included within the new discipline, the newly translated treatises offered conflicting notions of the method or methods by which it was to be pursued.

The first Western scholar to struggle seriously with the methodological issues thus raised was Robert Grosseteste (c. 1168–1253). Grosseteste accepted the lesson of his Arabic sources that optical questions responded most satisfactorily to a mathematical approach.[2] On the other hand, if he believed in the physical nature of light and thus its availability for analysis, he did not yet accept, as Bacon shortly would, "that light's physical nature would yield to geometrical analysis."[3] That the matter was still open to question by astute thinkers may be seen in the optical studies of Albertus Magnus (c. 1200–1280). Albertus worked with many of the same Greek and Arabic sources available to Grosseteste (e.g., Plato, Euclid, Alkindi, and Alhacen) without arriving at the same conviction, since he "refused to convert to the mathematical religion" then fueling the advances in optics.[4]

Although Grosseteste's and Albertus's ecclesiastical standing as theologians and high churchmen made them key figures for placing optical science in the mainstream of the new speculative philosophy without running afoul of the Church, their work does not attain the sustained power of originality and synthesis of their younger contemporary, Roger Bacon (c.1215–c.1292), especially in his *Perspectiva,* written in all probability in 1263.[5] By close theoretical analysis and adroit synthesis of his sources, Bacon transformed the way people thought about optical theory.[6] He did so by his painstaking demonstration of the geometrical basis of perspective, still a basic tenet of optics today.

Bacon uses geometry to elucidate the theory of direct vision, tracing the path of radiation through the humors of the eye; he develops a theory of binocular vision along geometrical lines, and rules of perspective; and he presents an exhaustive geometrical analysis of the propagation of light, including the phenomena of reflection and refraction.[7]

Let us be clear about his achievement. Bacon did not propound a truly modern science of optics. For one thing, he did not articulate and practice a truly experimental method.[8] On the other hand, he was the first to articulate a true geometrically based theory of perspective and was also the first Western philosopher to adopt the Arabic philosophers' practice of illustrating abstruse mathematical or geometric arguments with scientific diagrams.[9] No, his principal contribution, in the eyes of Lindberg, "was to take the disparate factual and theoretical content found in the [Greek and Arabic sources he inherited, particularly Alhacen] and mould it into a workable and convincing synthesis; this was a significant achievement, but a theoretical rather than an experimental one."[10]

It is less Bacon's place in the history of science that interests us here, however, than his very considerable role in shaping thirteenth-century attitudes toward vision and refraction. In this, he, through his theories of the consequences of perspective, played an incomparable role. From the outset, Bacon held that vision was preeminent among all the cognitive senses because it is the most perceptive of them all, and the one that leads most inexorably to wisdom. Rather than simply asserting this postulate, however, Bacon set forth his theory of geometric perspectivism, which allowed him painstakingly to analyze visual perception not as a unitary whole, but as a complex interaction of countless elements, both within the viewer and in the material conditions attendant on the act of viewing.

Ambivalence, ambiguity, and indeterminacy are as crucial to his account of perception as are his quite substantial explanations of what we do see. For he holds that any act of perception is, at best, only a partial recognition of the myriad stimuli that continually present themselves to the viewer's gaze. Bacon's efforts to illustrate what we do not see and why, or, the parallel case, of why we perceive an object incorrectly, turn out just as portentous for his contemporary readers as his lucid explanations of how we do see. For Bacon demonstrated that visual perception, like the predication of meaning in language, does not simply happen. It requires the collaboration or interaction of a number of variables, not the least fallible of which is the human perceiver on whose physical and psychic state so much depends.

Only by painstaking analysis of the mechanics of vision, Bacon holds, can one understand the way the mind comes to make judgments based on sensory data. Understanding vision, in short, yields insights into the arcane folds of our inner life. Ultimately, on Bacon's view, the mechanics of vision permits us to understand how we apprehend mentally or spiritually. It is but a step to postulate physical vision as akin to mental or spiritual vision—in essence of equating the eye and the soul—and Bacon does not shrink from taking that step.

First, however, he examines exhaustively the physiology of the eye and the mechanics of physical vision, particularly direct perception, refracted perception, and reflections. If the concept he engages is a sophisticated performative *mimesis*—showing how images are formed and transmitted—the principal tools are: *species,* variously represented as "likeness," "image," or as what we might conceive of as rays that convey bits and pieces of "likeness" from the surface of the object to the eye; and *speculum,* or "mirror," the reflecting surface by which *species* may also be conveyed from an object to the eye.

The eye, on Bacon's perspectivist view, is the apex of a visual triangle or cone whose base is the object whence emanate hundreds of species or rays, each conveying a piece of "likeness" from the object—color, shape, texture, size, and so on—to the eye, which aggregates and transmits to the mind or soul the plethora of species coming from the surface of the object. When processed they produce a reproduction or likeness of that object, its mental percept within the perceiver. Thanks to the multitude of species, each conveying the likeness of the part of the object whence it emanates, the percept resembles the object in all points except for size.

Bacon explains the disparity in the dimensions between the object and its visual image in terms of the physiology of the eye and perspectivist geometry. He conflates physiology and geometry ingeniously in answering the question "how can a large body be perceived—and thus to some extent contained—in a very small eye?" The response involves both the shape of their eyes—they must be round—and an explanation of perspectivist optics, which he illustrates diagrammatically (fig. 14.1).

> The first reason [that the eyes must be round] is to make possible its swift movement, so that sight (when we wish) can run from one visible object to another, in order that each object might be grasped with full certitude by such a swift motion; but no figure is better suited to motion than the sphere,

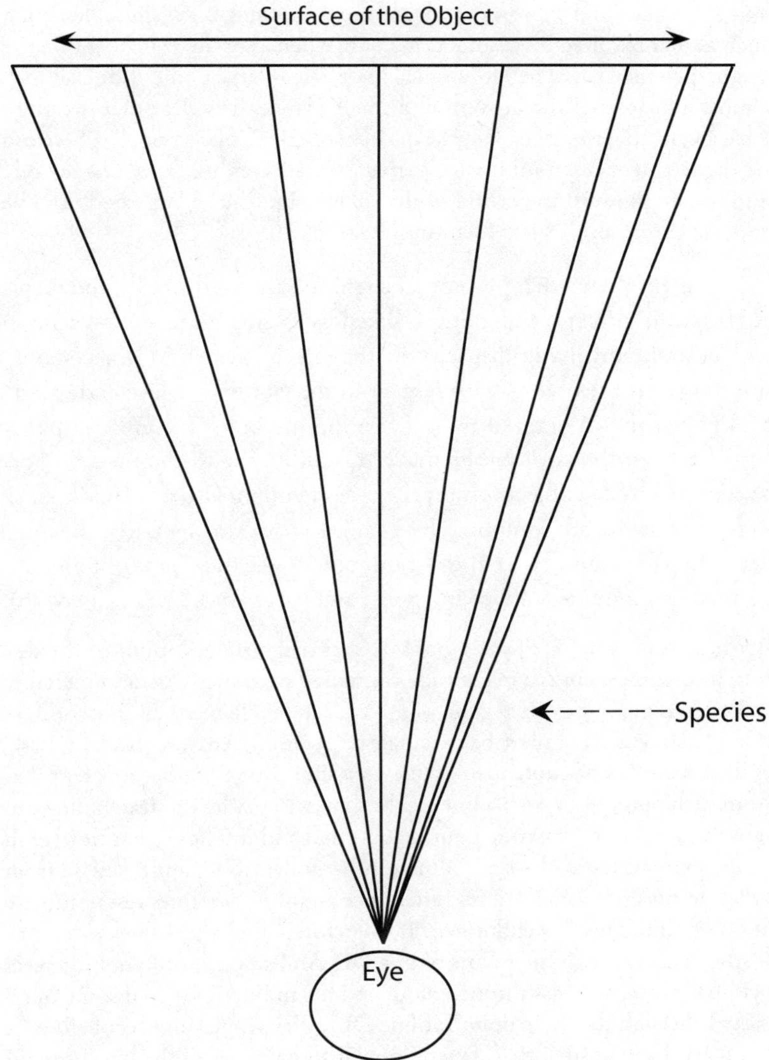

Figure 14.1. How a large body can be seen by a small eye. David C. Lindberg, *Roger Bacon and the Origins of "Perspectiva" in the Middle Ages* (Oxford: Clarendon Press, 1996), p. 59.

> and so the eye and its parts must be round. Second, . . . [s]ensible action such as that required by vision occurs only when a species is incident on the eye perpendicularly. Therefore, since the eye sees large bodies (for example, almost a quarter of the heaven) at a single glance, it is clear that it cannot have a flat surface nor be of any shape but spherical, since a small sphere can be the recipient of an infinity of perpendiculars coming from a large body and tending toward the centre of the sphere; and thus a large body can be seen by a small eye, as is evident in the figure.[11]

Pursuing his theme that perceptual cognition means disparity and displacement between percept and object—likeness is not sameness—Bacon next poses questions involving disparity in the size of perceived objects and the positioning of those objects with respect to the viewer. The eye and mind can as readily perceive "a grain of millet" as a mountain for the great disparity in volume between the two objects makes no difference to the process. Species will vector from each object toward the eye. He might also have said that since objects of great size are composed by a multitude of smaller parts, the grain of millet is but the smallest part of the mountain: to see the one as opposed to the other is simply a matter of viewing point and focus (figs. 14.2, 14.3a & 3b).

> Aristotle proves in his Physics, book 6, that magnitudes cannot be divided into indivisibles, nor is a magnitude composed of indivisibles; and therefore there are as many parts in a grain of millet as in the diameter of the world, as the figure reveals. Let there be a triangle or pyramid, ABC, with a large base, and let its vertex be subtended by the very short line ED; it is apparent that from each point of line AB a line can be drawn to C, since a straight line can [always] be drawn from one point to another; and it follows that from each of the extremities of the base a line can be drawn to C, and likewise from other points and from all of its parts, since an infinity of lines can terminate at one point. This is well known. If, therefore, all of these lines extend to C, they pass through the points of line DE. And since they do not intersect before C, they will pass through all the points in line DE, for if some or all passed through the same point [of line DE], they would intersect before C; but it has been posited that they do not. If all or some [of the lines] should intersect at some point of line DE, then doubtless after intersection they would separate from one another to infinity and never intersect in C, as is evident to sense in this shorter pyramid, FGH.[12]

Though preoccupied here by arguing the logic of geometric perspectivism, Bacon also demonstrates how crucial is the viewer's position vis-à-vis the object in order that correct vision may occur. What and how the viewer sees will depend in no small measure on his or her relationship to the thing viewed.

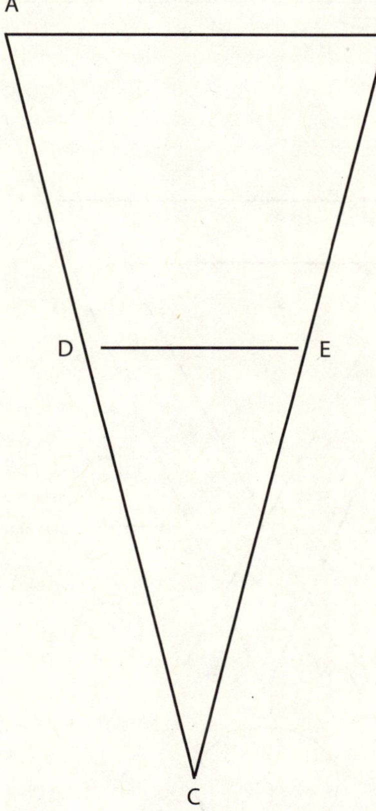

Figure 14.2. Visual pyramid: how the eye perceives objects of different magnitudes. David C. Lindberg, *Roger Bacon and the Origins of "Perspectiva" in the Middle Ages* (Oxford: Clarendon Press, 1996), p. 71.

In short, he raises the question of interference. And, although the physical relationships of object and eye concern him principally here, a reading of the whole treatise suggests his sense that interference can be psychic as well as physical.

In fine, Bacon distinguishes clearly between the physics and geometry of vision—how the eye perceives—and the visual judgment resulting from any given experience of sight. The former is invariable and scientifically determinate. The latter is contingent, situational, subjective, and therefore highly variable or relativistic. When he says that the "eye should perceive the thing

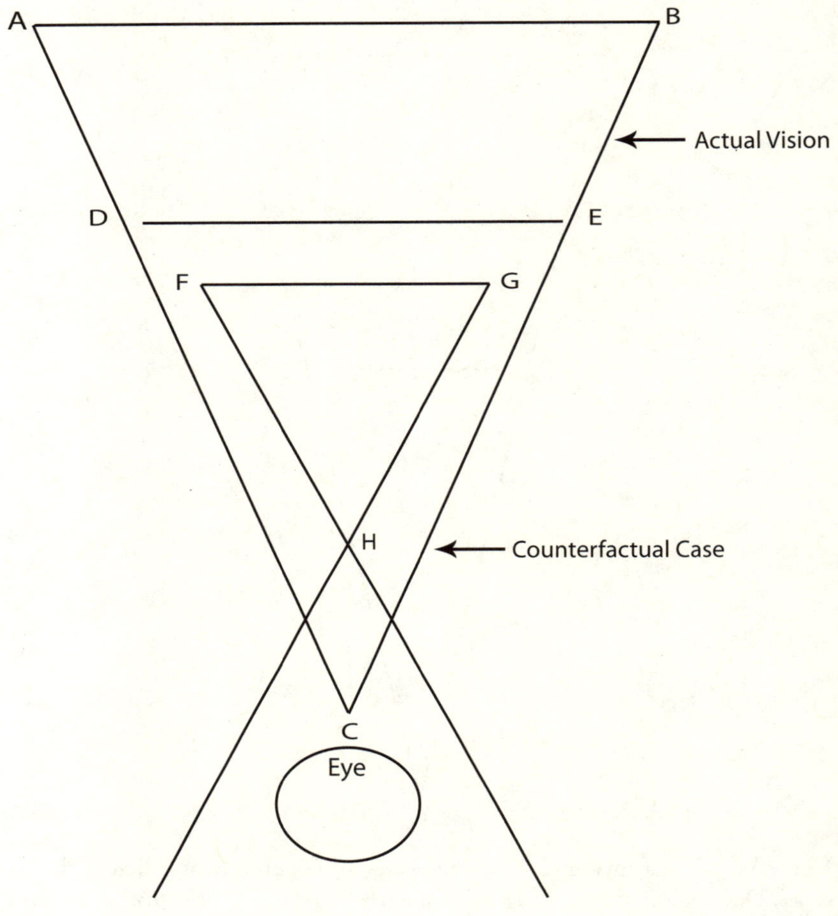

Figure 14.3a. Visual pyramids true and false. David C. Lindberg, *Roger Bacon and the Origins of "Perspectiva" in the Middle Ages* (Oxford: Clarendon Press, 1996), pp.71, 73.

itself, distinctly and sufficiently with certitude," he means that the fact of perception should correspond to this description. The nature of the visual judgment, that is how the individual perceiver interprets the sight, is another matter entirely. But more of this later.

The different angles by which rays reach the eye account for partial or

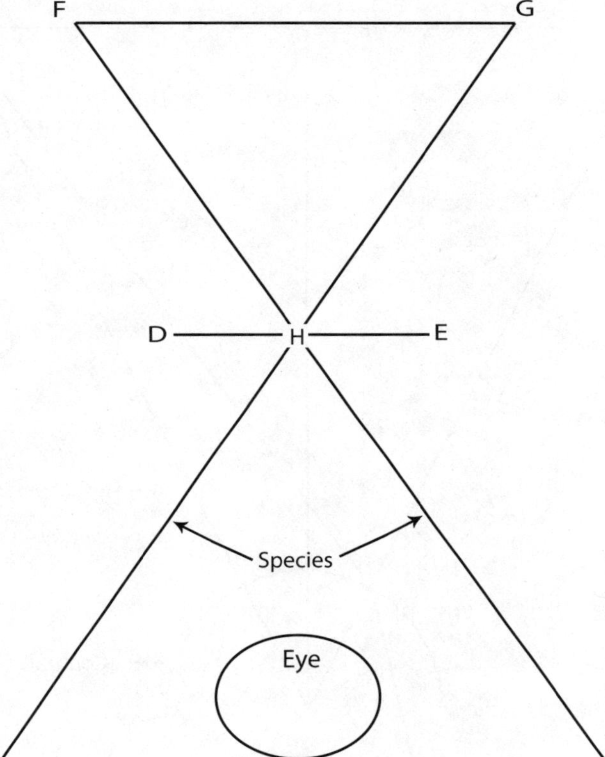

Figure 14.3b. Counterfactual case: lines intersect before C = no image. David C. Lindberg, *Roger Bacon and the Origins of "Perspectiva" in the Middle Ages* (Oxford: Clarendon Press, 1996), p. 73.

weakened images, or, indeed, the failure to perceive an object altogether that may, nonetheless, lie squarely within the visual field. The angle at which a ray reaches the eye determines its power. Rays that fall perpendicularly on the retina carry the most visual force; so much so that they may screen or block altogether rays that arrive on the retina from acute angles. Once again, a fact of physical nature carries implications for mimetic performance and visual judgment. First, let's look at the geometric description (fig. 14.4).

> Every point of the eye and cornea is truly the recipient of the vertex of a pyramid [emanating] from the whole object. In each of those points the species of all parts [of the visible object] are mixed. Nevertheless each point of the eye or cornea or aperture of the uvea is the recipient of a perpendicular

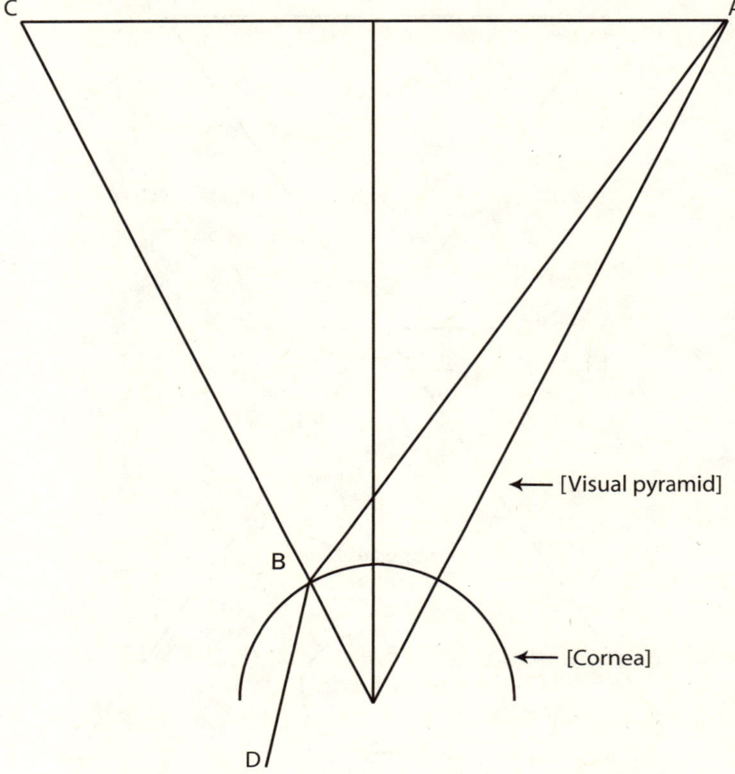

Figure 14.4. Refraction of perpendicular and oblique rays. David C. Lindberg, *Roger Bacon and the Origins of "Perspectiva" in the Middle Ages* (Oxford: Clarendon Press, 1996), p. 77.

species from only one point of the visible object, although that same point [of the eye] is the recipient of an infinity of oblique species. Therefore, since the body of the eye is denser than air, it is necessary, by the laws of refraction . . . for all of the oblique species to be refracted at the surface of the cornea. And since oblique incidence weakens a species, as does refraction, while perpendicular incidence is strong, therefore the perpendicular species conceals many weak lights; thus the light of the sun conceals an infinity of stellar lights. For example, to point B comes a perpendicular [ray] from C, and to the same point B comes [ray] AB, [evidently] non-perpendicular since it is not directed toward the centre of the eye. Therefore, the species of A is concealed, even though it can pass from point B to the [anterior] glacial humour along refracted line BD. It follows that the perpendiculars are respon-

> sible for [visual] judgement. And since perpendicular species are arranged distinctly and in proper order on the surface of the visual organ, therefore distinctions [among the parts of the visible object] can be made.[13]

In the physical world, Bacon argues, it is a fact that some species strike the eye with greater power than others thanks to the angle of perception. They may be so strong, in fact, as to conceal other rays altogether. That is the case in theory, or what we might call a neutral, or a zero degree of viewing. Bacon's diagram and explanation does show that the oblique species do reach the eye. And he does not rule out, indeed quite the contrary, that even if a perceiver receives a strongly imprinted visual impression that is perfectly coincident with the object, psychic interference may alter the viewer's visual judgment so that he or she experiences the weaker or distorted species more intensely than the stronger, perpendicular species. The effect on the viewer's visual judgment will be the same as if he had altered his viewing point. Bacon repeatedly speaks of the disparity in visual experiences, citing a variety of conditions that affect the relative accuracy of the likeness. Material or physical conditions that produce weak or distorted images are of particular concern, but he leaves no doubt that more subjective elements may also weaken or distort visual judgment. We shall return to this discrepancy between physical and psychic viewing in a moment.

First, however, let's consider one last case of vision, the most curious of all for the thirteenth century, apparently, because it was surrounded by myth and superstition of the sort then thought to be produced by mirrors. Unlike other forms of vision, Bacon begins his explanation of mirrors by attacking the common superstition that a mirror contains within it an image—or, with a nod to Ovid's (and Guillaume de Lorris's) Narcissus—some being. In short, reflection and refraction have not been well understood (fig. 14.5).

> Next we must carefully consider the fact that there is nothing in the mirror; nor does anything appear to be in it, as the vulgar judge. Rather, what is seen is the object from which the species comes, opposite the mirror, as Alhacen teaches in many ways in book 4. For just as the end of straight line OA, when vision occurs by means of this line, is itself the visible object A, so the end of the reflected line ODA will be A. Besides, a species is not seen except by chance and accidentally, as has been explained above. Furthermore, [if what is seen were actually in the mirror,] then a species would be like a blemish impressed in the mirror, or like some designated part of the mirror in which a species has been impressed. Consequently, the eye would not need to be in a particular location in order to see the blemish in the

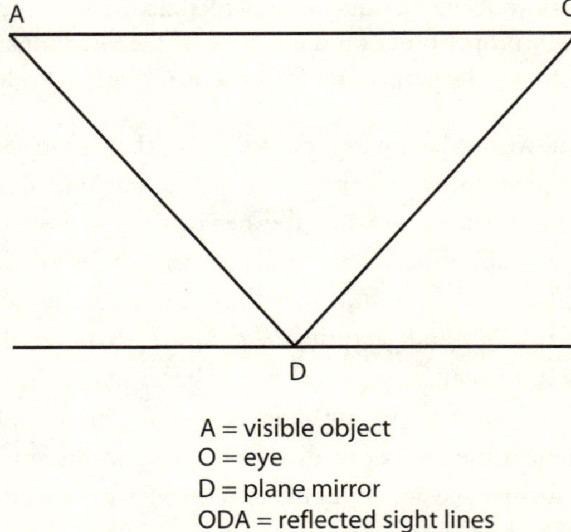

Figure 14.5. Plane mirror. David C. Lindberg, *Roger Bacon and the Origins of "Perspectiva" in the Middle Ages* (Oxford: Clarendon Press, 1996), p. 259.

> mirror or some designated part of it; therefore vision by reflection in the eye would not need to be located in a particular spot. But this is false, for unless the eye is at O, it will not see anything by reflection to that point; for if it were elsewhere, the reflected species would not reach it, owing to the requirement that the angles of incidence and reflection be equal. This can be demonstrated in many ways, but since it is most certain to all who know perspective, we need not dwell on it further. And from this the skilful investigator can infer an infinity of consequences. First of all, it follows that no species is impressed in the mirror or fixed in its substance, as the vulgar judge; but the species only has its direction reversed by the surface of the mirror, according to equality of the angles of incidence and reflection.[14]

While Bacon has no difficulty putting to rest vulgar superstitions regarding the suspect images purportedly harbored by mirrors, his assertion that the strongest images are those that reach the eye directly, that is, by a perpendicular trajectory, inevitably renders reflected and refracted images problematic. A reflected image can never be entirely straightforward:

> It must be known that an object seen by reflection does not appear in its true place, because sight is accustomed to seeing by means of straight lines and [to judging] visible things to be at the extremities of these lines, and therefore it does not perceive the bending that occurs in reflection. Consequently, it judges the visible object always to be on [the rectilinear extension

> of] the visual ray, and the place of the image, which we call the "appearance of the object," to be at one of its points. . . . Although the object does not always appear in the same place, in most cases it appears at the intersection of the visual ray and the cathetus [the perpendicular drawn from the visible object to the mirror]. However, sometimes it is not found at that intersection, but merely on the visual ray, which can be parallel to the cathetus [and thus never intersect it]; this can occur in a concave mirror, as will be explained. When the visual ray does intersect the cathetus, [the location of] this intersection varies in many ways. Sometimes the intersection is located behind the observer's head, sometimes in the eye, sometimes on the surface of the mirror, sometimes in [the body of] the mirror, sometimes behind the mirror, the latter in several different ways. For sometimes the object appears as far behind the mirror as it [actually] is in front of the mirror, and this diversity results from differences in the mirrors.[15]

Not only is the image not in the mirror, as simple people thought, but it is not even where the mirror shows it to be. Naïve visual judgment will inevitably "believe the mirror," and thus be led into error. This is a far from trivial observation, for if the signified object is not where it seems to be, it may also not be what or how it appears. We must conclude that mirrors are, for Bacon, Guillaume de Lorris, and Jean de Meun, just as perilous as they were for Narcissus. And for good reason.

When we consider that even with direct perception the viewer sees not the object, but the likeness of the object formed by the myriad species that convey its components to the eye, then it's not difficult to understand why the mirror image complicates the formula still further. It is after all but an image of an image. And even then, we can never be sure, as Bacon demonstrates, exactly where the reflected object may actually be found. While the plane mirror geometry of figure 14.5 may seem straightforward enough—rays reflected at a right angle—he shows that mirrors have a way of distorting even the simplest convention. And with convex mirrors (or concave), distortions increase even more considerably.

> Now the appearance of the image follows the nature of the reflecting surface. In convex mirrors, therefore, almost nothing appears as it truly is except the order of the parts, which is the same in the smaller [image] as in the object. The straight appears curved in convex mirrors, for since reflection takes place at a convex surface, the ends of the outermost rays are further from the centre of the eye than is the end of the middle ray, and from the orientation [of the rays] we judge the properties [e.g., curvature] of the object. . . . Again, it should be noted that in convex mirrors the distance of

the image from the mirror is smaller than that of the visible object, while in plane mirrors they are equal.[16]

While it is impossible to convey the complex and intricate arguments Bacon advances in support of his perspectivist optical theories in so compressed a form, I think that the foregoing at least conveys the gist of his ideas and methods. It does not, perhaps, prepare us for the abrupt shift of emphasis that occurs toward the end of the treatise. There, Bacon suddenly turns from the physical to the moral consequences of optics and boldly elaborates a poetics of vision. Having previously argued the primacy of sight among the senses—precisely because it is the most perceptive of them all, and the one that leads most inexorably to wisdom, he now urges a more abstract and moral inquiry.[17] He introduces the theme by quoting Psalm 17:8: "Preserve me, O Lord, as the pupil of your eye."

To our eyes it may seem strange that a treatise so resolutely dedicated to logical study of physical phenomena should quote scripture and spend its last four sections showing the relevance of science to divine wisdom. Nevertheless, he insists that such is his project: "Concerning the relationship of *perspectiva* to sacred wisdom and mundane utility, in four chapters."[18]

I have spoken of perspectival matters, insofar as they are required for the understanding of philosophical wisdom and mundane things. Now, in conclusion, I wish to reveal how this science has inexpressible utility with respect to divine wisdom.

In a radically daring move, Bacon, after acknowledging the role of divine wisdom as the principle governing this world, then goes on to assert that perspectivism unlocks the mysteries of divine intention. "The science of *perspectiva* is necessary [to the understanding and elucidation of scripture] . . . for in divine scripture, nothing is dealt with as frequently as matters pertaining to the eye and vision . . . and therefore nothing is more essential to a grasp of the literal and spiritual sense than the certitude supplied by this science."[19]

What he means, it quickly transpires, is that henceforth the literal meaning of scripture will equate with a scientific understanding of the physiology and physical function of scriptural reference. God's meaning, in short, is to be linked to a proper physical understanding of God's creation. Physical science now goes hand in hand with hermeneutics, or, rather, we see that physical science is a hermeneutics of the physical world.

For example, when it is said, "Preserve me, O Lord, as the pupil of your eye," it is impossible to know God's meaning in this phrase unless we first consider how the preservation of the pupil is achieved, to the point where God would consider it worthy to preserve us in a like manner. For when something is set forth as an example and similitude, that which is exemplified cannot be understood unless the nature of the example is grasped. For example, when the Lord says, "Let them be wise as serpents . . ." (Matthew, 10:16), he wants his disciples to consider the properties of a serpent in which its wisdom resides and the nature of a dove in which its agreeable simplicity is found. We cannot understand the preservation of the pupil except through the science of *perspectiva.*[20]

Bacon's hermeneutics of vision quickly spawned a tradition of moralizing or allegorical interpretations of the eye within a decade of the publication of his *Perspectiva.* From 1275 forward, Peter of Limoges's treatise, *De oculo morali,* not only popularized the allegorical interpretation of optical phenomena, but was also, thanks to its wide circulation, an important means of disseminating perspectivist optical theory.[21] But my interest does not lie in pursuing these matters, however interesting. Rather, I want to see how and why perspectivism, on Bacon's view, would logically lead to biblical hermeneutics. By understanding these questions, we may better grasp how they so quickly and thoroughly infiltrated the vernacular literary scene, particularly the *Roman de la Rose.*

The link between perspectivism and hermeneutics appears inevitable once one thinks about it. First of all, Bacon shows that images are dynamic, rather than static, since they evolve over time and through space as the species travel from the surface of the object to the eye. They do so because the eyes of the perceiver focus on the object, thereby establishing the visual pyramid that gathers and contains the species. The latter are encoded with a piece of visual information, each bearing the elements of likeness—color, texture, shape, details, and so on—of the part of the object whence it emanates. Since each species is thus an image, or fragment of an image, in its own right—like a tile from a mosaic—it has, as Bacon shows, materiality: "species have corporeal being and therefore material being."[22]

This is essential, for without corporeal and material being, they could not be perceived sensually. Yet the things we perceive often come initially to our preconscious perception so that we are not aware of any single stimulus, but only of the aggregate of sensations. When we "hear" a word, for example, no unitary auditory signal conveys the expression. Rather, we hear articulated sounds, packets of phonetically encoded information which ear and mind translate into the desired or expected word. If any part of the phonetically encoded chain goes astray, we cannot match the remaining sound patterns to the vocabulary known to us, and so we are obliged to request our interlocutor to repeat himself.

Bacon's concept of species is similar. His genius lay in recognizing that for species to convey likeness—that is, something recognizable—the coded visual data carried by the multitude of species contained in a single glance required a principle of "directional organization." Some mental process had to gather, bundle, and send them on a converging path toward the eyes. The latter, in turn, would receive the species as compressed data, which could then be processed into a surrogate of the object, or in short, an image. The visual cone that allowed for compression and transmission of the coded data or species was itself animated by the dynamic principle of geometric perspectivism, *perspectiva.*

Perspectiva does for the coded visual data or species what the speculative grammarians argued that syntax does for language. Syntax, they showed, organizes the many disparate words into a string of signifiers that reading translates into coherent meaning. Reading, of course, is itself a process of image coding and deciphering that unfolds in time and space. In this case, the folio or page with its writing, illuminations, rubrics, and décor. If we think of *perspectiva* as *a kind of "ocularist syntax,"* then one can readily see how, for Bacon, the reading process could explain the dynamics of image processing: the "bundled" species constitute the "text" to be processed by the eyes and mind in order to perceive the likeness of the object punctually encoded in the hundreds of species that constitute any representation.

The fact that we do not "see" the object itself, but rather a "text" of it made up of tiny bits of visual coding, explains why vision, that most brilliant "queen of the cognitive senses," is so fallible, so prone to error and misprision. Perspectivism emphasizes the crucial role of viewpoint or vantage point for vision and the judgment that accompanies it. If a viewer does not have the correct vantage point—the safest being the frontal rather than oblique perspective—it will not be possible to "see" the object correctly. And here, again, the analogy with reading holds true. One may "parse" a passage of text without fully comprehending it either through inattention, insufficient literacy, or because the context of the message is unclear.

By demonstrating the crucial role of perspective in determining clear vision and thus the judgments predicated on sight, Bacon arrives at an analogous analysis of the dynamics of perception, memory, and judgment as that adumbrated by Plato at *Philebus,* §38b–§39c. It's worth taking a moment to revisit Plato's argument. The comparison will help us to appreciate five crucial components of perception:

1. Western philosophy's perennial notion that vision is both a physical act and a psychic process whose consequences for moral thought must be understood in terms of the interaction of vision, memory, and judgment;
2. Time and space as dynamic components of this process, as much for the psychic as for the physical stages;
3. The tendency to equate the reception of perceptual signals with reading (texts/books), and consequently to analogize visual signals or species with language;
4. The converse notion, that words may be conceived as visual images, and writing as a kind of word painting (*ekphrasis*);
5. Finally, how Bacon's analysis of the mechanics of vision furthers our understanding of optics without necessarily eliminating either the ambiguity of perception or the uncertainty of judgment. Bacon shows, in short, what Plato intuits, namely, the subjective basis of perceptual imprecision.

Here is Plato's text from the *Philebus,* §38b–§39c:

Socrates: Now is it not always memory and perception that give rise to opinion and to the attempts we make to reach a judgment?
Protarchus: Certainly.
Socrates: Let me suggest what we must believe to occur in this connection.
Protarchus: Well?
Socrates: If a man sees objects that come into his view from a distance and indistinctly, would you agree that he commonly wants to decide about what he sees?
Protarchus: I should.
Socrates: Then the next will be that he puts [this] question to himself. . . . "What is that object which catches my eye there beside the rock under a tree?" . . . And then he would answer his own question and say, if he got it right, "It is a man." . . . Or again, if he went astray and thought what he was looking at was something made by shepherds, he might very well call it an image.
Protarchus: He might quite well.
Socrates: And if he had someone with him, he would put what he said to himself into actual speech addressed to his companion, audibly uttering those same thoughts, so that what before we called opinion has now become assertion.

Protarchus: Of course.

Socrates: Whereas if he is alone he continues thinking the same thing by himself, going on his way maybe for a considerable time with the thought in his mind.

Protarchus: Undoubtedly.

Socrates: Well now, I wonder whether you share my view . . . that at such times our soul is like a book.

Protarchus: How so?

Socrates: It appears to me that the conjunction of memory with sensations, together with the feelings consequent upon memory and sensation, may be said as it were to write words upon our souls. And when the experience writes what is true, the result is that true opinion and true assertions spring up in us, while when the internal scribe that I have suggested writes what is false we get the opposite sort of opinions and assertions.

Protarchus: That certainly seems right, and I approve of the way that you put it.

Socrates: Then please give your approval to the presence of a second artist in our souls at such a time. . . . A painter, who comes after the writer and paints in the soul pictures of these assertions that we make.[23]

The foregoing remarks should go some way toward explaining how naturally, even inevitably, Bacon would have made the link between geometrical perspectivism and biblical hermeneutics. While it is true enough that mainstream rhetorical treatises from antiquity to the Renaissance showed the proximity of word and image, particularly word-as-image, Bacon's geometrical optics injects a new dimension in the equation. In the face of his perspectivism, image takes on concrete materiality. Bacon and his contemporaries provide a new vocabulary and conceptual matrix for thinking about images, and more compelling still, a new and logical means for showing how optics, including reflection and refraction, can help explain more precisely the mix of physics and psyche in the viewer. What Bacon does, in effect, is to show logically how we think with images in much the same way as with language. He makes graphically apparent, in short, the self-consciousness and self-reflexivity of perspectivism.

Ultimately, however, Bacon's role lay more in formulating the new concepts on perspectivism than in applying them, apart, as we have seen, from his strained attempts to explore their import for biblical hermeneutics. Their application would lead to a new and rich vein of metaphorical and allegorical literary creation in the century that followed. Perhaps no work profited more from this standpoint than did the *Roman de la Rose.* It is no accident that this work, within a short time after its completion by Jean de Meun (c. 1285) generated a rich tradition of illuminated manuscripts, among the largest number of any vernacular work of the period.

More significantly, the illuminated manuscripts of the *Rose* develop a new phenomenology of the visual image, beginning with the incipit. This means simply that one finds a remarkable independence to the visual images in relationship to the original text. If images are often suggested by the text, in the sense that the pictures do depict something suggested in the poetry, they show great freedom in how they represent the text. We also find cases, particularly in the *bas-de-page,* where pictures bear no apparent relation to the poetry. That subject, however, will be developed in a subsequent study.

Notes

1. David C. Lindberg, *Roger Bacon and the Origins of "Perspectiva" in the Middle Ages: A Critical Edition and English Translation of Bacon's "Perspectiva" with Introduction and Notes* (Oxford: Clarendon Press, 1996), p. xxxvii.
2. Ibid., p. xxxvii.
3. Ibid., p. xxxix.
4. Ibid., p. xl.
5. "Bacon was born into a prosperous English family in an unknown place and at an unknown date, variously estimated to be about 1210, about 1214, or about 1220. [He is presumed to have died in 1292, or soon thereafter.] . . . We know nothing of Bacon's early education, but it is evident that his university studies were pursued at Oxford and Paris. After earning the M.A. degree at one or the other of those two universities (usually conjectured to be Oxford), Bacon taught in the faculty of arts at Paris, lecturing principally (but not exclusively) on Aristotle's libri naturales. This teaching apparently took place in the early to mid-1240s. Bacon claims to have seen Alexander of Hales, who died at Paris in 1245, with his own eyes; and this provides us with our first firm chronological anchor. There is great uncertainty about Bacon's movements in the late 1240s and 1250s. All we really know is that in 1251 he was in Paris, where he witnessed the uprising of the Pastoreaux rebels." Ibid., p. xvii.
6. "Bacon experienced a dramatic broadening of his philosophical outlook in he late 1240s, breaking out of the confines of Aristotelian philosophy and devoting himself for about two decades to the study of a variety of other sources available in translation from Greek and Arabic. These studies may have been inspired by the example of Robert Grosseteste, who was almost certainly not Bacon's teacher, but to whose works Bacon clearly had access; the outcome of these studies was a broad mastery of the materials that Bacon would eventually write about under the

rubrics of mathematical and experimental science (including geography, alchemy, astronomy, astrology, meteorology, and *perspectiva*). Bacon's claim to have spent two thousand pounds on books, instruments, and other scholarly necessities must apply to this period. The passage is worth quoting, since it bears on the scientific work to which the present volume is devoted. "For during the twenty years in which I have labored especially in the pursuit of wisdom, abandoning the opinions of the vulgar, I have spent more than two thousand pounds on these studies, for books of secrets, various experiences [*experientias*], languages, instruments, tables, and other things." Ibid., p. xviii.

7. Ibid., p. xliv.

8. For a revisionist discussion of Bacon's grasp and practice of experimental science, see ibid., pp. lii–lv.

9. "That Bacon found ways of applying geometry to optical questions is apparent from even a superficial examination of his works. Here, for the first time in the West, we find original optical treatises containing geometrical drawings in profusion. Bacon's *De multiplicatione specierum* contains thirty-nine such drawings, the *Perspectiva* fifty-one, and *De speculis comburentibus* twenty-eight. Nor are these drawings merely decorative; all of them support serious and sustained geometrical argumentation. Bacon uses geometry to elucidate the theory of direct vision, tracing the path of radiation through the humours of the eye; he develops a theory of binocular vision along geometrical lines, and rules of perspective; and he presents an exhaustive geometrical analysis of the propagation of light, including the phenomena of reflection and refraction." Ibid., p. xliv.

10. Ibid., p. lvii.

11. Roger Bacon, *Perspectiva,* I.4.4, in ibid., pp. 57–59. (All subsequent Bacon citations are from Lindberg, *Roger Bacon and the Origins of "Perspectiva."*)

12. *Perspectiva,* I.6.1, pp. 71–73.

13. *Perspectiva,* I.6.2, pp. 75–77.

14. *Perspectiva,* III.1.2, pp. 259–261.

15. *Perspectiva,* III.1.2, pp. 261–262.

16. *Perspectiva,* III.1.3, pp. 267–269.

17. "And if our deliberations to this point have been beautiful and delightful, the matters now to be considered are far more beautiful and delightful, because we take special delight in vision and because light and colour have singular beauty, exceeding all of the other things that are conveyed to our senses. . . . But concerning sight alone, and not the other senses, have philosophers developed a separate science, *perspectiva.* It follows that the wisdom gained through vision must have a special utility, not found in the other senses." *Perspectiva,* I.1.1, pp. 3–5.

18. *Perspectiva,* III.3.1. "et iam dictum est de rebus perspectivis prout ad sapientiam philosophie et rerum huius mundi cognitionem necessarie sunt. Volo nunc in fine innuere quomodo hec scientia habet ineffabilem utilitatem respectu sapientie divine."

19. *Perspectiva,* III.3.1, p. 323.

20. Ibid.

21. Lindberg, *Roger Bacon and the Origins of "Perspectiva,"* p. 390, n. 624.

22. *Perspectiva,* I.6.4, p. 87.

23. *The Collected Dialogues of Plato,* ed. Edith Hamilton and Huntington Cairns, Bollingen Series 71 (Princeton: Princeton University Press, 1961), pp. 1118–1119.

Contributors

Marina Brownlee is the Robert Schirmer Professor of Spanish and Comparative Literature at Princeton University. Her books on medieval topics include *The Status of the Reading Subject in the "Libro de buen amor"* and *The Severed Word: Ovid's "Heroides" and the "Novela Sentimental."* Volumes she has co-edited on medieval studies include *The New Medievalism* and *Boundary and Transgression in Medieval Culture.* She is currently writing on iconicity in fifteenth-century Spain.

Alison Calhoun is currently finishing her dissertation on Montaigne at the Johns Hopkins University under the direction of Michel Jeanneret. In 2006–2007, she was the Louis Marin Fellow at the École Normale Supérieure (Ulm) in Paris, and in 2005, the Johns Hopkins representative at the Institute for French Cultural Studies, held at Dartmouth College. She has presented papers on Montaigne, Abelard, and typologies of death in sixteenth-century France. Her general research interests include an interdisciplinary approach to Early Modern French literature integrating philosophy, travel narrative, music, and theater by focusing on issues of morality, gender, death, the self, and otherness.

Hans Ulrich Gumbrecht is the Albert Guérard Professor of Literature at Stanford University. Among his books on literary theory and literary and cultural history are *Eine Geschichte der spanischen Literatur* (Spanish translation forthcoming); *Making Sense in Life and Literature; In 1926—Living at the Edge of Time; Corpo e forma; Vom Leben und Sterben des großen Romanisten; The Powers of Philology; Production of Presence;* and *In Praise of Athletic Beauty.* Gumbrecht is a regular contributor to the Humanities section of the *Frankfurter Allgemeine Zeitung, NZZ* (Zürich), and the *Folha de São Paulo.* He is a member of the American Academy of Arts and Sciences, Professeur attaché au Collège de France, and has been a visiting professor at numerous universities on several continents, most recently at the Scuola Normale Superiore in Pisa.

Daniel Heller-Roazen is Professor of Comparative Literature at Princeton University. He is the author of *Fortune's Faces: The "Roman de la Rose" and the Poetics of Contingency* and *Echolalias: On the Forgetting of Language,* as well as the editor and translator of Giorgio Agamben's *Potentialities: Collected Essays in Philosophy.* His next book will be published in spring 2007: *The Inner Touch: Archaeology of a Sensation.* He is currently preparing the Norton Critical Edition of the *Arabian Nights.*

Andreas Kablitz is Professor of Romance Philology and head of the Romanisches Seminar of the Philosophische Fakultät of the Universität zu Köln. In 1997, he was awarded the distinguished Leibniz Prize for outstanding scholarship. An active and effective administrator, as well as scholar, Kablitz is Co-Director of a Special Research Group in Media Studies awarded by the Deutschen Forschungsgemeinschaft (DFG) at the Universities of Köln, Bonn, and Aachen. He is also a principal organizer of a proposed Center of Excellence also focused on media studies. A specialist in Romance studies, Andreas Kablitz has written on Dante, Petrarch, and other major Italian writers. He has published extensively on French literature from the Middle Ages to the twentieth century, without neglecting Spanish letters. An academic advisor to the Fritz Thyssen Stiftung (foundation), and a counselor for the DFG, Kablitz travels extensively in Europe and Asia evaluating programs. He also coedits, with Joachim Küpper, the prestigious *Romanistiches Jahrbuch.* He lectures extensively throughout Europe and North America as a visiting professor, as well as frequently organizing and participating in scholarly conferences.

Hildegard Elisabeth Keller is Professor of German Medieval and Early Modern Literature at the University of Zurich. She has also been a visiting professor in European and American universities: Konya (1992), Amsterdam (2000), Munich (2000/2001), and Indiana University in Bloomington (2005). She initiated and directs a research project to edit five volumes of writings by the Swiss surgeon Jakob Ruf, *Jakob Ruf: Leben, Werk und Studien.* Since 1998, together with students, colleagues, and professionals, she has produced and presented recordings and theatrical productions of and about medieval literature and culture. Her publications include: *Wort und Fleisch. Körperallegorien, mystische Spiritualität und Dichtung des St. Trudperter Hoheliedes im Horizont der Inkarnation; Jakob Ruf, ein Zürcher Stadtchirurg und Theatermacher im 16. Jahrhundert; My Secret Is Mine: Studies on Religion and Eros in the German*

Middle Ages; Stimmen aus mittelalterlichen Frauenklöstern, audiobook, ed. with Jeffrey F. Hamburger.

Joachim Küpper is Professor of Romance Literatures and Comparative Literature at the Freie Universität Berlin. His field of research covers medieval and early modern texts from the Iberian Peninsula and from Italy, the French and the Italian novel of the nineteenth century, and inter-art relations and problems of general aesthetic theory. Main publications include: *Balzac und der Effet de réel; Ästhetik der Wirklichkeitsdarstellung und Evolution des Romans von der französischen Spätaufklärung bis zu Robbe-Grillet; Diskurs-Renovatio bei Lope de Vega und Calderón; Zum italienischen Roman des 19. Jahrhunderts. Foscolo, Manzoni, Verga, D'Annunzio; Petrarca. Das Schweigen der Veritas und die Worte des Dichters;* "1437: The Beginning of Modern Thinking (Nicholas of Cusa)," in David E. Wellbery et al., eds., *A New History of German Literature;* "Was ist Literatur?" *Zeitschrift für Ästhetik und Allgemeine Kunstwissenschaft* 45, no. 2 (2001); "The Traditional Cosmos and the New World," *MLN* 118, no. 2 (2003).

Jan-Dirk Müller was an assistant professor in history at Heidelberg (1976 Habilitation) after studies in German literature and philosophy. He then taught at the Universities of Heidelberg (1970–1977), Bielefeld (1977–1981), Münster (1981–1984), Hamburg (1984–1991), and Munich (since 1991). He is an ordinary member of the Bavarian Academy of Science, corresponding member of the Göttingen Academy, member (till 2001 Speaker) of the Sonderforschungsbereich Pluralisierung und Autorität in der Frühen Neuzeit. His research is in Heroic epics, early German novel, courtly lyrics, humanism, and Renaissance literature.

Stephen G. Nichols, James M. Beall Professor of French and Humanities, heads the Department of German and Romance Languages and Literatures at Johns Hopkins University and specializes in medieval literature, art, and history. One of his books, *Romanesque Signs: Early Medieval Narrative and Iconography,* received the Modern Language Association's James Russell Lowell Prize for an outstanding book by an MLA author in 1984. In 1991, *The New Philology,* conceived and edited by Nichols for the Medieval Academy of America, was honored by the Council of Editors of Learned Journals. In 1992, the University of Geneva conferred on him the title of Docteur ès Lettres, *honoris causa,* while the French Minister of Culture made him chevalier de l'Ordre des Arts et Lettres in 1999. He is a Fellow of the Medieval Academy of America and a Senior Fellow of the School of Criticism and Theory, which he also directed from 1995 to 2001. Recent publications include *L'Alterité du Moyen Age; Medievalism and the Modernist Temper; The New Medievalism;* and *Mimesis: From Mirror to Method, Augustine to Descartes* (reprinted, 2004). Current projects include: *Laughing Matters: The Enigma and Exasperation of Laughter* and *Building History: The Politics of Medievalism in Restoration France.*

David Nirenberg received his BA in history from Yale University in 1986 and his PhD from Princeton University in 1992. He is Professor of History at the University of Chicago, where he moved in 2007 from Johns Hopkins University, where he was the Charlotte Bloomberg Professor of the Humanities and Director of the Leonard and Helen Stulman Jewish Studies Program. His research focuses on the relations, real and imagined, between Judaism, Christianity, and Islam. His books include: *Communities of Violence: Persecution of Minorities in the Middle Ages; A Man of Three Worlds: Samuel Pallache, a Moroccan Jew in Catholic and Protestant Europe;* and *The Body of Christ in the Art of Europe and New Spain, 1150–1800.*

Gabrielle M. Spiegel is Krieger-Eisenhower Professor of History, Chair of History, and Dean of Faculty of Johns Hopkins University. She has held a Guggenheim Fellowship, a Rockefeller Residency Fellowship in the Program in Atlantic History (Johns Hopkins), and a Fellowship at the Center for Advanced Study in the Behavioral Sciences, Stanford University. Her work focuses on French medieval history and historiography, literary and cultural theory, and postmodern historiography. She is the author of *The Chronicle Tradition of Saint-Denis: A Survey; Romancing the Past: The Rise of Vernacular Prose Historiography in Thirteenth-Century France; The Past as Text: The Theory and Practice of Medieval Historiography* (translated in Italian as *Il Passato come Testo. Teoria e pratica della storiografia medievale*); and *Practicing History: New Directions in Historical Writing after the Linguistic Turn.* With Stephen G. Nichols, she translated *Kantorowicz: Stories of a Historian,* by Alain Boureau.

Eugene Vance teaches French literature, comparative literature, and comparative religion at the University of Washington. Considering the restlessness of St. Augustine's writings as a radical challenge to the aspirations of the medieval mind, he writes about the destabilizing interplay between the discourses and forms—poetic, intellectual, spiritual—of medieval culture in its implacable search for certainty and transcendence. His books include: *Reading the Song of Roland; L'Archéologie du signe; From Topic to Tale: Logic and Narrativity in the Middle Ages; Mervelous Signals: Poetics and Sign Theory in the Middle Ages.*

Gregor Vogt-Spira was Professor of Classical Philology / Latin at the Ernst-Moritz-Arndt-Universität Greifswald (Germany). Currently, his research interest focuses on the historical epistemology of ancient poetics and literary theory and its transformation until the Renaissance, based on an extensive study of early, classical, and late Latin literature. He is editor of Julius Caesar Scaliger's *Poetices libri septem,* books 5 and 6 (1998; 2003), and heads an international research group investigating key concepts of ancient culture and its reception, like "the Archaic." An early book of his dealt with the role of chance in Greek culture (*Dramaturgie des Zufalls. Tyche und Handeln in der Komödie Menanders,* 1992). For many years he has been working in the area of orality and literacy; in this context, he has written a book on satire in the Roman republic (forthcoming) and edited five volumes in the series *ScriptOralia.*

Rainer Warning is Emeritus Professor of Romance and Comparative Literature at the University of Munich. He has written largely on literary theory and on the history of literature from the Middle Ages up to our century. His books include *Diderots Jacques le fataliste und Sternes Tristram Shandy; Funktion und Struktur. Die Ambivalenzen des geistlichen Spiels* (English translation, *The Ambivalences of Medieval Religious Drama*); *Rezeptionsästhetik; Lektüren romanischer Lyrik. Von den Trobadors zum Surrealismus; Die Phantasie der Realisten;* and *Proust-Studien.* At the moment he is preparing for publication a book on literary heterotopias.

Heather Webb, Assistant Professor of Italian at the Ohio State University, has published on Catherine of Siena's letters and has essays forthcoming on Dante: one on the *rime petrose,* one on ideas of vital heat in the *Commedia* and another on "Paradiso 25" that will appear in *California Lectura Dantis.* She is currently working on a book entitled *The Medieval Heart: Circulation before William Harvey.*

Michel Zink graduated from the École Normale Supérieure (1964) and from the Sorbonne (agrégation in classics 1967, PhD 1970, thèse d'Etat 1975). He was an assistant, then an associate professor of medieval French literature at the Sorbonne (1968–1976), a full professor first at the University of Toulouse (1976–1987), then at the Sorbonne (1987–1994). Since 1994 he holds the chair of Literatures of Medieval France at the Collège de France. Since 2000 he is a Member of the Institut de France (Académie des Inscriptions et Belles-Lettres). He is currently the vice-chairman of the Collège de France's board of professors. He has been a visiting professor in several American, European, and Japanese universities: Yale (three times), UC Berkeley, Penn, Johns Hopkins (two times), Columbia, Konstanz, Roma (La Sapienza), Napoli, Santiago de Compostela, Geneva, Waseda University, and National University at Tokyo. He is a Foreign Honorary Member of the American Academy of Arts and Sciences, a Corresponding Fellow of the Medieval Academy of America, a Doctor Honoris Causa of the University of Sheffield. He has published many books on medieval literature and got several awards in this field. He has also published novels and tales. He is chevalier de la Légion d'Honneur and officier des Palmes académiques.

Index

Page numbers in *italics* refer to illustrations.

Index